Chinese Traditional Herbal Medicine
Vol 2. Materia Medica and Herbal Resource

Michael Tierra, L.Ac., OMD, A.H.G.
and Lesley Tierra, L.Ac., A.H.G.

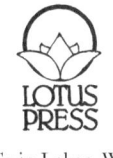

Twin Lakes, WI

DISCLAIMER

This book is a reference work, not intended to diagnose, prescribe or treat. The information contained herein is in no way to be considered as a substitute for consultation with a licensed health-care professional.

Copyright © 1998 Michael Tierra

All rights reserved. No part of this book may be produced in any form or by any electronic or mechanical means including information storage and retrieval systems without permission in writing from the publisher, except by a reviewer who may quote brief passages in a review. For inquiries contact

LOTUS PRESS
PO Box 325,
Twin Lakes, WI 53181 USA
Toll Free Order PH: (800) 824-6396
Office PH: (262) 889-8561
Office FAX: (262) 889-2461
Website: www.LotusPress.com
Email: lotuspress@lotuspress.com

First Edition 1998
Reprinted 2011, 2024
Printed in the United States of America

ISBN 978-0-9149-5532-0
Library of Congress Catalogue Number 98-66146

DEDICATION

To Dr. Miriam Lee, a courageous pioneer of Traditional Chinese Medicine in California. Suffering legal harassment in the early years, she most generously and openly shared her wisdom and skill with a whole generation of Western practitioners, who revere her with great honor and respect.

ACKNOWLEDGMENTS

Dr. Naixin Hu, TCM Doctor and former professor of herbal medicine at the Traditional Chinese Medical College in Shanghai, for critically reviewing and contributing many valuable suggestions.

Thomas Garan, who helped in research and editing many portions of the text.

Bill Schoenbart, TCM practitioner, who was able to bring his deep understanding of Traditional Chinese Medicine and his skill as an editor to this book.

Ewan Klein, TCM practitioner in Scotland, who helped review the manuscript.

CONTENTS

Foreword vi

Introduction 1

I

The Chinese Materia Medica 9

Herbs that Calm the Spirit 241
          Anchor and Settle 242
          Nourish the Heart 246
     Clear Internal Heat 44-87
          Clear Heat and Dry Dampness 62
          Clear Heat and Purge Fire 45
          Clear Heat and Relieve Toxicity 68
          Clear Summer Heat 82
          Cool the Blood 54
     Dispel Wind and Dampness 109
     Drain Dampness 96
     Drain Downward 87
          Purgatives 87
          Lubricating Laxatives 91
          Cathartics 92
     Expel parasites 260
     External application 263
     Open the Orifices 250
     Pacify Internal Liver Wind 253
     Release the Exterior 23
          Cool/Acrid 35
          Warm/Acrid 24
     Regulate Blood 150
          Invigorate the Blood 158
          Stop Bleeding 151
     Regulate Qi 141
     Relieve Food Stagnation 137
     Stabilize and Bind 229
     Stop Tremors 253
     Tonics 180
          for Deficient Blood 192
          for Deficient Qi 183
          for Deficient Yang 202
          for Deficient Yin 218
Transform Dampness, Aromatic 132
Transform Phlegm and Stop Cough 116
     Cool 117
     Relieve coughing and wheezing 128
     Warm 124
Warm the Interior/Expel Cold 25, 173

2
The Use of Chinese Herbal Formulas   272

3
Treatment of Specific Disease   371

Bibliography   420

Glossary   425

General Index   429

Index of Herbs by Latin Name   449

Index of Herbs by Chinese Name   453

Index of Chinese Herbal Formulas   457

Index for Chapter 3:   462
Treatment of Specific Disease

FOREWORD

Chinese Herbal Medicine, one of the most precious resources from my mother country, is finally beginning to achieve the recognition it deserves in the Western world. Today we see how not only acupuncturists, but a wide range of health care practitioners, including medical doctors, herbalists, chiropractors, nutritionists, and midwives, are increasingly using Chinese herbs for their patients. Acupuncture has been well known for some time as an independent health care method, but people are just now beginning to understand more clearly that acupuncture and herbal medicine are the two parts of a complete system of healing, called Traditional Chinese Medicine (TCM).

The organization of training in Chinese medical universities can give some insight into the scope and depth of TCM, and the balance between the different parts of TCM. Each province in China has one government sponsored University of TCM. The largest in Beijing has a staff of several thousand, maintains a large hospital, and runs more than a dozen independent research institutes.

There are usually three departments: Materia Medica, Acupuncture and Herbal Medicine. The Materia Medica department is concerned with pharmacological and botanical descriptions of the herbal medicines, plant collection, storage and preparation. Graduates get four years of training, and occupy positions similar to pharmacists here. They also carry out scientific research to ensure safety and efficacy of the herbal materials. They do not prescribe. Students in the acupuncture department study for 5 years, with the same basic medical theory as herbal doctors, but with more attention on needling and less on herbs. Their training is similar in format to graduates of American acupuncture schools, but one to two years longer. The department of herbal medicine is by far the largest university department, typically occupying approximately 60% of the classroom space, compared to 25% for materia medica, and perhaps only about 15% for acupuncture. This is quite the reverse in the West where acupuncture has thus far defined the public and legal recognition of TCM.

It is my one sadness that Chinese herbalism has not yet achieved its own independent prominence, as befits its stature in China. Only recently with the separate certification by the National Commission for the Certification of Acupuncturists (NCCA) has there been a separate testing and certification procedure for the certification of Chinese herbalists. While not officially recognized in all states, it nevertheless easily establishes the possibility for the recognition of a professional class of herbalists in America, albeit Chinese herbalists. It is up to the new generation of herbalists to form these laws.

TCM students of the herbal medicine department major in herbal medicine, minor in acupuncture, and, after graduation, prescribe herbal medicines to their patients. Unlike in the West—where there is huge schism between traditional medicine and conventional Western allopathic medicine—TCM doctors occupy positions equal in stature to the Western style family doctors. They practice side by side as equals in all Chinese hospitals under the combined Western/TCM system throughout China. What a great benefit to our Western patients if there was greater acceptance, respect and dialogue between Western and Traditional doctors. If more Western doctors could learn to embrace the well established efficacy of TCM, there would be much less abuse of extreme therapeutic procedures and the use and the unnecessary use of conventional Western drugs for conditions that herbs or acupuncture could better treat. After all, Chinese herbs excel at nourishing and detoxifying the body at a deep and fundamental level, and supported in this way the body has a much greater capacity to heal itself; can anyone deny this truism? Western medicine, in contradistinction, is powerful and heroic, and able to maintain life in times of severe crisis or dysfunction. Yet it is difficult to name a single prescription pharmaceutical which can nourish the lungs, the kidney, the heart or the Spirit in order to prevent the onset of crisis.

From my years of teaching herbal medicine to Europeans studying at the Chengdu University of TCM (Sichuan province), and my more recent experiences treating Westerners at Chrysalis Natural Medicine Center in Wilmington, Delaware, I have become acutely aware of the problems confronting Western students of Chinese Herbal Medicine. Even for the Chinese student, it is a formidable task, requiring 5 years of medical school, with 6-8 hours a day of study, six days a week. Their training covers TCM medical theory, pharmacology, acupuncture, internal medicine, diagnostics, and prescription formulation. Students must be able to read, comprehend, and recite passages from the ancient textbooks (many written in our classical language), and know the properties and uses of over 1,000 herbal medicines and hundreds of formulas. Recently standards have been increased, with several years of postgraduate study, including study of Western medicine, necessary to become a doctor. How much more difficult it must be for the Westerner, who does not have direct access to the literature, the herbal medicine university, or the teaching hospital. But Chinese Medicine has faced many challenges over the centuries, from political opposition in the past to the recent opposition of those claiming that it has no basis in science. Yet it has met and overcome all of those challenges, and is now flourishing all over the world, in large part due to the efforts of the many pioneers who have striven, at great cost and effort to themselves, to bring the knowledge of the healing powers of Chinese herbs to the aid of those who are suffering and sick.

I consider my close friends and colleagues Michael Tierra and Lesley Tierra to be two of those pioneers. Michael, after distinguishing himself more than thirty years ago in the field of Western herbalism, was among the small group of visionaries who recognized the importance of Chinese herbalism at that time, and along with his wife, Lesley, were among the handful who have steadfastly pursued the arduous task of mastering the essence of that knowledge. Their new work, written in their characteristically clear and lucid style, will bring a wealth of traditional knowledge to all those fortunate enough to realize its significance.

Naixin Hu, OMD
L.Ac. Co-director of Chrysalis Natural Medicine Center
Former Acupuncturist to the Royal Family of Egypt

INTRODUCTION

In the first volume we presented the theory, principles and diagnostic methods that are an essential part of the practice of Traditional Chinese Medicine (TCM). This second volume is a practical manual that includes an extended Materia Medica of the most common TCM herbs, a formulary that categorizes traditional formulas into three levels of usage and a section on the treatment of some of the most common diseases according to Western pathological classification. There are also chapters on Chinese food therapy and accessory healing therapies that are traditionally part of the practice of Chinese herbal medicine.

This second volume should prove to be a practical reference for both the student and practitioner as well as the increasing numbers of health professionals who are interested in integrating Chinese herbal medicine as part of their practice and lay persons who, for various reasons, are curious to know more about the practice of Chinese herbal medicine.

As with all 'holistic' systems of healing, Traditional Chinese Medicine (TCM) is an integration of all aspects of body-mind health with lifestyle, emotions and diet considered along with treatment using herbs, acupuncture, massage or other therapies. In books of this type, with the voluminous amount of material related to the practice of Chinese herbal therapy, it is not possible to fully represent the integration of all other factors that are important to the process of healing. Indeed, with over 5000 years of collected experience, it is also a part of Taoism, which forms a philosophical basis for Traditional Chinese Medicine.

Taoism views physical imbalances to be the result of inherited tendencies, lifestyle (which includes emotional and physical stress, diet and work) and fate. The principle of transformation and change, exemplified in the philosophy of Yin and Yang as complementary polar opposites, views all negative and positive aspects of life as part of one's 'Tao' or path.

Just as the procession of day into night and the seasons with their different climates occurs with orderly predictability, one's life unfolds into different periods of alternating positive and negative cycles. Through methods of self reflection, TCM facilitates an appreciation of our uniquely inherited limitations as well as acquired factors which may aid us on our path. By understanding the unique cycles of our life unfoldment, Traditional Chinese Medical Diagnosis is able to intuitively extend beyond the realm of the limits of momentary physical analysis.

The Four Diagnoses: interrogation, observation, palpitation and listening, presented in volume one, includes observing various aspects of our physical appearance, pulse and tongue diagnosis. This differential method, which is an approach of examining various parameters to determine what is and is not in agreement with each other, actually allows the traditional practitioner to form an understanding not only of our current state, but inherited strengths and weaknesses which if not attended to in the present, are likely to influence and to some extent determine the quality of our life in the future. It is the first job of the traditional Chinese healer, therefore, to serve as a guide and teacher in order to help us to achieve inner harmony as peace of mind and outer harmony as physical well being.

Perhaps one of the most important considerations about Traditional Chinese Medicine is that it is a system where all aspects of diagnosis, herbal and food classifications and treatment are interdependent upon each other. As soon as one posits a diagnosis of, for instance, external Cold, immediately there is available in one's mind a number of herbs and formulas classified as external warm and used to treat external Cold. This same interconnected approach extends to all diagnostic patterns such as heat, dampness, wind, phlegm, restless spirit and so forth.

It is for this reason that TCM is said to have both a philosophy and a system of health and healing. It is also the reason that it is very difficult to extrapolate a single herb or treatment modality for use in a system such as Western medical science that tends to follow a linear approach, with each part having little relation to the whole. However, it is possible to utilize the knowledge and elements of Western physiology and biology to conform to a more functional or energetic orientation similar to TCM.

Starting from the known to the unknown, all the aspects of TCM diagnosis permit an evaluation based first on what is empirically observed and known, reaching out to further realms of subtle awareness to include one's destiny or fate. The ancient oracle called the I-Ching exemplifies the Chinese preoccupation with fate and right action. An examination of the pulse, for example, offers a degree of verifiable evidence concerning the relative strength of the heart, the nervous system and the blood. However, patients are often amazed at the wide range of information concerning the condition of individual organs, the past and future that an experienced practitioner is able to discern. Another example is tongue diagnosis: Because it can be seen and observed one might think that it represents a higher degree of diagnostic certainty. Again, the practitioner when diagnosing a red tongue signifying heat, for instance, must

differentiate it from the various shades of pink which may be within the normal range. A still greater degree of ambiguity is reflected in the reading of various signs on particular areas of the tongue that are designated to correspond to individual Internal Organs. Do such seeming inaccuracies and contradictions of which any advanced student-practitioner of TCM is well aware, represent flagrant inaccuracies and vagaries. Or is it an inherent encouragement to an intuitive process that has and will always be a significant part of the high practice of all forms of medicine?

It is a fundamental difference that, unlike Western diagnostic approaches, where specific pathologies are described and named, Chinese medicine views disease as a state of imbalance. Therefore, the TCM healer engages the methods of traditional differential diagnosis to evaluate aspects of both our physical and mental health as well as the use of various methods to help determine our fate in order to offer guidance, foods and herbs that can help us to achieve maximum harmony through all stages of life.

TCM CASE STUDIES

The following cases are offered to exemplify the mind-body approach of TCM in clinical practice: A woman diagnosed with Lupus erythematosus (LE), an autoimmune disease, characteristically exhibited red, scaling discoloration on both her lower legs. Of major concern, however, was a 4 inch circumference ulcer on her left leg that for months had failed to respond to any medication her doctors prescribed. From the Traditional Chinese Medical perspective, this condition could be described as blood Stagnation with damp heat and wei qi (immune system) deficiency. The therapeutic principle, therefore, is to remove blood Stagnation and damp heat, promote healing and tonify the Wei Qi. Many herbs and formulas could be considered for this condition. Indeed, Chinese herbal therapy had a very positive effect on her symptoms. During the second session, it was revealed that her mother had experienced similar physical problems at different times in her life pointing to a possible inherited predisposition to the disease. Since there were times of greater and lesser aggravation, however, the fact that she had recently moved to North America from a strife ridden European country left her with stressful concern and worry over her aging parents and her brother with Down's syndrome living in her native land. The TCM perspective states that excessive sadness, worry, stress and guilt injures the spleen, lungs and kidneys. Regardless of any physiotherapy it was crucially important to facilitate and guide the process of emotional

resolution and give herbs to calm and nourish her nerves. It was remarkable to see how a process of mental transformation effected the physical. By reminding her of the difference between love and worry and not to worry over that for which she had no direct responsibility or control, came noticeable healing of the leg sore.

Another case was a man in his mid twenties who had developed a chronic sinus infection following an improperly treated upper respiratory tract infection some months previous. His constitution was of a Yin type, thin, somewhat timid and soft spoken. Though he was cold sensitive, he had a flushed appearance on his cheeks and face which represents metabolic stress and weak heat caused by deficiency. In addition to his primary sinus complaint, he commented how his minor wounds and injuries were slow to heal, suggesting nutritional deficiencies, specifically insufficient protein. Because of his religious beliefs, he had been a vegetarian for many years. Experience has shown that Westerners, especially of Northern European ancestry, who adopt a strict vegetarian diet, often with a noticeable lack of protein and the overuse of raw foods, are in danger of seriously injuring their digestive and assimilative capacities. As a result, such individuals are unlikely to respond to herbs alone without their diet being adjusted to include more cooked foods and possibly some animal protein. I recommended that he have organic chicken soup twice a day and take an herbal formula that included magnolia flowers to break up sinus congestion and Gypsum to clear internal stomach heat. His condition was 90% resolved within the first week and he commented how his sinuses tended to clear even while drinking the tea. He then wanted to focus on a treatment for chronic childhood eczema that was localized to his ankles and knees. Upon studying the formula, I found that it could be modified slightly to treat his eczema as well. The diet was of such key importance that when he arbitrarily failed to take the chicken soup for only two days, the effect of the herbal treatment was significantly compromised. Healing for this man involved not only treating physical symptoms but an adjustment of his philosophical outlook that could reflect the needs of his physical constitution. From the Chinese perspective, true fulfillment in life is only achieved when we adopt a path, that includes diet, that is in harmony with all aspects of our being, our ancestry, life work, the availability of quality foods and other specific physical requirements.

One of the most common diseases for which conventional Western medicine has little satisfactory answer is in the category of arthritic and rheumatic complaints. These can have many TCM causes and are broadly categorized as '*Bi*' pains caused by blockage. It so happens that TCM is

very effective in treating most of these conditions but once again, factors of lifestyle including diet and stress must be addressed.

While Western medicine tends to focus primarily on the removal of pain and inflammation, usually with antibiotics or steroids, TCM sub-classifies arthritic conditions into various types including 1) fixed pain aggravated by wind, cold and dampness which can be treated with herbs and formulas that resolve wind, cold and dampness; 2) migratory pains treated with warming, circulating and antispasmodic herbs; 3) pains caused by inflammation which are treated with anti-inflammatory herbs; 4) pains caused by chronic hormonal deficiencies categorized as liver and kidney Qi deficiency treated with herbs and formulas that contain kidney and liver tonics.

Because of the endless variety of disease patterns, the Chinese Materia Medica is arranged to accommodate the treatment of all possible patterns of imbalance. Like the colors of an artist's palette or the notes of the musical scale, when a certain color is missing or certain notes of the musical scale are unavailable, the artist/musician is limited in his/her artistic expression. Similarly, the TCM practitioner is limited when certain herbs in the Materia Medica are unavailable. This may seriously compromise one's ability to treat certain conditions. I say this in light of the current question around banning certain herbs such as Ephedra (Ma Huang) or Aconite (Fu Zi) from availability. Perhaps these may be regulated from popular consumption but certainly not from the practice of a trained Chinese herbal practitioner.

So long as the classification of herbs and therapeutic substances includes the traditional classification according to energies, flavors, organ-meridians affected, dosage, indications and contraindications, it is possible to arrive at the appropriate treatment for most diseases. For this reason, it is important to spend the requisite time to gain as full a mastery of the Materia Medica as possible. Study and review must be ongoing, since one is more likely to become self limited in the usage of only a few herbs and formulas at the exclusion of others based on the frequency of indication and usage.

For simple diseases one or two herbs can be used, but with more complex problems, many herbs are combined in formulas to form unique interactions with each other as well as treat the various physiological functions and organs that contribute to the disease process. The classical formulas have been passed down, studied and refined for millennia by literally thousands of master herbalists. Many, originally created to treat a specific condition, have over time been successfully employed for a much wider scope of applications. The formula known as Rehmannia

Eight (Jin Gui Shen Qi Wan or Ba Wei Wan), for instance, was originally intended for the treatment of impaired childhood development but over the course of nearly 2000 years, its scope has broadened to include most diseases associated with Coldness, deficiency of yang and conditions associated with degeneration and aging.

Bob Flaws describes TCM as it is practiced today as a "blend of both rational and empirical methodologies"[1]. He describes how the Chinese practice according to *bian bing* and *bian zheng* diagnosis. *"Bian bing* means to differentiate various named diseases and recognized pathological signs and symptoms. *Bian zheng*, on the other hand, means to discriminate various recognized patterns of disharmony." He then quotes: *Tong bing yi zhi, Yi bing tong zhi.* One disease, different treatments; Different diseases, same treatment.

From this we recognize that in TCM we may see the same recognized disease with various patterns of hot, cold, excess, deficiency, internal, external, yin, yang, dry, damp, etc., so a different approach to treatment with different herbal formulas is indicated for the same disease based on the different patterns of each. Similarly, a dietary approach and single herbal formula based on a particular pattern of hot or cold, for instance, can be beneficial for many different diseases.

In the first volume, we will discuss the principles of differential diagnosis and the recognition of patterns and corresponding treatment approaches and herbal formulas. In the second volume we classify most of the common diseases and their respective patterns with corresponding herbal treatments.

THE LANGUAGE BARRIER

Without understanding the language and subtle meaning associated with Chinese characters, it is very difficult if not impossible for the student and practitioner of Chinese herbalism to gain full understanding of the characteristic diagnostic terminology that describes the various patterns of imbalance. This certainly does not mean that a non-Chinese speaking Westerner is unable to be an effective practitioner of Chinese herbology and acupuncture. For the non-Chinese speaking practitioner, of which I am one, it is vitally important to transform the concepts and terms of TCM into Western thought processes. This means, among other things, examining traditional concepts in terms of Western physiology.

For the time being limitations are often overcome by classifying diseases according to conventional Western medicine with corresponding patterns of Chinese sub-classifications. Practically speaking, this is quite effective and affords the added advantage of improved communication

with Western medical doctors and patients who understand their diseases according to named pathologies, however limited this may be in the practice of Traditional Chinese Herbalism.

HERBOLOGY OR HERBALISM

The reader may notice the tendency to refer to the terms 'herbology' and 'herbalism'. There are positive and negative connotations to each. 'Herbology' suggests a more purely scientific approach without a pre-established world view that includes the more intuitive aspects of practice that is, to my mind, better expressed by the term, 'herbalism'. 'Herbalism', on the other hand, has cultist negative connotations that may justifiably form a barrier to understanding by many who would otherwise be more open to explore the profound value and significance of Traditional Chinese Medicine.

Whether 'herbology' or 'herbalism', in the short span of time since the lifting of the "Bamboo Curtain" in 1972, Traditional Chinese Medicine continues to gain the respect of Western medical researchers, doctors and other practitioners and millions of patients each year. In the mid 1970's to 1980's there were only a small handful of TCM practitioners in the North America. Today there are thousands throughout all of the states.

CHINESE HERBALISM:
A FULLY DEVELOPED PROFESSION

At its inception in the west, Traditional Chinese Medicine has been known primarily by only one of its branches, namely acupuncture. As a result, many of the first practitioners had no formal training in the far more difficult Chinese herbal medicine. The state and national board examinations only included a few herbal related questions. This is rapidly changing and the National Association for the Certification of Acupuncturists has extended its scope to include the certification of Chinese herbalists. It is important that herbal medicine and the herbal branch of Traditional Chinese Medicine be recognized on their own merit.

TOWARDS A PLANETARY HERBOLOGY

Eventually there will come a time when the distinction between ethnocentric systems of medicine will become less differentiated. Western herbalism, striving to maintain acceptance with the rise of allopathic medicine over the last two hundred years, has lost much of its traditional basis which extends back to European folk medicine and Greek and

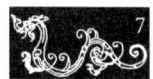

Roman times where herbs and diseases where similarly energetically classified at least in terms of their 'hot and cold' atmospheric energies. The Western herbal Materia Medica has, for the most part, been fragmented as a result of the deletion of important botanicals deemed too potent and dangerous for use by the inexperienced or through practitioner neglect.

Even a mere four or five hundred years ago, in the time of Shakespeare, the Materia Medica used by his physician son in law, John Hall, included a wide variety of herbs, minerals, insects and animal parts, each energetically classified according to therapeutic usage similar to herbs in the Traditional Chinese Materia Medica. As a result of a strange turn of fate, and the propensity of the Chinese to preserve and honor their past and ancestors, China, the oldest surviving civilization of the world, increasingly is able to bestow its priceless gift of healing and herbal medicine to the West and the entire world.

Once on a visit to Thailand, I was curious to learn of indigenous Thai herbal medicine. It was a native Thai gentleman who directed me to a clinic a little away from the main street in Cheng Mai, to a Chinese herbalist. He explained that in his opinion and indeed the opinion of people throughout the Asian world and Africa that Traditional Chinese Medicine is the most effective. The high degree of effectiveness and accuracy of Traditional Chinese Medicine does not lie solely in its indigenous herbs or a specific healing modality, but in the all inclusive strength of its theoretical and diagnostic system.

In conclusion, I don't think that as Traditional Chinese Medicine is disseminated throughout the world, it will remain a purely ethnic phenomenon unto itself. Rather, as it integrates with other cultures and with Western medical science, it will transform into different patterns according to different customs and terms. The result, however, is that we will all benefit as heirs of one of the most powerful holistic healing systems ever evolved.

ONE
THE CHINESE MATERIA MEDICA

Mastering the Chinese Materia Medica is perhaps second only in importance to TCM diagnosis. Without a TCM diagnosis, it would be very difficult to prescribe an accurate treatment; with a diagnosis, one must have sufficient mastery of basic traditional formulas and their individual herbs to achieve a successful treatment protocol.

The Materia Medica is organized into approximately 18 primary categories and various subcategories. Each herb is classified according to its energies, flavors, Organ meridians, actions, indications, contraindications and dosage. Whenever uniquely appropriate, methods of preparation are also given.

There are differences in the selection and number of herbs between one source and another, but the traditional Chinese Materia Medica is remarkably consistent and lists approximately 250 to 300 herbs in relatively common clinical use. Herbs, in this sense, refers to medicinal substances derived not only from plants but the mineral, animal and insect kingdoms as well. Because plants predominate in the text, for over 3000 years the term "Pen T'sao," or herbal, has been used.

Various methods are used to study the Materia Medica. To begin, one should learn all the herbs in relationship to their basic categories. Next, focus more closely on the more specific indications of the herbs that commonly reoccur in the most representative classical formulas. This may reduce the list of herbs to begin memorizing to around 50 to 100. With experience, the remainder of the herbs that are less commonly used can be memorized. To facilitate this process for the student, we have indicated the most representative herbs numbered one to three in order of importance and use for each category. With 250 to 300 or more herbs, and literally thousands of ancient classical formulas from which one begins by learning the most representative 70 to 100 formulas, mastering this body of knowledge is, indeed, a formidable and proud achievement.

ORGANIZING AND DESCRIBING HERBS IN THE MATERIA MEDICA

The way herbs are classified in both the traditional Chinese and Western systems reflects the fundamental difference of philosophy and approach between the two systems. Traditional systems are not based upon pharmacological constituents, but rather according to the system of diagnosis and usage. Western herbals do use broad therapeutic property descriptions such as diaphoretics, laxatives, or diuretics, but this again only indicates a mechanical therapeutic effect which may not necessarily correspond to a specific Organ meridian or functional imbalance. The Chinese Materia Medica utilizes a more holistic application, classifying herbs according to flavors, energies, Organ meridians affected, as well as traditional actions, indications, dosage and contraindications. This allows for a deeper conceptualization of the indications and contraindications of each herb according to individual requirements.

A few examples might elucidate the difference between the two systems. Cinnamon twigs (Ramulus Cinnamomum) and Mint (Mentha haplocalyx) both induce perspiration and have a spicy flavor; Cinnamon twigs, however, are classified as spicy-warm, while Mint is classified as spicy cool. The first is useful for individuals who have a greater sensitivity to chill and cold while the second is used for fevers associated with a greater degree of Heat and inflammatory symptoms. Both the herbs Dianthus chinensis (Qu mai) and Poria cocos (Fu ling) are classified as diuretics in Western herbalism. They are, however, used very differently. Dianthus has a Cold energy and a bitter flavor and is used for clearing Damp Heat from the Heart, Kidney, Small intestine and Urinary bladder Organ meridians. The bland or slightly sweet flavor of Poria has a more tonic effect on the Spleen as well as the Lung, Heart and Urinary Bladder. In other words one is Colder and clears Heat and inflammation, while the other is more tonic and supportive.

Such delineations allow for greater precision of application, which is extremely important when using herbal medicines that have broader and milder actions than drugs. In this way, an herb is like an individual color on an artist's palette or a note in the musical scale. To remove certain colors or notes from an artist's or musician's resources is to severely limit the final artistic result. Similarly, as an artist or musician combines colors and forms, notes and rhythms for certain artistic expressions, an herbalist most often combines herbs in different combinations and proportions to balance physiological processes and energies according to the individual and his or her specific condition.

THE NAMES OF HERBS

Herbs are listed according to their pharmaceutical name, Mandarin Chinese name, full Latin binomial and their common name. The pharmaceutical name first identifies in Latin the part used, then its most common Latin name. Following is a list of the common pharmaceutical names of the parts of herbs used:

Herba — the whole plant
Folia — the foliage only
Cortex — the bark of a tree or root
Ramulus — the twigs or branches
Flos — the flowers
Fructus — the fruit
Semen — the seed
Pericarpium — the husk of the fruit
Radix — the root
Rhizoma — the underground rhizome

In addition, corresponding animal parts are also similarly listed with a few examples as follows:

Concha — the shell
Penis et testis — the male genitals
Endothelium Corneum — chicken gizzard
Periostracum — the molted shell of the cicada, for instance
Cornu — the antler

Common Name
Relying solely on either the Western or Chinese common names, while more convenient, can also be both confusing and misleading. First, on occasion, many herbs share the same common name, which is fine for local parlance but not for national or international delineation. Secondly, different species of the same herb often have different properties and still share the same common name. This necessitates that one be either aware of these differences or use the more specific botanical Latin binomial.

Botanical family
Knowing the botanical families of herbs can be a help, since within the same family herbs often share similar biochemical characteristics which would allow them to have similar uses. However, for a variety of reasons botanists seem to have a need to change previously well known Latin names and even the families of certain plants. For those of us who

have difficulty remembering or pronouncing Latin names, this can go from bad to worse. One example is the change of the herb Siler divaricata to Ledebouriella seseloides. The fact that both names still appear in texts suggests a certain resistance among herbalists to adopt the clumsy second name.

ENERGIES AND FLAVORS

The two most important considerations in determining the application of a specific herb or formula is its energy and flavors.

The energies describe the overall strength of an herb as well as its relative degree of Heat or Cold. One of the fundamental principles of treatment is to give Cold herbs for Hot or inflammatory conditions and Hot herbs for Cold or hypo-tonic conditions.

What does this mean physiologically? Essentially all diseases and conditions can be classified as Hot or Cold. This means they are either caused by a hyper-metabolic or hypo-metabolic condition. Herbs that are Cold or Cool help lower a hyper-metabolic condition referred to as Heat, while herbs that are Hot or Warm help raise a hypo-metabolic condition referred to as Cold.

For instance, if one tends towards constipation with blood in the stool, a Warm natured anti-diarrhea herb such as Nutmeg or Cinnamon bark would aggravate the inflammation. On the other hand if one had Cold, weak digestion with diarrhea as a result of weakness and Coldness, Nutmeg or Cinnamon bark would be most appropriate. These are some of the basic strategies that are available when one is first able to understand the Heating or Cooling energies of an herb.

Simply to say that one has caught a cold makes it very difficult to find an appropriate treatment according to the present philosophical intention of Western medicine. Treatment with drugs tends to be purely suppressive or symptomatic, i.e. decongestant or fever reducing, for instance. Such symptomatic approaches, characteristic of Western medicine, are useful for crisis conditions but can be harmful to the core energy of an individual if inappropriately or too casually applied.

Another example is the use of antibiotics for infections. Western antibiotics would be energetically classified as Cold. Because they are so strong, they are usually capable of overcoming whatever degree of Heat or Coldness an individual exhibiting symptoms may have as their core energetic state. Generally, individuals who eat animal protein have a tendency towards more Heat while those who eat more vegetable-based foods have a tendency towards Coolness. Antibiotics tend to destroy not only the harmful bacteria of the body but the desirable bacteria as well.

Individuals who consume animal protein tend to respond and fare better in the long run with the use of antibiotic drugs than does the average vegetarian.

The flavors represent the traditional way of practically understanding and utilizing the biochemical constituents of herbs. Each of the Five Flavors indicates possible biochemical components. For example, herbs with a sour flavor contain acids or fermentive components; bitter herbs may indicate alkaloids and bitter glycosides; sweet herbs indicate the presence of plant sugars, saponins, or nutritional components; spicy or pungent herbs have volatile oils; salty herbs such as seaweeds contain various mineral salts, and so forth.

The flavors are used therefore not only according to their intrinsic sensory impression, but more important, according to their therapeutic effects. As an example, the sweet flavor usually indicates a tonic nutritive property. Qi tonics are all classified as sweet with various sub-flavors indicating other biochemical constituents. Most individuals tasting the medicinal herb for the first time would hardly consider Ginseng (Ren shen) as sweet, even though in Chinese herbalism that is its primary flavor because it is a Qi tonic. The Qi tonic, Atractylodes (Bai zhu), has barely any sweet flavor and it is classified as primarily bitter, but because it is used as a Qi tonic, it is assigned a secondary sweet flavor in the Materia Medica. Interestingly, a closely related Atractylodes species, A. Lancea (Cang zhu), is used in the category of herbs that Transform Cold and Damp, which includes rheumatic diseases. While it is definitely less sweet than its Qi tonic counterpart, it is defined as having an acrid, bitter flavor with no sweet sub-flavor at all. Interestingly, both herbs share many of the same biochemical constituents, but it is the difference of their usage as much as any other factor that points to their differing biochemistry.

ORGAN MERIDIANS AFFECTED

The adaptation of classifying herbs in the Organ-meridians is unique to Chinese herbalism and relatively more recent historically. As a result there are differences according to various sources. The classification according to affected Organ meridians first appeared in the Song dynasty in the *Zhen Lei Pen T'sao* (Materia Medica Arranged According to Pattern, 1108) by Tang Shen-Wei. However it was Zhang Yuansu in his *Yixue Qiyuan* (Explanation of Medicine), published in 1186, that firmly upheld the idea that herbs had a specific effect as 'entering' each of the various Organ meridians.

In most cases, the assignments are obvious, being based on the relationship of the Five Flavors to each of the Organ meridians, as well as therapeutic actions that would tend to more directly affect a specific Internal Organ. This would include the assignment of the sweet flavor to the Spleen Organ meridian, the spicy flavor to the Lung Organ meridian and so forth. Obviously herbs that exert a profound stimulation or activity of an Organ may also be thought to enter a specific Organ meridian.

Herbs that seem to have a specific effect on an Organ meridian can not only be themselves employed in the treatment of a specific imbalance in the corresponding system, but can be used in small amounts as a conductor of other non-related herbs to that system.

Following is a list of Organ meridian directing herbs:

Organ Meridian	Organ Meridian Directing Herbs
Heart and Heart Meridian	Coptis (Huang Lian) and Asarum (Xi Xin)
Small Intestine	Ligusticum (Chuan Xiong) and Phellodendron (Huang Bai)
Kidneys	Cinnamon bark (Rou Gui), Anemarrhena (Zhi Mu) and Asarum (Xi Xin)
Bladder	Notopterygium (Qiang Huo)
Lungs	Platycodon (Jie Geng), Cimicifuga (Sheng Ma), Angelica dahurica (Bai zhi)
Large Intestine	Angelica dahurica (Bai Zhi) and Cimicifuga (Sheng Ma)
Spleen	Cimicifuga (Sheng Ma), Atractylodes (Bai Zhu), Pueraria (Ge Gen) and White peony (Bai Shao Yao)
Stomach	Angelica dahurica (Bai Zhi), Cimicifuga (Sheng Ma) and Pueraria root (Ge Gen)
Pericardium	Bupleurum (Chai Hu) and Moutan (Mu Dan Pi)
Gallbladder	Bupleurum (Chai Hu) and Aurantii Immaturus (Zhi Shi)
Liver	Bupleurum (Chai Hu), Aurantii Immaturus (Zhi Shi), Evodia (Wu Zhu Yu) and Ligusticum (Chuan Xiong)
Triple Warmer	Upper Warmer: Forsythia (Lian Qiao), Bupleurum (Chai Hu), Lycii bark (Di Gu Pi); Middle Warmer: Aurantii Immaturus (Zhi Shi); Lower Warmer: Aconite (Fu Zi)

DETERMINING QUALITY OF HERBS

Chinese herbs are commercially sold in several grades and qualities. Quality is determined by a variety of factors, the most important being

the history of its growth and harvesting. Generally wild herbs are considered to have stronger properties. However, due to ecological concerns it may not be advantageous to continue our dependence on the availability of certain high grade herbs that are still harvested in the wild (such as American Ginseng, Goldenseal or Echinacea). The area, climate and soil where an herb is found or cultivated can have a profound effect on its ultimate potency. Another factor that determines potency is the time of harvest, which should be at the time the desired part of the herb is at its peak. This means roots should be harvested in the early spring before the plant begins to develop or in the fall when its life force has retreated back down into the earth. Barks should be harvested in the spring or fall as well. Leaves should be harvested before the flower buds appear. Flowers and fruits are harvested in their prime, and so forth.

Certain herbs are perennials, such as Ginseng, Astragalus and Dang gui, and must remain in the soil for a minimum number of years for them to maximize their potency. Quality of most herbs is otherwise based upon size, shape, appearance, color, odor and flavor. The determination of herb quality is a skill depending on both knowledge and experience. One must become familiar with the individual standards and characteristics of each herb.

Unless the crude botanical is immediately extracted in alcohol, for instance, it must be dried and properly stored for use. Methods of storage vary, but the basic intention is to protect the dried and prepared botanicals from moisture, air, light and bug infestation. The last can be the source of considerable loss and degradation. Because of this, some herbs have been sprayed, fumigated or treated to help them maintain color and deter insect infestation (See chapter 14).

This does not mean that Chinese herbs are universally of substandard quality. If this were the case, millions of Chinese and other people around the world would not use them. The demand for efficacy will always necessitate a certain standard for cultivation, and historically Chinese agricultural practices in regard to the cultivation of medicinal plants, optimizing the concentration of specific biochemical constituents and properties, are far in advance of those in the West. The reason for this is the same as that for the superiority of Chinese herbalism. Unlike the West, the Chinese have a long standing unbroken tradition in all aspects of herbalism, including methods of cultivation.

PREPARING HERBS FOR MARKET

The purpose of preparation is to alter or modify the nature and action of herbs to render and adjust them for the needs of pharmacy.

Following is an outline of a few of the more common methods of preparation and processing:

A) Basic Preparations

This includes cleaning, sifting, winnowing or 'garbling' and/or removing any undesirable parts. The object is to render the herb in a form that will maximize surface area for extraction. As such, they may be available in either a 'cut and sifted' mode which are in nondescript pieces, as Western herbs are commonly sold at this time, or in pieces and slices that aid in the process of easier identification and quality evaluation, which is more typical of the commercial presentation of Chinese herbs. This latter method attempts to approximate a standard size and weight, and since the roots are typically diagonally sliced, it also helps in the process of extraction.

Herbs and various minerals may also need to be ground into a fine powder. This is especially true of minerals, since powdered botanicals prepared in this way must be used before 3 months as they tend to oxidize and lose potency at a far more rapid rate.

B) Basic Processing of Herbs

Herbs can be dry fried to make them Warmer and drier. This makes them more suitable for strengthening Spleen Yang and Qi. They can also be fried with honey to make them sweeter and more tonic. Frying in salt gives them a more downward energy to benefit the Kidneys. Frying with vinegar makes them more astringent, pain relieving, blood moving and anti-toxic. This is because the acidic nature of vinegar tends to neutralize, to some degree, potentially toxic alkaloids. Fried with Ginger juice, herbs are Warmer and more assimilable and beneficial for the Stomach. Fried with wine, herbs will be more beneficial for circulation and useful for relieving pain.

Calcined or charred herbs are made by placing them either directly over a flame or in an oven. The reasons for this method are to a) make them more brittle and able to be pulverized or powdered, b) use the ashes of certain herbs and substances to inhibit hemorrhage, c) to counterbalance the Cold energy of certain shells and minerals.

Herbs can also be prepared with alcohol as an extractive. Usually, strong rice wine is used in the preparation of Chinese herbal extracts. The herbs are simply macerated in approximately 50 proof alcohol or high proof rice wine for a period of two weeks to a year. This is then strained and taken internally as a tonic or used topically as a liniment to relieve pain. Certain herbs, such as prepared Rehmannia and Dang gui

(Angelica sinensis), are alternately sprayed with wine and dried several times to alter the energy and function and to extract the active ingredient in the herb itself. Such herbal alcoholic extracts have a very long shelf life.

DOSAGE

Historically, weights varied at different periods. Since the Tang dynasty, one liang equaled 31.25 grams. This being an awkward number, the People's Republic of China standardized modern equivalents as follows:

1 liang = 30 grams
1 chien = 3 grams
1 fen = 0.3 grams
1 li = .03 grams

Most average strength Chinese herbs are 6-9 grams dosage. Herbs that are light in weight or strong are 3-6 grams. Heavier minerals and herbs are precooked and range from 9 to 30 grams. If one is studying Japanese-Chinese herbalism (Kampo), the average dose is approximately one third that of the Chinese.

Dosage was originally determined according to the patient's condition and tolerance. The following can be considered a guideline to proper dosing:

1. Strong and toxic substances, such as cinnabar, should be prescribed in the smallest possible dose.
2. Heavy roots are taken in higher dosage than light flowers or leaves.
3. Most heavy minerals and shells are used in still higher dosage.
4. Tonics, sedative, tranquilizing herbs are prescribed in higher doses, while sweating, qi moving (carminative), blood moving, drying and fragrant herbs are prescribed in smaller doses.
5. A single herb or substance is generally prescribed in higher dosage than when it is in a formula. However, the primary herb(s) in a formula is always prescribed in a higher dose relative to the assistant and counter-assistant herbs.
6. Fresh herbs containing more water need to be taken in double the indicated dose.
7. The dose for a more serious disease should be as high as the patient can tolerate.
8. For children under one year the dose is 1/10 that of an adult dose; From 2-3 years the dose is 1/4 the adult dose; from 3-6

years it is 1/3 the adult dose; from 10 years to adult the dose is approximately 1/2 the adult dose.

METHODS OF PREPARING AND TAKING CHINESE HERBS

Herbs can be taken in many forms. Some of these reflect the form that is optimum for absorption, others are more a matter of convenience. Chinese herbs are available in decoctions, pills, alcoholic liquors, macerations, pastes and extracts.

Water decoction is generally the best medium for absorption for most herbs. There are many methods used for decoctions. One is to use approximately 20 times by volume the amount of water to herbs. First immerse the herbs for a half hour or so in the water then slowly raise the temperature to boiling. Reduce the flame to lessen the loss of volatile oils from the herbs. The volume of liquid is reduced to approximately two or three cups of tea. One cup is taken two or three times daily.

Heavier minerals and roots are preferably decocted first for a longer period of time. Aromatic herbs or lighter leaves and flowers with important volatile oils are added toward the end of the process of decoction or infused in the hot tea that is covered to prevent their loss.

A strong decoction is made by twice or thrice cooking the herbs as a double or triple decoction respectively. After each cooking, the tea is set aside and more water is added for subsequent cooking. When the various stages of decoction are completed all the resultant teas are mixed together which usually results in approximately two or three cups.

Pills, capsules and alcoholic preparations are easy to overdose. In general, always begin with the minimum indicated dose on the label and increase as individual tolerance will allow. If one is taking a formula for the Kidneys it is good to take it with a pinch of salt or soya sauce to help carry the action of the herbs to the Kidneys. If one is taking a preparation for arthritic or rheumatic problems, taking it with a teaspoon of rice wine or alcohol will help carry it into the blood more effectively. A Spleen Qi tonic is more effective if it is taken with a small amount of honey, barley malt or rice. This is all in accord with the flavors according to the Five Elements. Herbs taken to cleanse the liver should not be taken as an alcoholic extract. If one desires to take a tincture without the alcohol, most of it can be evaporated by putting the appropriate amount of extract in a cup of boiling water for a few minutes.

Concentrated extracts of Chinese herbs are very convenient to dispense and have much wider patient acceptance. Most traditional classical formulas can be obtained from a variety of manufacturers.

They have a further convenience of taking up very little space in the pharmacy. They can be taken as a powder or granule simply eaten or mixed with water or they can be put into gelatin capsules. Dosage for most conditions is 500 mg. per 20 pounds of body weight. For acute conditions more should be taken for one to three days, then tapered off as the symptoms subside.

HOW AND WHEN TO TAKE HERBS

Metal cooking vessels are never used to prepare medicinal herbal teas. This is because metals, such as iron, copper, brass or aluminum, and to a lesser extent other types of metals, can react with and alter the chemistry of herbs. Instead, glass or ceramic containers are used.

There are many methods of preparing herbal teas, called "tangs" (literally translated as "soups" or decoctions) based upon the predilection of the herbalist. One standard method is to combine the ingredients of each formula in 3 to 4 cups of water. This is then brought to boiling and allowed to slowly simmer for approximately 45 minutes to an hour or until the original volume of fluid has been reduced to approximately 2 cups. One cup is taken morning and evening. The remaining strained herbs of the original tea can be cooked again the next day using two cups of water which is cooked down to one so that one dose of herbs can make three servings.

There are many other methods, including presoaking heavier roots, barks and substances for an hour or two before bringing to a boil, further decocting or reducing the herbs even a third time, and so forth. However, the method described is the one we have used for years with good results.

Certain ingredients require different cooking times and processes. For instance, some herbs, especially the surface relieving diaphoretics whose potency is dependent upon volatile oils, are volatilized and destroyed in a lengthy decoction process and are added last to be steeped after the heavier ingredients have been extracted. These include herbs such as mint, chrysanthemum flowers, fresh ginger and cinnamon twigs. On the other hand, heavier herbs, especially minerals such as dragon bone, oyster shell and iron, require longer extraction, up to one or two hours of preparation. In the case of toxic herbs, such as unprepared aconite, it is required to slowly simmer them at least an hour in boiling water to lessen or neutralize their toxicity. This is even recommended for the preparation of prepared or previously detoxified herbs such as prepared aconite (Fu zi).

In cooking a formula that combines minerals or toxic herbs with those that have volatile oils, one needs to first decoct the longer cooking herbs and then progressively add the other herbs which need less cooking time. Those that need to be steeped are added at the end with the heat turned off and allowed to sit and infuse for the last 10 or 15 minutes.

Tonics are generally taken before meals. Herbs that are cooling and detoxifying can be more irritating and may be taken after meals. Purgatives and anthelmintics should be taken on an empty stomach for maximum effect. Sedative and tranquilizing herbs should always be taken before rest and at least three times throughout the day to support and strengthen the nervous system which is necessary for proper rest to occur in the evening. Pain-relieving herbs can be taken as often as needed.

Herbs should be taken warm for Cold conditions and cool for Hot conditions such as fevers. Individuals who experience nausea should take the herbs in small repeated dosages according to tolerance.

Both for convenience and therapeutic efficacy, Chinese herbs can be taken in many forms. Powders, called "san", are taken by simply mixing them with a little warm water. Another method is to mix the herbal powders with honey to form either several small pills, called "wan", or one large pill mass. Because honey is sweet, it is a good method for taking herbal tonics. The average dose for most herbal powders is approximately 6 grams at a time at least twice a day, more or less according to constitution, body size, age and sensitivity.

Alcoholic extracts, called "chih", are usually made with a high alcoholic potency rice wine. To make these, the whole or powdered herbs are allowed to macerate in the rice wine or alcohol for six months to a year.

Chinese herbs are also taken as nutritive tonics in soup, or in a rice soup, called "congee", using herbs such as Jujube dates, Astragalus root, Dioscorea, Lycii berries, Ginseng or Codonopsis root. These are commonly cooked with glutinous sweet rice using one part (by volume) rice to 7 to 10 parts water. This is cooked slowly for 8 to 10 hours and is taken in the morning or at various times throughout the day as an easily digested porridge. Other foods, such as meat and various appropriate root vegetables, can be added. This method is least likely to generate an adverse reaction and is particularly good for those who have poor digestion or are wasting, thin, emaciated and/or weak. Today it is most convenient to use a timed "slow cooker" or high quality stainless steel rice cooker for these kinds of preparations.

A popular innovation is the use of concentrated powdered extracts. These are made through a special closed extraction process where the

herbs are decocted in an enclosed vessel so as to fully capture their volatile components, which are then reintroduced back into the final dry concentrate. Depending upon the quality of the original herbs, they can be quite good, representing a concentration of approximately 5 parts herb down to one part of the powdered extract. Many of the classic formulas are available in this form as well as single herbs to prepare individual formula combinations. The ready availability of these products in many Western countries makes them convenient for practitioners and students with limited funds and space for storing a pharmacy of 250 or so herbs. They are also highly convenient and easy for patients to take on a regular basis.

In general, teas and congees or soups are the most highly assimilable forms for taking herbs. Alcoholic extracts are also readily assimilable, however they are inappropriate for those with Liver Fire or Damp Heat. Pills and powders take more digestive capacity to metabolize.

Contraindications and Incompatibilities

Any substance is contraindicated if it is not needed. Conversely, even toxic substances may not have toxic effects if they are needed or somehow used by the body to foster normalcy. Herbs may be added to a formula to counteract its undesirable properties as well.

Contraindications are usually an obvious matter of common sense, especially when a particular herbal property is prescribed in relation to the TCM pattern of disharmony. For instance, Excess Yang Heat would be aggravated by herbs that Warm and tonify. Yin Deficiency, characterized by wasting Heat, is aggravated by herbs with a Warm or Hot energy. Herbs that are moist aggravate Dampness.

The Nineteen Antagonisms and Eighteen Incompatibles

Traditionally there is a list of combinations that are considered incompatible. In all cases they involve the combination of herbs that one never finds together in traditional formulas or have properties that are directly opposite or antagonistic to each other. This is one of the many reasons that one would begin the study and practice of TCM with the use of the classical formulas.

Nineteen Antagonisms
Sulfur (Liu Huang) is antagonistic with Sal glauberis (Po Xiao).
Hydragyrum (Shui Yin) is antagonistic with Arsenicum (Pi Shuang).
Radix Euphorbiae (Da Ji) is antagonistic with Lithargyrum
(Mi Tuo Seng).

Semen Croton tiglii (Ba Dou) is antagonistic with Semen pharbitidis (Qian Niu Zi).
Nitrum (Ya Xiao) is antagonistic with Rhizoma sparganii (San Leng).
Flos caryophylli (Ding Xiang) is antagonistic with Tuber curcuma (Yu Jin) and Radix curcuma (Jiang Huang).
Radix aconiti (Wu Tou) is antagonistic with Cornu rhinoceri (Xi Jiao).
Radix Ginseng (Ren Shen) is antagonistic with Excrementum trogopteri seu pteromi (Wu Ling Zhi).
Cortex Cinnamomum (Rou Gui) is antagonistic with Halloysitum Rubrum (Chi Shi Zhi).

Eighteen Incompatibles
Radix glycyrrhizae uralensis (licorice) is incompatible with:
Euphorbiae kansui (Gan Sui)
Radix euphorbiae seu knoxiae (Da Ji)
Flos daphne genkwa (Yuan Hua)
Herba sargassi (Hai Zao)

Radix aconiti (Wu Tou) is incompatible with:
Bulbus fritillaria (Bei Mu)
Fructus trichosanthes (Gua Lou)
Rhizoma pinellia ternata (Ban Xia)
Radix ampelopsis (Bai Lian)
Rhizoma bletilla striata (Bai Ji)

Rhizoma et radix veratri (Li Lu) is incompatible with:
Radix ginseng (Ren Shen)
Radix adenophorae seu glehniae (Sha Shen)
Radix salvia miltiorrhiza (Dan Shen)
Radix sophorae flavescentis (Ku Shen)
Herba cum radice asari (Xi Xin)
Herba paeonia lactiflora (Bai Shao)

In a world that accepts strong drug medicines with a plethora of adverse reactions, radiation and chemotherapy as acceptable treatments, modern research in China has exposed no serious side effects for most, if not all, of the above combinations.

Dietary Restrictions
Certain foods tend to be contraindicated with some herbs and formulas. In most cases this means the avoidance of foods that would aggravate a previous imbalance such as raw, cold foods for conditions of

Coldness; hot, spicy foods, heavy, sweet foods and richly nutritious animal protein foods for conditions of Excess; greasy and mucilaginous foods for conditions of Dampness; and foods that are heavy and hard to digest for conditions of Food Stagnation and digestive weakness.

In addition, there are certain herbs that are prohibited to be taken simultaneously with various foods. For instance neither Licorice (Gan Cao), Coptis (Huang Lian), Platycodon (Jie Geng) nor Mume (Wu Mei) can be taken with pork. Mint cannot be taken with turtle meat nor Poria mushroom with vinegar.

Contraindications During Pregnancy
Certain substances can induce miscarriage or damage to the fetus. These are generally herbs that have strong Blood and Qi moving properties and herbs that are toxic or have strong heating properties. Following is a representative group of herbs that are prohibited during pregnancy: Croton (Ba Dou), Pharbitidis (Qian Niu Zi), Euphorbiae (Da Ji), Mylabris (Ban Mao), Phytolaccae (Shang Lu), Moschus (She Xiang), Cyperus (Xiang Fu), Zedoariae (E Zhu), Hirudo (Shui Zhi).

Following is a representative list of herbs that should be used with great care during pregnancy: Rhubarb root (Da Huang), Aconiti (Fu Zi), Ginger (Gan Jiang), Pinellia (Ban Xia), Cinnamon bark (Rou Gui), Abutili (Dong Kui Zi), Carthamus (Hong Hua), Persicae (Tao Ren).

HERBS THAT RELEASE THE EXTERIOR

Herbs that release the Exterior treat acute External conditions affecting the upper respiratory tract, including eye, ear, nose and throat diseases and the skin. This category is further subdivided as External Cold and External Heat. The concept of Wind associated with this category refers to the tendency for such infectious and inflammatory diseases to react and change quickly and proliferate.

The Lungs, skin, and pores are regarded as the domain of the Wei Qi, which corresponds to the immune system. In turn, this energy is sustained and nourished with the assimilation of food, water and air by the acquired energy of the Spleen-Stomach and the inherited constitutional Qi of the Kidney-adrenals. External diseases such as colds, flu, allergies and skin diseases, therefore, while directly caused by bacteria or viruses, are only able to penetrate when we are overwhelmed by environmental stress or in a debilitated state.

The light acrid or spicy flavor characteristic of all herbs in this category is surface dispersing. Most enter the Lungs because the Wei Qi emanates from that Organ system. They may also enter the Bladder

Organ meridian because this is the representative Organ associated with the Tai Yang. Being the longest meridian of the body, the Bladder meridian runs from the inner canthus of the eye over the top of the head and down both sides of the spine to the feet. Literally, when we catch a chill, we can feel the reaction along the neck and upper spine, which is the area of attack. Still others, such as fresh Ginger (Sheng Jiang), enter the Stomach and Spleen because this is the area of acute gastrointestinal diseases. Finally, a number of them such as Bupleurum (Chai Hu) and Mint (Bo He) enter the Liver and Gallbladder because they treat External Wind and also calm the Liver.

Wind represents not only the proliferating aspect of disease but the neurological aspect of tension and spasm. It is this reactive phase of acute External disease that causes the pores to contract, for instance, and literally causes the body to lock the disease inwards.

As a result, the primary intention of therapy is to release the Exterior by inducing sweating. This is primarily done in two ways: one is through the use of Warm stimulating herbs that increase surface capillary circulation and thus increase perspiration. The other method is through the use of cooling diaphoretics that relieve surface tension, allowing the pores to dilate freely. Thus the two subcategories are Warm Surface Relieving herbs that treat Coldness and Cool surface relieving herbs that treat Heat.

Because depth and location is a defining aspect of this category, External surface relieving herbs are primarily used to treat the early stage of External disease.

WARM/ACRID RELEASE THE EXTERIOR

Ephedra Sinica   Ma Huang   (1)

Common Name: Ephedra, Ma Huang

Part Used: Aerial portion (Herba)

Family: Ephedraceae

Energy and Flavor: bitter, acrid and Warm

Organ Meridians Affected: Lung and Urinary Bladder

Actions: 1. Releases the surface, 2. Promotes the circulation of Lung Qi, 3. Promotes urination.

Indications: 1. For Greater Yang stage (Tai yang) disease with chills, fever, headache and lack of sweating; 2. Relieves cough, wheezing and asthma; 3. Clears edema.

Contraindications: Not for those with high blood pressure nor those with insomnia or spontaneous sweating. Use of this herb for extended periods of time is not recommended.

Dosage: 3 - 9 grams

Notes: For Wind-Cold-Exterior syndrome with chills, fever, headache, general aches, upper respiratory congestion, absence of sweating, thin and white tongue coat with floating and tight pulse, combine with Cinnamon Twigs (Gui Zhi) in Ephedra Tea Combination (Ma Huang Tang); for the common cold, cough and asthma Ephedra is combined with Apricot seed, Gypsum and Licorice root; for edema it is combined with White Atractylodes and Poria cocos.

There are many Ephedra species that grow in diverse areas of the world, including the Southwestern high desert of the North American continent. Chinese Ma Huang, however, originating in inner Mongolia, has the greatest concentration of ephedrine and pseudoephedrine alkaloids. Somehow the Chinese have known for centuries that the highest concentration of the active principle is in the portion of the stem between the joints. For this reason, the best quality has the joint cut away. This is becoming less available because of the labor intensive factor. Interestingly, the root (Ma Huang Gen) has exactly the opposite property and is used for excessive perspiration and diarrhea.

This herb has been much abused in the western marketplace as a stimulant. Individuals, seeking to commercialize on its stimulant properties, make it into a highly concentrated extract which is then sold as an energy stimulant, dietary weight loss product and even as a recreational drug. This moves it beyond the realm of a whole herb to the level of a drug that exceeds the traditional contraindications for Ephedra. Individuals who are at risk with potential coronary heart disease should avoid these type of Ma Huang products.

Cinnamomum Cassia   Gui Zhi   (1)

Common Name: Cinnamon Twig

Part Used: Branches (Ramulus)

Family: Lauraceae

Energy and Flavor: sweet, acrid and Warm

Organ Meridians Affected: Lung, Heart and Urinary Bladder

Actions: 1. Adjusts the nutritive Ying and defensive Wei Qi when sweating does not relieve External disease; 2. Warms and disperses Cold; 3. Removes obstruction of Yang; 4. Promotes the circulation of Yang Qi in the chest; 5. Regulates and moves blood.

Indications: 1. For External Cold, Deficient patterns; 2. Warms the channels and relieves Cold, Damp Wind arthritic and rheumatic conditions; 3. Resolves Cold Damp Phlegm; 5. Relieves Blood Stagnation, treating dysmenorrhea and lower abdominal masses.

Contraindications: Do not use for those with Warm febrile diseases, those who are showing Heat signs, and should be used with caution for women who are pregnant or are bleeding heavily.

Dosage: 3 - 9 grams

Notes: For Wind-Cold-Exterior Conditions such as the common cold without sweating, combine with Ephedra (Ma Huang); for Wind-Cold-Exterior-Deficiency with abnormal sweating, aversion to wind and fever combine with White Peony (Bai Shao) in Cinnamon Twig Combination (Gui Zhi Tang); for rheumatic and arthritic pains aggravated by Wind-Cold-Damp combine with Prepared Aconite (Fu Zi); for palpitations, shortness of breath and edema caused by Deficient Yang of the Heart and Spleen combine with Poria (Fu Ling) and Atractylodes (Bai Zhu); for angina combine with Macrostem Onion (Xie Bai) and Trichosanthes fruit (Gua Lou); for amenorrhea with abdominal pain caused by Cold Blood Stagnation combine with Peach Seed (Tao Ren), Poria (Fu Ling) and Moutan (Mu Dan Pi) in Cinnamon and Poria Combination (Gui Zhi Fu Ling Tang).

This herb is used as a warm circulatory tonic producing movement of Qi (neurological energy) and Blood and consequent warmth, and it is also diuretic. Cinnamon twigs spread the Yang of the Heart and can be used to warm the extremities. On the North American continent, sassafras, also in the Lauraceae family, has similar properties but is not nearly as warming as cinnamon.

Zingiberis Officinalis   Sheng Jiang   (1)

Common Name: Fresh Ginger

Part Used: Rhizome (Rhizoma)

Family: Zingiberaceae

Energy and Flavor: acrid and Warm

Organ Meridians Affected: Lung, Stomach and Spleen

Actions: 1. Relieves the Exterior and disperses Cold; 2. Warms and circulates Qi in the Middle Burner; 3. Calms a restless fetus and treats morning sickness; 4. Treats seafood poisoning.

Indications: 1. Treats External Wind, Cold disease with symptoms of fever, chills, headache, nasal congestion and cough; 2. Warms the center, promotes appetite, digestion and relieves nausea; 3. For morning sickness; 4. For seafood poisoning.

Contraindications: Do not use for symptoms of Exterior Deficiency with sweating or for Damp Heat conditions.

Dosage: 3 - 9 grams

Notes: For nausea and vomiting caused by a Cold Stomach, combine with Pinellia (Ban Xia). If the vomiting is caused by Heat, combine with Bamboo Shavings (Zhu Ru) and Coptis (Huang Lian).

In Ayurveda, both an immediate flavor and a post digestive flavor are assigned to an herb. Fresh Ginger is classified as having an initial spicy energy and a post digestive sweet energy, which means that it is beneficial for digestion and assimilation (goes to the Stomach and Spleen). Dry Ginger is hotter and more of a metabolic stimulant. Fresh Ginger has many uses both internal and external. Internally, any food or milk heated and taken with the addition of a few slices of fresh Ginger will make it more thoroughly assimilable and therefore more tonic. Fresh Ginger tea with honey is one of the best treatments for children or adults who are beginning to show signs of mucus and phlegm which often precede a cold. Externally, dipping a cloth in fresh Ginger tea and applying it to spasms, sprains and chronic pains and injuries offers tremendous symptomatic relief by promoting better circulation.

Magnolia Liliflorae   Xin Yi Hua   (3)

Common Name: Magnolia Flower

Part Used: Flower (Flos)

Family: Magnoliaceae

Energy and Flavor: acrid and Warm

Organ Meridians Affected: Lung and Stomach

Actions: 1. Releases the Exterior and disperses Cold; 2. Opens the nasal passages.

Indications: 1. Treats External Wind for Wind-Cold diseases with obstruction of the nasal passages, headache and rhinitis.

Contraindications: This herb should not be used by those who are Yin Deficient with signs of Heat as it is very drying. Overdose may cause dizziness and/or red eyes.

Dosage: 3 - 9 grams

Notes: The flowering bud of this herb is unique in its effect of warming and opening the sinuses of the nasal passages. As with many of the External releasing diaphoretic herbs described, it should never be boiled, but only added at the end of decoction and steeped to prevent the loss of essential volatile oils.

Perillae Frutescens   Zi Su Ye   (2)
Common Name: Perilla Leaf
Part Used: Foliage (Folium)
Family: Labiatae
Energy and Flavor: acrid, Warm and aromatic
Organ Meridians Affected: Lung and Spleen

Actions: 1. Relieves the Exterior and disperses Cold; 2. Promotes the circulation of Spleen and Stomach Qi; 3. Calms a restless fetus; 4. Detoxifies seafood poisoning.

Indications: 1. Treats External, Cold diseases such as common cold, chills and headache; 2. Warms the center and promotes appetite and digestion, relieves nausea and vomiting; 3. For morning sickness; 4. For food poisoning.

Contraindications: This herb should not be used by those who have External diseases where there is already sweating nor by those who have a Damp-Heat condition.

Dosage: 3 - 9 grams

Notes: Sometimes called "Japanese Sweet Basil", since it is often used as a healthful condiment called "shiso" in traditional Japanese cooking. Eating the raw leaves is especially effective for relieving toxic poisoning from eating shell fish and fish. It is also taken with Citrus peel and Cardamon seed to relieve the symptoms of morning sickness and prevent miscarriage.

For Wind Cold cough and bronchitis, 9 grams of dried Perilla leaf (more if fresh), 9 grams Apricot seed and 6 grams Citrus peel (Chen pi) are decocted in water. Enough water and sweet glutinous rice are used to cook into a porridge consistency (congee).

Schizonepetae Tenuifolia   Jing Jie   (1)
Common Name: Schizonepeta, Chinese Catnip
Part Used: Aerial portion and Flowers (Herba seu Flos)
Family: Labiatae
Energy and Flavor: acrid, neutral and aromatic
Organ Meridians Affected: Lung and Liver

Actions: 1. Relieves the Exterior and disperses Cold or Heat depending on the other herbs used; 2. Releases the Exterior for measles; 3. Stops bleeding; 4. Abates swellings.

Indications: 1. Treats External Wind, for disease of Wind Cold or Wind Heat depending on the other herbs used in the formula; 2. Treats External Wind to express ailments such as rashes or measles; 3. For blood in the stool or uterine bleeding; 4. Treats abscesses and other swellings.

Contraindications: This herb should not be taken by those with spontaneous sweating or with Liver signs such as headache, especially when there is a Deficiency. It should not be used for skin diseases that have become full blown.

Dosage: 3 - 9 grams

Notes: Also known as Japanese Catnip, this herb is presently under cultivation in the West. It has many uses ranging from the treatment of fevers, headache and sore throat, to various eruptive skin diseases including boils and abscesses. It is also antispasmodic and is useful for the treatment of rheumatic complaints as well as facial paralysis, symptoms of stroke, stiffness of the neck and spine.

Schizonepeta Congee is used to treat Wind Cold, the common cold and flu. Combine 9 grams of Schizonepeta, 3 grams Bo He Mint (Spearmint will also do), 9 grams fermented Black soya beans (black beans can also be used) and 100 grams of sweet glutinous rice. Decoct the first three ingredients for 5 to 10 minutes in a covered pan. Cook sweet glutinous rice with the Black soya beans in enough water to make a porridge consistency. Towards the end of cooking mix in the tea of the first three herbs.

For measles, skin eruptions and itching, Schizonepeta is combined with Cicada slough (Chan Tui), Arctium (Niu Bang Zi) and Mentha (Bo He).

Notopterygium Incisum   Qiang Huo   (2)

Common Name: Notopterygium

Part Used: Root and Rhizome (Radix et Rhizoma)

Family: Umbelliferae

Energy and Flavor: acrid, bitter, Warm and aromatic

Organ Meridians Affected: Kidney and Urinary Bladder

Actions: 1. Relieves the Exterior and disperses Cold and Dampness; 2. Relieves Wind-Damp-Cold painful obstruction; 3. Directs Qi to the Greater Yang (Tai Yang) channel and the Governing Vessel.

Indications: 1. Treats External Wind, for Cold diseases such as chills, headache and the common cold;

2. Disperses Cold and Dampness for symptoms such as rheumatic pains of the joints; 3. Directs herbs of a formula to the Greater Yang (Tai Yang) channel and the Governing Vessel.

Contraindications: This herb should not be used by those with Yin or Blood Deficiency conditions or arthritis caused by Blood Stagnation.

Dosage: 6 - 12 grams

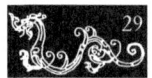

Notes: The umbelliferae group of medicinal herbs include the various Angelicas, Lovage, a Southwestern Native American herb called "Osha" (Ligusticum porteri), Chinese Bupleurum, Ledebouriella and Lomatium species. These herbs share similarities in their ability to drive the circulation and relieve various types of Stagnations (Qi, Blood and Cold) that can eventually lead to toxicity.

Combined with Ledebouriella (Fang Feng) and Turmeric (Jiang Huang) for Cold Wind Dampness diseases associated with headaches and arthritic and rheumatic conditions, especially of the upper back and shoulders. For Exterior symptoms of Cold with chills, fever, headaches and general pain, it can be combined with Ledebouriella (Fang Feng), Angelica Dahurica (Bai Zhi) and Black Atractylodes (Cang Zhu).

Ledebouriella Divaricata   Fang Feng   (1)

Common Name: Ledebouriella, Siler

Part Used: Root (Radix)

Family: Umbelliferae

Energy and Flavor: acrid, sweet and Warm

Organ Meridians Affected: Lung, Liver, Spleen and Urinary Bladder

Actions: 1. Relieves the Exterior and disperses Cold; 2. Relieves Wind-Damp-Cold painful obstruction; 3. Disperses Wind.

Indications: 1. Treats External Wind, for common cold, stiff neck, chills and headache; 2. Disperses Wind, Dampness and Cold for symptoms such as rheumatic pain, arthritis and other painful obstructions where Wind is predominant; 3. Treats conditions of Wind in combination with other herbs for symptoms such as tremors, intestinal Wind and migraine headaches.

Contraindications: This herb should not be used by those who are Yin Deficient or those with Blood Deficiency or by those with Heat signs associated with Yin Deficiency.

Dosage: 3 - 9 grams

Notes: The Chinese name literally means "Preventing Wind" and indicates its primary use as an antispasmodic, especially for the treatment of tension type headaches. Wind generally refers to diseases that are adversely influenced by climatic wind and dampness, which can include various types of arthritic aches and pains and spasms. A more serious Internal Wind disease is stroke.

To prevent colds and flu, combine with Astragalus (Huang Qi) and Atractylodes (Bai Zhu) in Jade Screen Combination (Yu Ping Feng San); for Wind Heat conditions with fever, sore throat, eye redness and

headaches, combine with Schizonepeta (Jing Jie), Scutellaria (Huang Qin), Mentha (Bo He) and Forsythia (Lian Qiao).

Angelica Dahurica   Bai Zhi   (2)
Common Name: Angelica, Angelica Dahurica
Part Used: Root (Radix)
Family: Umbelliferae
Energy and Flavor: acrid and Warm
Organ Meridians Affected: Lung and Stomach
Actions: 1. Relieves the Exterior and disperses Wind; 2. Disperses Wind and Cold from the Yang Brightness channels; 3. Relieves Wind-Damp-Cold painful obstruction; 4. Dries Dampness and pus and reduces swelling; 5. Opens the nasal passages.
Indications: 1. Treats External Wind for common cold and allergies; 2. Warms the Yang Brightness channels and circulates Qi for headaches and nasal congestion with pain; 3. Warms the joints, dries Dampness and relieves painful blockage obstruction (Bi Pain); 4. For sores and swellings before or after the pus has formed to reduce swelling or drain the pus; 5. For nasal congestion.
Contraindications: This herb should not be used by those with Yin or Blood Deficiency.
Dosage: 3 - 9 grams
Notes: For Wind-Cold-Exterior syndrome with headache and upper respiratory congestion combine with Green Onion (Cong Bai), Prepared soybean (Dan Dou Chi) and Fresh Ginger (Sheng Jiang); for rhinitis, nasosinusitis and upper respiratory allergies combine with Xanthium (Cang Er Zi) and Magnolia Flower (Xin Yi) in Xanthium Combination (Cang Er Zi San).

Ligusticum Sinense   Gao Ben   (3)
Common Name: Chinese Lovage, Ligusticum
Part Used: Rhizome and Root (Rhizoma et Radix)
Family: Umbelliferae
Energy and Flavor: acrid and Warm
Organ Meridians Affected: Urinary Bladder and Lung
Actions: 1. Relieves the Exterior and disperses Wind; 2. Disperses Cold and relieves pain; 3. Disperses Wind-Damp-Cold painful obstruction.

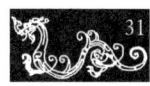

Indications: 1. Treats Externally contracted Wind-Cold symptoms such as headache and pain of the mouth; 2. Relieves pain from Cold such as headache, toothache and abdominal pain; 3. Expels Wind, Damp and Cold for painful obstruction such as rheumatism and arthritis.

Contraindications: This herb should not be used for those who are Yin Deficient with Heat signs nor by those with Blood Deficiency.

Dosage: 3 - 9 grams

Notes: Commonly used for the treatment of Wind Cold pains of the upper body, especially headaches, for which it can be combined with Angelica Dahurica (Bai Zhi) and Ligusticum (Chuan Xiong).

Allium Fistulosi   Cong Bai   (1)

Common Name: Green Onion, Scallion

Part Used: Bulb (Bulbus)

Family: Liliaceae

Energy and Flavor: acrid and Warm

Organ Meridians Affected: Lung and Stomach

Actions: 1. Relieves the Exterior and disperses Wind-Cold; 2. Vitalizes the Yang Qi and disperses Cold; 3. Removes toxicity of swellings

Indications: 1. Treats early stages of External Cold diseases such as common cold; 2. Warms the channels and relieves pain of the abdomen and nasal passages; 3. Applied topically to toxic swellings for abscess and open sores.

Contraindications: This herb should not be used when there is spontaneous sweating.

Dosage: 3 - 9 grams, should be added near the end of the decoction

Notes: Onions have similar but milder properties to garlic. They have a Warm circulating energy with detoxifying properties. The green onion is the mildest in the family, having less of a metabolic push than garlic, so it is used for the initial stages of External Cold diseases.

One of the most common treatments for the beginning of the common cold is Glutinous Rice and Scallion Congee. This is made by first cooking the glutinous rice into a porridge. While it is still hot, stir in finely chopped scallions and bring briefly to a boil. Allow to cool and eat on an empty stomach. This will help overcome the cold by inducing perspiration. To loosen phlegm in the chest and mobilize Yang, combine Allium with Trichosanthes (Gua Lou).

Elsholtziae Splendens   Xiang Ru   (3)

Common Name: Elsholtzia, Aromatic Madder, Madder

Part Used: Aerial portion (Herba)

Family: Labiatae

Energy and Flavor: acrid, Warm and aromatic

Organ Meridians Affected: Lung and Stomach

Actions: 1. Relieves the Exterior and disperses Summer-Heat; 2. Induces urination and reduces swellings.

Indications: 1. Treats conditions of Wind-Cold in the summer; 2. Reduces edema and swellings.

Contraindications: This herb should not be used by those with Deficiency with sweating. This herb should be taken cool (not hot) or taken with other cooling herbs.

Dosage: 3 - 9 grams

Notes: This herb is primarily used for Summer Heat syndromes with symptoms of Dampness with chills and fever. For this it is commonly combined with Agastache (Huo Xiang) and Dolichoris (Bian Dou).

Asarum Sieboldi   Xi Xin   (2)

Common Name: Wild Ginger, Asarum

Part Used: Herb and Root (Herba cum Radice)

Family: Aristolochiaceae

Energy and Flavor: acrid and Warm

Organ Meridians Affected: Lung and Kidney

Actions: 1. Relieves the Exterior and warms the Yang; 2. Expels Cold and relieves pain; 3. Warms the Lung and reduces Phlegm; 4. Moves the Qi and disperses Phlegm to open the nasal passages.

Indications: 1. Treats External Wind-Cold with underlying Dampness and/or Yang Deficiency; 2. Relieves pain from Cold obstructing the channels, usually associated with Wind-Cold, with symptoms of toothache, headache and general body aches; 3. For Cold Fluids stuck in the Lungs with symptoms of thin copious sputum or chronic bronchitis; 4. For nasal congestion with Cold associated ailments.

Contraindications: This herb should not be used by those who are Qi Deficient with sweating nor by those with headache due to Blood or Yin Deficiency. It should also not be used for Lung conditions when there is thick yellow Phlegm. It should be avoided during pregnancy.

Dosage: 1 - 3 grams

Notes: Wild Ginger is a strong warming and circulation promoting herb and is sometimes classified under Internal Warming Stimulant. Various species are found growing throughout the world. One (Asarum canadensis) in the Pacific Northwest of North America is somewhat

milder and traditionally used as a tea for colds as well as a treatment for cold and damp sensitive rheumatic complaints.

Asarum can be used for various Wind-Cold conditions such as coughing, joint pains, cramps, numbness and pain of the extremities. For Cold Phlegm attacking the Lungs with symptoms of cough, asthma, abundant clear phlegm, combine it with Ephedra (Ma Huang) and Dried Ginger (Gan Jiang); for upper respiratory allergies with clear nasal discharge, combine it with Angelica Dahurica (Bai Zhi), Magnolia Flower (Xin Yi) and Mentha (Bo He); for Wind-Cold-Damp joint pains, combine it with Notopterygium (Qiang Huo), Ledebouriella (Fang Feng) and Cinnamon Twigs (Gui Zhi). Western Asarum (A. Canadense) can be used as a Blood moving emmenagogue for dysmenorrhea and amenorrhea.

Coriander   Hu Sui

Botanical Name: Coriandrum Sativum

Common Name: Coriander

Part Used: The herb

Family: Umbelliferae

Energy and Flavors: Spicy and Warm

Organ Meridian Affected: Lungs and Stomach

Actions: 1. Promotes sweating; 2. Brings rashes to the surface

Indications: Use with Cicada (Chan Tui), Schizonepeta (Jing Jie) and Arctium (Niu Bang Zi) for early stages of measles and other eruptive diseases. The tea can also be applied topically to help erupt rashes to the surface of the skin.

Notes: Coriander herb, also known in Spanish as Cilantro, is used as a condiment in both East Indian and Central American cuisine. Apart from the classification as Warm by the Chinese, in cooking it is used to counteract the heating effects of strong spicy foods.

Discrimination:

Ephedra (Ma Huang) – used to treat Cold natured lung diseases, asthma and cough.

Cinnamon Twig (Gui Zhi) – warming and circulating, moves the Yang, harmonizes the Nutritive Ying and Wei, disperses External Cold.

Fresh Ginger (Sheng Jiang) – benefits digestion, harmonizes and warms the Stomach and Spleen.

Wild Ginger (Xi Xin) – benefits circulation, opens the meridians and treats Coldness caused by Kidney Yang Deficiency.

Ligusticum (Gao Ben) — specifically useful for headaches.

Notopterygium (Qiang Huo), Angelica (Bai Zhi) along with Ledebouriella (Fang Feng) — relieve Wind-Cold-Dampness in the meridians and muscles and treat acute arthritic and rheumatic pains.

Schizonepeta (Jing Jie) — treats skin diseases and when charred is used to stop bleeding.

Magnolia Flower (Xin Yi Hua) — specifically used to clear the head and sinuses.

Elscholtziae (Xiang Ru) — used for Summer Heat diseases associated with Internal Dampness.

Bulbus Alii (Cong Bai) — treats colds and, when externally applied, ripens and resolves toxic swellings and sores.

Perilla Leaf (Zi Su Ye) — treats gastrointestinal diseases and seafood poisoning.

Coriander Herb (Hu Sui) — brings rashes to the surface.

COOL/ACRID RELEASE THE EXTERIOR
Arctium Lappa   Niu Bang Zi   (1)

Common Name: Burdock Seed, Arctium Fruit

Part Used: Fruit (Fructus)

Family: Compositae

Energy and Flavor: bitter, acrid and Cold

Organ Meridians Affected: Lung and Stomach

Actions: 1. Relieves the Exterior and disperses Heat; 2. Allows the release of toxicity from the surface and clears Heat; 3. Reduces swelling and clears pathogenic Heat; 4. Lubricates the Intestines.

Indications: 1. Treats External Wind-Heat with fever and sore throat; 2. For all Wind-Heat skin ailments such as measles and rashes; 3. For swollen throat and swellings on the skin; 4. For constipation due to Wind-Heat.

Contraindications: This herb should not be used by persons with diarrhea.

Dosage: 3 - 9 grams

Notes: One of the most important and versatile herbs. The root is called "gobo" and cooked (usually sauteed) as a part of traditional Japanese diet. Burdock, along with all other herb seeds, when used medicinally, should be crushed to release their contents into decoction. The seeds are one of the best treatments for skin diseases, while the root is useful as a general detoxifier and blood purifier. The root is effective for a wide variety of chronic degenerative diseases such as arthritis and as an

anticancer herb. I use it extensively for the treatment of cancer. I remember a 94 years young woman who visited my clinic one day and spoke of using it on and off for over twenty years to control her cancer and dissolve tumors as they would arise.

To ripen measles and rashes combine with Cimicifuga (Sheng Ma), Mentha (Bo He) and Pueraria (Ge Gen); for sore throat, combine with Platycodon (Jie Geng), Schizonepeta (Jing Jie) and Mentha (Bo He).

Mentha Haplocalyc   Bo He   (1)
Common Name: Chinese Field Mint
Part Used: Aerial portion (Herba)
Family: Labiatae
Energy and Flavor: acrid, Cool and aromatic
Organ Meridians Affected: Lung and Liver

Actions: 1. Relieves the Exterior and disperses Wind-Heat; 2. Clears Wind-Heat from the head, eyes and throat; 3. Allows the release of toxins from the skin; 4. Moves Stagnant Liver Qi

Indications: 1. Treats External Wind-Heat conditions such as the common "cold" with fever, headache and sore eyes; 2. Treats all conditions of Wind-Heat with symptoms of headache, red eyes and sore throat; 3. For the onset of measles and rashes; 4. For stifling feeling in the chest, mood swings and irregular menstruation due to Liver Qi Stagnation.

Contraindications: Mint should be used with caution by those with Yin Deficiency Heat and spontaneous sweating. This herb should not be used by nursing mothers as it may slow lactation.

Dosage: 2 - 6 grams

Notes: Considered to be similar to the wild variety called "horse mint" that grows in the mountains. This herb is easy to grow but it is the most aggressive and invasive of all the mints. Generally, one can substitute Western lemon balm (Melissa officinalis) or Spearmint (Mentha arvensis) in formulas calling for this herb. Like many of the surface relieving herbs whose active principles are dependent upon the volatile oils they contain, all of these, and especially mint, should only be infused in a covered pot after the decoction is prepared.

This herb is commonly used for Exterior Wind Heat with symptoms of headache, colds, sore throat, aversion to wind and coldness with Chrysanthemum (Ju Hua), Platycodon (Jie Geng) and Arctium fruit (Niu Bang Zi).

Cryptotympana Atrata   Chan Tui   (2)
Common Name: Cicada

Part Used: The molted skin (Periostracum) or slough

Family: Cicadidae

Energy and Flavor: sweet, salty and Cold

Organ Meridians Affected: Lung and Liver

Actions: 1. Clears Wind-Heat and benefits the throat; 2. Allows the release of toxins from the skin and relieves itching; 3. Arrests Wind and relieves spasms and convulsions associated with Heat.

Indications: 1. For Externally contracted Wind-Heat with symptoms of sore throat and loss of voice; 2. For initial stages of skin eruptions, especially with itching associated with the condition; 3. For convulsions and spasms due to Warm febrile diseases, especially useful for children.

Contraindications: Cicada should not be used by pregnant women.

Dosage: 3 - 9 grams

Notes: A perfect example of the so-called Doctrine of Signatures where something is useful for that which it resembles. The cicada skin that is seasonally shed represents change (like Wind) of the insect and is used for skin diseases. For itching caused by External Wind combine with Schizonepeta (Jing Jie), Tribulus (Bai Ji Li) and Arctium (Niu Bang Zi).

Chrysanthemum Morifolium   Ju Hua   (1)

Common Name: Chrysanthemum Flower

Part Used: Flower (Flos)

Family: Compositae

Energy and Flavor: bitter, sweet, acrid and Cold

Organ Meridians Affected: Lung and Liver

Actions: 1. Relieves the Exterior and clears Heat; 2. Relieves Wind-Heat from the Liver channel and clears the eyes; 3. Cools Heat of the Liver and Kidney due to Yin Deficiency; 4. Relieves patterns of Liver Yang rising.

Indications: 1. Treats External Wind and clears Heat for common "cold" with fever and headache; 2. For Wind-Heat affecting the Liver channel with symptoms of red, painful swollen eyes; 3. For blurry vision and dizziness due to Yin Deficiency of the Liver and Kidney; 4. Treats internally contracted Wind and Liver Yang rising with symptoms of headache, dizziness and hypertension.

Contraindications: Not for those with Qi Deficiency with diarrhea and/or no appetite.

Dosage: 5 - 15 grams

Notes: This is like "Chinese chamomile" because it is one of the most common beverages used by the Chinese. It is the most balancing tea to consume cool to protect the Yin and Blood in warm weather, perhaps

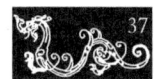

with the addition of a teaspoon of unrefined sugar. It is good for a number of conditions including Summer Heat, digestive upset, the common cold, conjunctivitis, hypertension and headache.

For Wind Heat with symptoms of fever, headache, chills and sore throat, combine with Platycodon (Jie Geng), Mentha (Bo He) and Mulberry leaf (Sang Ye); for Liver and Kidney Yin Deficiency combine with Lycii Berries (Gou Qi Zi), Ligustrum (Nu Zhen Zi); for high blood pressure combine with Cassia seed (Jue Ming Zi), White Peony (Bai Shao) and Uncaria (Gou Teng).

Morus Alba (Leaf)   Sang Ye   (3)
Common Name: White Mulberry Leaf
Part Used: Foliage (Folium)
Family: Moraceae
Energy and Flavor: bitter, sweet and Cold
Organ Meridians Affected: Lung and Liver

Actions: 1. Relieves the Exterior and clears Heat; 2. Clears Heat in the Lung with associated Dryness; 3. Clears the Liver for either Wind-Heat or Yin Deficient Heat; 4. Cools the Blood.

Indications: 1. Treats the Exterior and clears Heat for common "cold" with fever, headache and sore throat; 2. For Hot dry cough or thick yellow Phlegm due to Lung Heat; 3. For Liver Heat with Wind-Heat invasion of the Liver channel causing eye symptoms such as acute conjunctivitis, painful red eyes, dry eyes or seeing spots in the vision; 4. For blood in the vomit caused by Heat in the blood.

Contraindications: This herb should not be used by those who have weakness and Cold in the Lungs.

Dosage: 5 - 15 grams

Notes: The mulberry tree is a virtual pharmacy in itself. Perhaps because of the long respect for silk produced by the silkworm, the Chinese learned of the many therapeutic benefits of the tree including the use of the leaves, branches, bark and roots. The leaves are used for influenza, cough, conjunctivitis the branches for rheumatism and arthritis and lower back ache the roots for cough and edema and the fruit as a food and nourishing Blood tonic. For Wind-Heat influenza, combine it with Mentha (Bo He) and Schizonepeta (Jing Jie); for coughs combine the Mulberry leaves with Platycodon (Jie Geng); for External Wind Heat with fever, sore throat, chills and red eyes, combine with Chrysanthemum (Ju Hua), Forsythia (Lian Qiao), Mentha (Bo He) and Platycodon (Jie Geng).

Viticis Rotundifolia   Man Jing Zi   (3)
Common Name: Vitex Fruit
Part Used: Fruit (Fructus)
Family: Verbenaceae
Energy and Flavor: acrid, bitter and Cool
Organ Meridians Affected: Liver, Stomach and Urinary Bladder
Actions: 1. Relieves the Exterior, scatters Wind and clears Heat; 2. Clears Wind-Heat associated with the Liver; 3. Clears Wind-Damp painful obstruction.
Indications: 1. Treats the Exterior and relieves Eternally contracted Wind-Heat with symptoms of headache and eye pain; 2. For Wind-Heat invading the Liver channel with symptoms of internal eye pain, headache, excessive tearing and spots in the vision; 3. For Wind-Damp painful obstruction with symptoms of cramping, numbness and a heavy feeling in the limbs.
Contraindications: This herb should be used with caution by those with Blood, Yin or Stomach Qi Deficiency.
Dosage: 5 - 15 grams
Notes: While related to the Western Vitex Agnus-castus, this is a different species with a different use. For Wind-Heat colds combine Vitex (Man Jing Zi), Perilla leaves (Zi Su Ye), Mentha (Bo He), Angelica dahurica (Bai Zhi), Chrysanthemum flowers (Ju Hua); for migraine headaches use it with Ligusticum (Gao Ben), Ledebouriella (Fang Feng), Gentianae Qinjao (Qin Jiao) and Pueraria root (Ge Gen).

Puerariae Lobatae   Ge Gen   (1)
Common Name: Kudzu, Kuzu, Pueraria
Part Used: Root (Radix)
Family: Leguminosae
Energy and Flavor: acrid, sweet and Cool
Organ Meridians Affected: Spleen, Stomach and Urinary Bladder
Actions: 1. Relieves muscle tension especially in the neck and shoulders; 2. Relieves the Exterior and scatters Wind; 3. Supports the Fluids and eases thirst; 4. Assists in the expression of measles; 5. Relieves diarrhea; 6. Relieves hypertension.
Indications: 1. Treats muscle tension when there is invasion of either External Wind-Heat or Wind-Cold as with the case of the common cold or influenza; 2. Treats the Exterior and relieves Externally contracted Wind-Heat or Wind-Cold; 3. For thirst due to Stomach Heat or Externally contracted Heat as with febrile diseases; 4. For the incomplete expression of measles to speed recovery; 5. For diarrhea associated with Heat or Spleen Deficiency; 6. For hypertension with symptoms of headache or dizziness.

Contraindications: Pueraria should not be used by those with Cold in the Stomach and excessive sweating.

Dosage: 5 - 15 grams

Notes: Pueraria is a versatile and important herb because of its ability to counteract and adjust acute diseases and symptoms caused by stress and tension due to either Wind-Heat or Wind-Cold. At the same time it is demulcent and soothing to the Stomach and Intestines, and can be used for diarrhea. Because of its upward antispasmodic property, it is specific for stiff neck and shoulders. For External, Wind-Cold conditions as well as tension and spasms of the upper back and neck, combine Pueraria with Cinnamon twigs (Gui Zhi), Ephedra twigs (Ma Huang) and White peony (Bai Shao Yao). Pueraria Combination (Ge Gen Tang) is also good for various skin conditions such as eczema.

Bupleurum Chinense   Chai Hu   (1)

Common Name: Bupleurum, Hare's Ear

Part Used: Root (Radix)

Family: Umbelliferae

Energy and Flavor: acrid, bitter and Cool

Organ Meridians Affected: Liver, Gallbladder, Pericardium and Triple Warmer

Actions: 1. Relieves fever associated with Lesser Yang diseases; 2. Moves the Liver Qi and relieves Liver Qi Stagnation; 3. Lifts the Yang Qi of the Spleen and Stomach.

Indications: 1. For successive fever and chills associated with Lesser Yang diseases, with symptoms of bitter taste in the mouth, irritability, vomiting or congested feeling in the chest; 2. For Liver Qi Stagnation with symptoms of menstrual difficulties, mood swings, dizziness or pain in the chest or flanks; 3. For prolapse of anus or uterus due to Deficiency of the Yang Qi of the Spleen or Stomach; 4. For diarrhea due to Deficient Spleen Qi.

Contraindications: This herb should not be used by those with Yin Deficiency or by those with extreme headaches or eye diseases such as conjunctivitis when caused by Liver Fire.

Dosage: 3 - 12 grams

Notes: This herb is represented in an entire group of harmonizing formulas that treat a combination of Cold and Heat, External and Internal, Deficient and Excess, classified as Shao Yang formulas. Some individuals are sensitive to Bupleurum because it can cause feelings of anger since, as some Chinese practitioners believe, "Chai Hu consumes the Yin". This may only happen in a small percentage of patients but is the reason that many Chinese herbalists, despite its wide recommendation

in the Shang Han Lun, tend to not use Bupleurum as much as the Japanese. Another reason is that the system of Japanese Kanpo medicine uses about a third of the dose of most Chinese herbs. In any case, for those with Blood Deficiency, Bupleurum should always be combined with Angelica Sinensis (Dang Gui) and/or Lycii berries (Gou Qi Zi).

For Half External and Half Internal conditions as well as bitter mouth taste, throat irritation, dizziness, a feeling of chest fullness, combine Bupleurum with Scutellaria (Huang Qin); for menstrual irregularity with depression and moodiness, combine it with White peony (Bai Shao Yao). For prolapsed Qi, despite the fact that Bupleurum has a Cold energy, it also has an upward energy and is added because it helps raise the Qi. For the treatment of prolapsed Qi, combine with Codonopsis (Dang Shen), Atractylodes (Bai Zhu) and Astragalus (Huang Qi) in the formula called Ginseng and Astragalus Combination (Bu zhong yi qi tang).

Cimicifuga Foetida   Sheng Ma   (2)

Common Name: Chinese Black Cohosh, Cimicifuga

Part Used: Rhizome (Rhizoma)

Family: Ranunculaceae

Energy and Flavor: sweet, acrid, slightly bitter and Cool

Organ Meridians Affected: Lung, Spleen, Stomach and Large Intestine

Actions: 1. Relieves the Exterior, scatters Wind and clears Heat; 2. Allows the release of toxicity from the skin and clears Heat; 3. Raises the Yang associated with Middle Qi Deficiency; 4. Directs herbs upwards 5. Cools the Blood.

Indications: 1. Treats the Exterior for externally contracted Wind-Heat with symptoms of headache and sore throat; 2. For incomplete expression of measles to speed recovery; 3. For prolapse of rectum, uterus or veins; also for shortness of breath and tiredness associated with this type of Deficiency; 4. Used to direct herbs upward when there is cause to do so; 5. For toxins in the Blood causing symptoms of tooth and gum aches, headache, Stomach inflammation or rashes due to Warm febrile diseases.

Contraindications: Chinese Black cohosh should not be used by those who have full blown measles or by those with Yin Deficiency. It should also not be used by those with Excess in the upper regions and Deficiency in the lower part of the body.

Dosage: 3 - 9 grams

Notes: Like Bupleurum, Cimicifuga has a clearing and upward Qi and is another one of the ingredients in Ginseng and Astragalus Combination (Bu zhong yi qi tang), whose major function is to raise the clear Yang.

For Wind Heat symptoms of fever, sore throat, chills and red eyes, it can be taken with Arctium (Niu Bang Zi), Isatis (Da Qing Ye) and Mentha (Bo He).

Equiseti Hiemalis   Mu Zei   (3)

Common Name: Horsetail, Shave Grass, Scouring Rush, Equisetum

Part Used: Aerial portion (Herba)

Family: Equisetaceae

Energy and Flavor: sweet, bitter and neutral

Organ Meridians Affected: Lung and Liver

Actions: 1. Disperses Wind and Heat; 2. Relieves the eyes; 3. Stops bleeding; 4. Diuretic.

Indications: 1. For fever with associated eye problems; 2. For eye difficulties associated with Heat, reduces pterygium, treats conjunctivitis and inflammation of the tear ducts; 3. For bleeding associated with Heat in the Blood; 4. For urinary problems associated with Heat.

Contraindications: Use with caution during pregnancy or by those who are weak, with symptoms of excessive Dryness or frequent urination.

Dosage: 3 - 9 grams

Notes: Horsetail, as it is commonly known throughout the world, is an ancient plant that dates back to the Jurassic period when they were much larger and assumed treelike proportions. In Western herbalism, its primary use is as a diuretic for urinary tract infections. David Winston, a North American east coast herbalist, uses an apple cider vinegar extract of horsetail topically applied for all tineas and fungal infections.

Sojae Praeparatum   Dan Dou Chi (2)

Common Name: Fermented Black Soybean

Part Used: Seed (Semen)

Family: Leguminosae

Energy and Flavor: sweet, slightly bitter and Cold

Organ Meridians Affected: Lung and Stomach

Actions: 1. Relieves the Exterior and scatters Wind, Cold and Heat, especially when there is Yin Deficiency; 2. Relieves stuffy sensation in the chest and irritability.

Indications: 1. Treats the Exterior for externally contracted Wind-Heat or Wind-Cold with symptoms of fever, common cold or headache; 2. For irritability, stuffy sensation in chest and insomnia that comes in the wake of febrile diseases.

Contraindications: Mothers who are nursing should not use this herb as it may inhibit lactation.

Dosage: 12 - 15 grams

Notes: Like all soya beans, Black soya bean contains genistein which is an estrogen precursor and tumor inhibitor. The pharmaceutical product is cooked and prepared with various ingredients. Depending on what herbs are used in their preparation, Black soya beans are either cool or warm. Cool Black soya beans are called Qing Dou Chi. These are prepared with Semen Glycinis Hispidae (Hei Dou), Folium morus (Sang Ye), and Artemisia apiaceae (Qing Hao). Warm natured Black soya beans are called Wen Dou Chi. They are prepared with Ephedra (Ma Huang), Perilla leaf (Zi Su Ye) and Bulbus Allium (Cong Bai) or Chinese leek. When combined with Gardenia fruit (Zhi Zi), it relieves irritability and insomnia that may occur after a prolonged fever.

For the treatment of colds, fevers and influenza, Prepared soya bean is especially good for children because they are nutritive and not so unpleasant tasting as many other herbs for similar conditions. Sprouted soya beans are neutral and can be used for rheumatic conditions, edema and swelling of the whole body and knees.

Spirodela Polyrrhiza   Fu Ping   (3)

Common Name: Duckweed, Spirodela

Part Used: Aerial portion (Herba)

Family: Lemnaceae

Energy and Flavor: acrid and Cold

Organ Meridians Affected: Lung and Urinary Bladder

Actions: 1. Relieves the Exterior and disperses Heat; 2. Relieves Wind and vents rashes; 3. Reduces water and lessens swellings.

Indications: 1. Treats the Exterior for symptoms of common cold with head and body aches; 2. For the incomplete expression of rashes such as measles and Wind-associated rashes; 3. For Hot swellings, especially in the upper part of the body, and difficulty in urination.

Contraindications: This herb should not be used by those who are weak with spontaneous sweating or any other disorders where there is sweating.

Dosage: 3 - 6 grams

Notes: Duckweed, a common pond or lake weed, is used as a diuretic and diaphoretic and to promote the eruption of measles and other rashes. Chinese herbalists have reasoned that since it floats on the surface of the water, it is especially effective for relieving surface conditions and

promoting perspiration. It can be used alone by powdering the dry herb and mixing it with honey to form pills.

Discrimination:

These herbs clear External Wind Heat as well as:

Bupleurum (Chai Hu) – a primary herb for treating Liver Stagnation and Regulating Qi, it is particularly used for all Shao Yang (Lesser Yang) diseases, it has an ascending energy and raises Spleen and Stomach Qi upwards.

Cimicifuga (Sheng Ma) – promotes the eruption of measles and other eruptive diseases, like bupleurum it has an ascending energy and can be used in small amounts to raise Spleen Yang upward and direct the energy of herbs in a formula upward.

Mentha (Bo He) – used for depression and diseases of the head and eyes, directs the energy of herbs upward to the brain.

Pueraria (Ge Gen) – relieves spasms of the neck and shoulders, lubricates the Intestines and raises the Clear Yang.

Arctium Seeds (Niu Bang Zi) – treats sore throat, swollen glands and non-erupted sores and rashes.

Chrysanthemum Flower (Ju Hua) – clears Heat, relieves headache and fevers, mildly nourishes Liver Yin.

Cicada Periostracum (Chan Tui) – treats sore throat, erupts rashes and measles, relieves spasms.

Mulberry Leaf (Sang Ye) – clears Lung Heat.

Prepared Soya Bean (Dan Dou Chi) – can be used for both External Hot and Cold conditions, mild Yin nourishing properties, relieves restlessness and irritability.

Vitex fruit (Man Jing Zi) – relieves headaches and eye pain.

Equiseti (Mu Zei) – used externally as an eyewash for conjunctivitis.

Spirodelae (Fu Ping) – treats colds and Heat rashes, reduces swelling and promotes urination.

HERBS THAT CLEAR INTERNAL HEAT

Herbs in this category are used to clear Internal Heat, which refers to inflammatory and infectious conditions. By implication, therefore, most of the herbs in this category will have both antibacterial and antiviral properties and are traditionally described as alteratives, blood purifiers or cooling herbs. They are further subdivided into five subcategories: 1)

Purge Fire, 2) Cool Blood, 3) Clear Damp Heat, 4) Clear Toxic Heat, 5) Clear Summer Heat.

Heat is the result of Stagnation. Stagnation can occur either as a result of Excess or Deficiency. However, most of the herbs in these categories are used to treat Excess Heat while a few are used to clear Heat caused by Deficiency. Imagine a car that overheats because it is being run at high RPM's with overly rich fuel and another because the engine is worn down and perhaps struggling with a steep uphill grade. Both require a very different approach to correct the problem. To remedy the first problem, the approach is to cool the engine's Heat by lowering the RPM's and using a lighter fuel mix. This is comparable to fasting and/or taking cooling and purifying herbs that purge Heat, clear Damp Heat and clear Toxic Heat such as Cassia Seeds (Jue Ming Zi), Gardenia fruit (Zhi Zi), Coptis (Huang Lian), Gentiana (Long Dan Cao), Fraxini (Qin Pi), Sophora (Ku Shen), Lonicera (Jin Yin Hua), Forsythia fruit (Lian Qiao), Taraxacum (Pu Gong Ying), Oldenlandia (Bai Hua She She Cao) and Pulsatilla root (Bai Tou Weng) to name a few. The second requires richer fuel and better lubrication and rebuilding of vital engine parts, which would be comparable to taking Yin nourishing tonics and using Heat clearing herbs such as Moutan peony (Mu Dan Pi), Phellodendron (Huang Bai), Anemarrhena (Zhi Mu), unprepared Rehmannia (Sheng Di Huang), Rhinoceros horn (Xi Jiao) (substitute water buffalo horn), Scrophularia (Xuan Shen), to name a few.

In most cases, herbs that clear Heat will have a bitter flavor. The bitter flavor, while assigned to the Chinese Fire element, ultimately strengthens the clear Yang, or Ministerial Fire (representing overall metabolic processes of the individual Organs), by clearing the impure Fire and Heat from the body.

CLEAR HEAT AND PURGE FIRE

The substances in this category have a wide range of flavors and Organ meridians they enter. The two substances most commonly used are Anemarrhena (Zhi Mu) and Gypsum (Shi Gao) which are used to treat Yang Ming, or Stomach Heat type fevers in the Qi stage.

Gypsum Fibrosum   Shi Gao   (1)
Common Name: Gypsum
Chemical Name: Calcium Sulfate
Part Used: The finely powdered stone
Energy and Flavor: acrid, sweet and very Cold

Organ Meridians Affected: Stomach and Lung

Actions: 1. Clears Heat and drains Fire; 2. Clears Lung Heat; 3. Relieves thirst and restlessness; 4. Clears Stomach Heat; 5. Cools Heat when applied externally.

Indications: 1. For high fever without chills, irritability, excessive thirst, profuse sweating, flooding and rapid pulse, a red tongue with a yellow coat; 2. Relieves coughing and wheezing with thick Phlegm; 3. For thirst and restlessness caused by Heat; 4. For severe headaches, toothache, gingivitis caused by Stomach Fire; 5. Applied as a powder or paste externally for wounds and burns.

Contraindications: Because this is a heavy substance, do not use for those with a weak Stomach or without true Heat.

Dosage: 10 - 50 grams

Notes: Gypsum is one of the most potent herbs for lowering fevers caused by Heat in the Lungs and Stomach. Despite this action, it has little or no antibiotic properties, so for fevers with accompanying infections, it should be combined with antibiotic herbs such as Anemarrhena (Zhi Mu). These ingredients are in turn combined with Oryza (Jing Mi) and Licorice (Gan Cao) to protect the stomach from the coldness of the two chief herbs in the formula called White Tiger Decoction (Bai hu tang). This formula is one of the most reliable formulas for most children's fevers. Because it is a Cold natured formula, if there is any sign of Deficiency, Ginseng (Ren Shen) is added.

This formula was used for a woman who presented an extreme, mask-like, reddening of the face caused by food allergies. The formula worked very well but since her condition tended to recur whenever she ate certain foods, she was able to maintain equally good results by substituting Dendrobium (Shi Hu) which is better for long term usage. In 1953, Russians who visited China developed encephalitis with a very high temperature. The condition persisted for two weeks, when the Chinese finally resorted to the use of Gypsum, which lowered their fever within three days.

Gypsum can be used for Excess type asthma because it is very potent for clearing Lung Heat. It can also be powdered and topically applied to burns, eczema and boils with suppuration of pus and fluids. For this it can be used alone or with other herbs.

Besides severe high fevers associated with encephalitis and meningitis, Gypsum formulas can also be considered for fevers with headache, heat in the skin and muscles, excessive perspiration without the fever going down, thirst, and severe sore throat. It has been used to clear toxic fluid accumulation in the pleural lining of the lungs.

Generally, in decoctions, because it is a mineral, it should be boiled alone, ideally for up to 2 or 3 hours before adding the other herbs (in emergency cases, we have boiled it for only 30 to 45 minutes with good results).

Gardenia Jasminoidis   Zhi Zi   (1)

Common Name: Gardenia, Cape Jasmine Fruit
Part Used: Fruit (Fructus)
Family: Rubiaceae
Energy and Flavor: bitter and Cold
Organ Meridians Affected: Heart, Liver, Gallbladder, Lung, Stomach and Triple Warmer
Actions: 1. Clears Heat and calms spirit; 2. Drains Damp-Heat affecting the Liver and Gallbladder; 3. Clears Heat in the Blood and stops bleeding; 4. Anti-inflammatory.

Indications: 1. For pathogenic Heat which causes high fever, which results in insomnia, irritability or delirium; 2. For Damp-Heat in the Liver and Gallbladder or other Lower Burner Organs such as the Urinary Bladder; where there are Damp-Heat sores affecting the face, including the mouth and eyes, or difficult urination or urinary tract infection; 3. For bleeding due to Heat in the Blood with symptoms of blood in the urine or stool, vomiting blood or nose bleed (Notes: When used to stop bleeding this herb is charred); 4. Used externally to move blood and reduce inflammation due to an injury; for this it is mixed with egg white and applied topically.

Contraindications: This herb should not be used by those who have diarrhea or those with Cold and Deficiency.

Dosage: 3 - 12 grams

Notes: The fruits of Gardenia seem only to occur in certain climates. It is sometimes called the "happiness herb" because it relieves the irritability associated with Heat and Liver Stagnation. Of the Heat clearing herbs, Gardenia also promotes blood circulation and is used in formulas and external liniments when both a detoxifying and pain relieving, blood moving herb is needed. It can be calcined and applied topically or taken internally for sprains and bleeding caused by Heat. It is also used for conditions of Liver Heat with Dampness for symptoms of jaundice, hepatitis, red inflamed boils and sores.

For high fevers with delirium and unconsciousness, combine with Scutellaria (Huang Qin), Forsythia (Lian Qiao) and Prepared Black Soybean (Dan Dou Chi); for jaundice with fever and blood in the urine, combine with Capillaris (Yin Chen Hao) Phellodendron (Huang Bai) and Rhubarb (Da Huang). To Cool the Heart and sedate the mind,

combine with Dragon Bone (Long Gu); to Cool the Liver and Blood, combine with Red Peony (Chi Shao).

Prunella Vulgaris   Xia Ku Cao   (3)
Common Name: Prunella, Self Heal, All Heal
Part Used: The flowering spike (Spica)
Family: Labiatae
Energy and Flavor: sweet, acrid, bitter and Cold
Organ Meridians Affected: Liver, Gallbladder, Lung

Actions: 1. Clears Liver Heat that affects the eyes; 2. Clears Heat and reduces nodules; 3. Calms Liver Fire and ascendant Yang.

Indications: 1. For Liver Heat that rises to the eyes causing swollen, red and painful eyes and headache; 2. For Stagnant Hot Phlegm which causes nodules in the neck such as goiter, or other areas involving the lymph; 3. For hypertension caused by Liver fire rising or ascendant Yang patterns.

Contraindications: This herb should not be used by those with a weak Stomach or Spleen associated with Coldness.

Dosage: 9 - 18 grams

Notes: While the flowering spike is the favored part, the whole plant is also used. Like Schizonepeta, this herb often appears unfresh and old. However, this is the stage when both of these herbs are therapeutically most beneficial. It commonly grows in Europe as well as North America. Its two major indications are for Heat associated with swellings and lumps such as goiter and certain types of cancers, and for conjunctivitis and eye pain. It is also commonly used as an adjunctive herb for softening hard nodules, swollen lymph and thyroid glands and tumors of cancer. Prunella is mildly antihypertensive with broadly antibacterial and antifungal properties against *Shigella spp., Salmonella typhi, E. coli, Pseudomonas aeuruginosa, Mycobacterium tuberculosis,* and *Streptococcus* along with many other pathogenic fungi and bacterium.

Nelumbinis Nucifera (Plumula)   Lian Xin   (3)
Common Name: Lotus Plumule
Part Used: Plumule (Plumula)
Family: Nymphaeaceae
Energy and Flavor: Cold, bitter
Organ Meridians Affected: Heart, Pericardium
Actions: 1. Drains Heart Fire; 2. Stops bleeding; 3. Restrains Essence.

Indications: 1. Confusion, delirium, restless mind, insomnia, vomiting of blood, blood in the urine, abnormal discharges such as leukorrhea and spermatorrhea.

Contraindications: Not for conditions of constipation or abnormal masses.

Dosage: 3 - 12 grams

Notes: This herb is used to clear Heat from the Heart with accompanying symptoms of mania, insomnia and delirium.

Calcitum   Han Shui Shi   (3)

Common Name: Calcite, Calcitum

Part Used: The finely powdered mineral

Energy and Flavor: acrid, salty and Cold

Organ Meridians Affected: Heart, Stomach and Kidney

Actions: 1. Clears Heat and drains Fire; 2. Expels Summer-Heat; 3. Cools Hot sores and burns; 4. Reduces edema.

Indications: 1. For pathogenic Heat with fever, thirst and irritability; 2. Treats Summer-Heat with symptoms of high fever, thirst, a thick yellow tongue coat and a rapid pulse; 3. Applied topically for hot infected sores, especially of the mouth, and burns; 4. Treats edema.

Contraindications: Calcite should never be used by those with Coldness and Deficiency of the Spleen and Stomach.

Dosage: 9 - 30 grams

Notes: This mineral has a very similar usage to the more commonly used Gypsum. It can be combined with Gypsum and other herbs for infectious diseases, Summer Heat conditions with symptoms of yellow coated tongue and fast pulse.

Phragmites Communis   Lu Gen   (2)

Common Name: Phragmitis, Reed Rhizome

Part Used: Rhizome (Rhizoma)

Family: Gramineae

Energy and Flavor: sweet and Cold

Organ Meridians Affected: Lung and Stomach

Actions: 1. Clears Heat and promotes the generation of Fluids; 2. Dispels Lung Heat; 3. Dispels Stomach Heat; 4. Promotes urination and clears Heat in the urinary tract.

Indications: 1. For Heat which causes thirst, fever and dehydration; 2. For Lung Heat with symptoms of abscesses and cough with thick yellow sputum; 3. For Stomach Heat with symptoms of vomiting and belching; 4. Treats acute urinary tract infections with symptoms of burning urination, blood in the urine and dark yellow and scanty urination.

Contraindications: This herb should not be used when there is weakness in the Spleen and Stomach caused by Cold.

Dosage: 9 - 30 grams

Notes: This common reed is often mistaken for bamboo. It grows along riversides or watery areas. The fresh roots are the most effective. Because it is Cold and moist, it is good for coughing with thick and sticky yellow colored phlegm. It can also be used for Stomach Heat with symptoms of vomiting and extreme thirst associated with heat stroke in the Summer.

For feverish diseases with symptoms of thirst and irritability, combine with Gypsum (Shi Gao), Ophiopogon (Mai Men Dong) and Trichosanthes (Tian Hua Fen); for Stomach Heat combine with Loquat Leaf (Pi Pa Ye), Fresh Ginger (Sheng Jiang) and Bamboo Shavings (Zhu Ru). A basic combination to Cool Heat in the Lung and Stomach is with Imperata (Bai Mao Gen).

Cassia Obtusifolia   Jue Ming Zi   (3)

Common Name: Cassia Seed

Part Used: Seed (Semen)

Family: Leguminosae

Energy and Flavor: sweet, bitter, salty and Cool

Organ Meridians Affected: Liver, Kidney, Large Intestine and Gallbladder

Actions: 1. Calms ascendant Liver Yang and brightens the eyes; 2. Expels Wind-Heat affecting the eyes; 3. Moistens the Intestines; 4. Lowers both blood pressure and serum cholesterol.

Indications: 1. For ascendant Liver Yang with symptoms of red painful eyes with excessive tearing and sensitivity to light and headache; 2. For Externally contracted Wind-Heat with red, itchy and painful eyes where there is also a sensitivity to light; 3. For constipation or slow evacuation due to dry Intestines or Liver Yin Deficiency; 4. For the treatment of atherosclerosis, as it lowers both blood pressure and serum cholesterol.

Contraindications: Cassia Seeds should not be used by those with diarrhea or lethargy and should not be used with Cannabis Seed.

Dosage: 6 - 12 grams

Notes: Cassia tora seed is a household herb that can be pan roasted and ground to a powder and used as a coffee substitute for individuals with hypertension.

Anemarrhena Asphodeloides   Zhi Mu   (2)

Common Name: Anemarrhena

Part Used: Rhizome (Rhizoma)

Family: Liliaceae

Energy and Flavor: sweet, bitter and Cold

Organ Meridians Affected: Stomach, Lung and Kidney

Actions: 1. Clears Heat and Fire from the Qi level; 2. Clears Heat and Fire from the Lung and Stomach; 3. Clears Heat and tonifies the Yin.

Indications: 1. Treats Heat and Fire in the Qi level with symptoms of high fever, thirst or acute infectious disease and a full and rapid pulse; 2. Treats Heat and Fire in the Stomach and Lungs with symptoms of thirst or cough with thick yellow Phlegm; 3. For signs of False Heat due to Lung or Kidney Yin Deficiency with symptoms of night sweats, low back pain, low-grade fever, bleeding gums, nocturnal emissions or abnormally high sex drive.

Contraindications: This herb should not be used by those with Spleen Deficiency with loose stools and/or diarrhea. It should also be avoided for Yin Deficiency Heat (because it clears Excess) and should only be used for Wind-Heat conditions.

Dosage: 6 - 12 grams

Notes: Anemarrhena is broadly antibiotic against *Staphylococcus aureus, Salmonella typhi, Bacillus subtilis, Vibrio cholerae* along with many other pathogenic agents. This is characteristically a Heat clearing herb with some Yin moistening properties, so it is added to formulas commonly with Gypsum for infectious fevers and with Phellodendron (Huang bai) when there is Yin Deficiency with Heat. It has a downward energy and helps to lubricate the Kidneys. It is used for conditions of Heat with restlessness and extreme thirst that is not relieved by drinking water. It is also combined with Coptis for clearing Heat and inducing saliva.

Lophatherum Gracilis　　　　　Dan Zhu Ye　　(3)

Common Name: Lophatherum

Part Used: Aerial portion (Herba)

Family: Gramineae

Energy and Flavor: sweet, bland and Cold

Organ Meridians Affected: Heart, Stomach and Small Intestine

Actions: 1. Clears Heat and aids thirst; 2. Aids urination and drains Damp-Heat.

Indications: 1. For Heat affecting the Stomach or Heart meridians with symptoms of irritability, thirst and swollen and painful gums; 2. Treats painful and difficult urination associated with Damp-Heat in the Small Intestine with a tongue with a dark red tip.

Contraindications: This herb should not be used by pregnant women.

Dosage: 6 - 12 grams

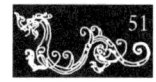

Notes: Chinese medicine maintains that Heat originates in the Heart. Symptoms of Heart Heat include mania and delirium, for which Bamboo leaves and/or shavings are often used. Because it clears Heat from the Stomach, Bamboo leaves are also used for mouth ulcers and sores. This herb can also be used to treat bladder infections. For fevers with thirst and irritability, combine with Gypsum (Shi Gao) and Anemarrhena (Zhi Mu).

Buddleia Officinalis   Mi Meng Hua (3)

Common Name: Buddleia Flower Bud

Part Used: Flower (Flos)

Family: Loganiaceae

Energy and Flavor: sweet and Cool

Organ Meridians Affected: Liver

Actions: 1. Clears Liver Heat and brightens the eyes.

Indications: 1. For Liver Heat rising with symptoms of red, swollen and painful eyes with excessive tearing or sensitivity to light; has also been used for cataracts and other ophthalmologic diseases.

Contraindications: None noted

Dosage: 4 - 12 grams

Notes: This herb is used for various eye diseases caused by Heat, such as cataracts, sore, swollen eyes and photophobia. For these conditions, it can be combined with Chrysanthemum (Ju Hua), Abalone Shell (Shi Jue Ming) and Tribulus (Bai Ji Li); for eye problems caused by Liver Yin Deficiency with symptoms of hypertension, dizziness, blurred vision, dry eyes and cataracts, combine with Lycii Berries (Gou Qi Zi). It can also be used for symptoms of heat and inflammation of the face, head, throat, teeth and gums.

Vespertilionis Murini (Excrementum)   Ye Ming Sha (3)

Common Name: Bat Feces

Part Used: the excrement (Excrementum)

Family: Vespertilionidae

Energy and Flavor: acrid and Cool

Organ Meridians Affected: Liver

Actions: 1. Clears Heat in the Liver and brightens the eyes; 2. Nutritional supplement.

Indications: 1. For Liver Heat patterns with night blindness, spots in the vision and cataracts; 2. For malnutrition; especially useful for children.

Contraindications: This substance should not be used by pregnant women.

Dosage: 3 - 9 grams

Notes: Bat feces contains a high amount of vitamin A and is specifically beneficial to improve vision, night blindness, photophobia and visual obstructions. Because of its high nutritional content, it is effectively used for children's malnutrition. For night blindness and other vision weakness problems, take it in capsules along with animal liver. For children's malnutrition, combine with digestive tonic and Qi regulating herbs such as the Six Gentlemen Combination (Liu jun zi tang). For Blinding Heat associated with anger it can be taken with pulverized Abalone shell (Shi Jue Ming); for visual weakness caused by Liver and Kidney Deficiency (often associated with aging), combine with Lycii berries (Gou Qi Zi), Cuscuta (Tu Si Zi) and Rehmannia (Shu Di Huang).

Celosia Argentea   **Qing Xiang Zi**

Part Used: the seeds

Family: Amaranthaceae

Energy and Flavor: sweet and Cool

Organ Meridians Affected: Liver

Actions: 1. Clears Heat in the Liver and brightens the eyes; 2. For hypertension caused by ascendant Liver Yang.

Indications: 1. For swollen, red eyes and visual impairment especially caused by hypertension. 2. For hypertension.

Contraindications: Because it drains Heat, it should not be used for glaucoma caused by Liver and Kidney Deficiency.

Dosage: 3 - 15 grams

Notes: For Excess Liver Heat that affects vision, combine with Chrysanthemum flowers (Ju Hua) and Gentian (Long Dan Cao). It can also be combined with other Heat clearing herbs for the eyes such as Cassia Tora (Jue Ming Zi) and Buddleae (Mi Meng Hua).

Discrimination:

All herbs purge Fire as well as:

Anemarrhena (Zhi Mu) – clears Lung Heat, moistens the Yin and Clears Deficiency Fire.

Gypsum (Shi Gao) – treats Yang Ming or Qi stage high fevers, Stomach Heat, externally for burns.

Gardenia (Zhi Zi) – clears Heat from the Triple Warmer, relieves irritability, promotes circulation and charred it is used to stop bleeding.

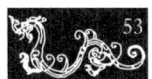

Phragmites (Lu Gen) — lubricates and clears Lung and Stomach Heat.

Lophatherum (Dan Zhu Ye) — clears Heat from the Heart, relieves irritability.

Cassia Seeds (Jue Ming Zi) — has purgative properties, lowers blood pressure and clears vision.

Prunella (Xia Ku Cao) — clears Liver and Gallbladder Heat, clears vision, dissipates nodules and treats cancer.

Buddleia Flower (Mi Meng Hua) — clears Heat from the eyes, treats light sensitivity and cataracts.

Celosia (Qing Xiang Zi) — clears Heat from the eyes and drains Liver Fire.

Bat Feces (Ye Ming Sha) — clears Liver Heat, improves vision, treats cataracts, improves nutrition.

HERBS THAT COOL THE BLOOD

Herbs in this category treat high fevers with symptoms of bleeding, known as Blood and Ying stage fevers. They are indicated when symptoms of bleeding accompany fevers. These are usually very serious, and call for formulas using rhinoceros horn as one of the ingredients. In no way do we endorse the use of rhinoceros horn but would either recommend the substitution of 3 to 4 times the amount of water buffalo horn or recommend patients with this type of fever to standard medical care.

Rhinoceri Unicornis   Xi Jiao   (1)

Common Name: Rhinoceros Horn

Part Used: Horn (Cornu)

Family: Rhincerotidae

Energy and Flavor: salty, bitter and Cold

Organ Meridians Affected: Heart, Liver and Stomach

Actions: 1. Cools the Blood, drains Fire and stops reckless movement of Blood; 2. Clears Heat and Fire and stops tremors and convulsions; 3. Cools Fire and expels toxins.

Indications: 1. Treats febrile diseases in which the pathogen has entered the Blood or Nutritive level with symptoms of high fever, delirium, thirst, vomiting of blood, nosebleed and convulsions; 2. For febrile diseases where the pathogen has entered the Blood or Nutritive level with symptoms of very high fever, convulsions, tremors, loss of consciousness or other types of impaired consciousness; 3. For infections with extreme Heat signs.

Contraindications: This substance should not be used by pregnant women or those with Cold conditions or when the Heat is not caused by a pathological factor. Caution: This substance should not be used with Aconite.

Because the rhinoceros is an endangered species, the horn of the water buffalo (Shui Niu Jiao) must be substituted in place of rhinoceros horn. All references in this text for the use of rhinoceros horn is based on its wide use in classical prescriptions and the reader is expected to substitute water buffalo (Cornu Bubali) in its place. When using water buffalo, six times the normal dosage of rhinoceros horn needs to be used in powder form while 3 to 4 times the amount should be used in decoction.

Dosage: 1 - 2 grams in powder; 1.5 - 6 grams in decoction

Notes: While Rhinoceros horn should no longer be used for medicine, it is, however, the most representative herb in the category and must be described as a point of education.

For fever and Blood Heat with hemorrhagic symptoms of epistaxis, vomiting blood, subcutaneous bleeding, combine with Unprepared Rehmannia (Sheng Di Huang), Moutan (Mu Dan Pi) and Red Peony (Chi Shao); for fever, unconsciousness, delirium and convulsions combine with Antelope's Horn (Ling Yang Jiao), Gypsum (Shi Gao) and Isatis Leaf (Da Qing Ye).

Calculus Bovis   Niu huang

Common Name: Ox Gallstone

Part Used: Gallstone

Family: Bovidae

Energy and Flavor: bitter, sweet and Cool

Organ Meridians Affected: Heart and Liver

Actions: 1. Clears Heat and Detoxifies; 2. Calms Liver Wind; 3. As an aromatic it opens the cavities to expel phlegm.

Indications: 1.Use for high fever with accompanying delirium and convulsion; 2. For chronic sore throat, internal abscesses that have ruptured.

Contraindications: This substance should not be used by pregnant women or those with Spleen and Stomach Coldness and Deficiency.

Dosage: 0.15 to 0.3 grams

Notes: This substance is extremely expensive and practically speaking, primarily used as a relatively inexpensive patent called Niu Huang Jie Du Pian which can be used for all of the above mentioned conditions as well as mouth sores. The combination of Niu Huang with Rhinoceros or Water Buffalo Horn can be a life saver for the treatment of Legionnaire's disease, meningitis and encephalitis.

Rehmannia Glutinosa   Sheng Di Huang   (1)

Common Name: Raw Rehmannia, Chinese Foxglove

Part Used: Root (Radix)

Family: Scrophulariaceae

Energy and Flavor: sweet, bitter and Cold

Organ Meridians Affected: Heart, Liver and Kidney

Actions: 1. Expels Heat by Cooling Blood; 2. Tonifies Yin by promoting Fluid production; 3. Soothes the Heart by calming Blazing Fire; 4. Cools and nourishes.

Indications: 1. For febrile diseases in the Nutritive or Blood level with symptoms of high fever, extreme thirst, reckless movement of Blood, a red tongue and a rapid pulse; 2. For Heat signs associated with Yin Deficiency with symptoms of low-grade fever, thirst, red tongue body and a thin rapid pulse; 3. For Deficiency of Heart Yin with symptoms of oral sores, insomnia, low-grade fever or irascibility with a red tipped tongue; 4. For chronic diseases where there is Yin Deficiency and Heat, such as wasting and thirsting disorders and diabetes mellitus.

Contraindications: This herb should not be used by those with Spleen Qi or Yang Deficiency especially when there is Dampness in conditions such as diarrhea, lack of appetite or Excess Phlegm. It should also be avoided by pregnant women.

Dosage: 9 - 30 grams

Notes: Unprepared rehmannia has antifungal and antibacterial properties and is used for symptoms of Yin Deficient Heat with bleeding. It has also been found to be effective in normalizing blood sugar levels for the treatment of diabetes. In addition, Rehmannia is commonly used to stimulate the new growth of flesh, muscles and bones for the healing of injuries and fractures. For External Heat invading the Blood and Nutritive (Ying) levels combine with Rhinoceros Horn (Xi Jiao), Scrophularia (Xuan Shen) and Ophiopogon (Mai Dong).

Scrophularia Ningpoensis   Xuan Shen   (2)

Common Name: Chinese Figwort, Scrophularia

Part Used: Root (Radix)

Family: Scrophulariaceae

Energy and Flavor: bitter, sweet, salty and Cold

Organ Meridians Affected: Lung, Stomach and Kidney

Actions: 1. Expels true or Internal Heat and cools the Blood; 2. Tonifies the Yin; 3. Reduces inflammations and drains Fire toxicity; 4. Reduces hard nodules, especially associated with the lymph.

Indications: 1. For Heat which has entered the Blood level in febrile diseases with symptoms of reckless movement of Blood, Dryness, insomnia and fever; 2. In the wake of febrile diseases where the Yin has been consumed with symptoms of insomnia, constipation, irritability or dizziness; 3. For toxic Heat and inflammation with symptoms of sore throat, boils, swollen and red eyes or other infections affecting the skin; 4. For Stagnant Phlegm conditions associated with Fire with symptoms of neck lumps, goiter, as well as severe swollen and sore throat.

Contraindications: This herb should not be used by those with Spleen or Stomach Deficiency or Dampness especially when there is diarrhea. Caution: Scrophularia should not be used with Radix Veratri.

Dosage: 9 - 30 grams

Notes: Scrophularia is less nutritive than Unprepared Rehmannia (Sheng Di Huang) but is more beneficial for the treatment of swollen and inflamed glands. While Rehmannia is used for conditions involving the Liver, Kidneys and Heart, Scrophularia is used for conditions affecting the Stomach and Lungs.

For sore throat caused by External Wind Heat combine with Arctium (Niu Bang Zi), Platycodon (Jie Geng) and Licorice (Gan Cao); for Heat attacking the Nutritive (Ying) level with high fever, thirst, insomnia, red tongue with little or no coat, combine with Anemarrhena (Zhi Mu), Gypsum (Shi Gao) and Rhinoceros horn (Xi Jiao).

Paeonia Suffruticosa   Mu Dan Pi   (1)

Common Name: Moutan Peony

Part Used: Root bark (Cortex)

Family: Ranunculaceae

Energy and Flavor: acrid, bitter and slightly Cold

Organ Meridians Affected: Heart, Liver and Kidney

Actions: 1. Cools the Blood; 2. Clears Yin Deficiency Heat; 3. Moves Blood and breaks up Blood stasis, thus clearing Heat; 4. Topically assists in pus drainage and is anti-inflammatory.

Indications: 1. For febrile diseases where the pathogen has entered the Blood level and there is reckless movement of Blood such as nosebleed, coughing or vomiting of blood or excessive menstruation due to Heat in the Blood; 2. For Heat due to Yin Deficiency (False Heat), and is especially useful when there has been a febrile disease that has caused the Yin Deficiency; 3. For Liver Heat caused by Blood stasis with symptoms of amenorrhea, dysmenorrhea, abdominal lumps such as tumors or from injury; 4. For hard sores that are not draining, it can be applied topically; it can also be used internally for intestinal abscesses.

Contraindications: This herb should not be used by women who are either pregnant or during excessive menstrual flow. It should be avoided when there are Cold signs or Yin Deficiency with excessive sweating.

Dosage: 3 - 9 grams

Notes: Moutan peony is commonly added as an assistant herb to formulas such as Rehmannia Six (Liu Wei Di Huang Wan) to clear Deficient Heat from the Liver and Kidneys. Its blood circulating properties are similar to Cinnamon twig (Gui Zhi) but it is not Warm. For this reason, it is used to open blood circulation and release either the congested Cold or Heat in the Blood. It has a strong downward direction and should not be used for Wind-Heat patterns or Heat in the Qi level as it can drive the Heat deeper into the body. It can be used for amenorrhea or dysmenorrhea but not when there is associated anemia. It can also be used for traumas and bruises with ecchymotic blood.

For the late stage of feverish diseases when the body is exhausted of fluids with Yin Deficiency, high fever at night and subsiding in the morning, red tongue with scanty coat, and thin, rapid pulse, combine with Anemarrhena (Zhi Mu), Unprepared Rehmannia (Sheng Di Huang), Turtle shell (Bie Jia) and Sweet Wormwood (Qing Hao); for Blood Stagnation with symptoms of amenorrhea and dysmenorrhea, combine with Peach Seed (Tao Ren), Cinnamon Twigs (Gui Zhi), Red Peony (Chi Shao) and Poria (Fu Ling) in the formula Cinnamon and Poria Combination (Gui zhi fu ling wan).

Lithospermi seu Arnebiae seu Macrotomia   Zi Cao (2)

Common Name: Groomwell, Lithospermum

Part Used: Root (Radix)

Family: Boraginaceae

Energy and Flavor: sweet, bitter and Cold

Organ Meridians Affected: Heart, Liver and Pericardium

Actions: 1. Expels Heat, moves and Cools the Blood; 2. Helps the incomplete expression of rashes and removes toxins from the Blood; 3. Applied topically it clears Damp-Heat and moves Blood; 4. Unblocks the Intestines.

Indications: 1. For toxic buildup in the Blood with Heat signs such as rashes and sores, especially those that are very dark in color; 2. For incomplete expression of rashes, chickenpox and measles; 3. Applied topically it can be used for Damp-Heat conditions such as burns, eczema and vaginal itching; 4. For mild cases of constipation.

Contraindications: This herb should not be used when there is diarrhea due to Deficiency of Spleen or Intestines. It only seems to be effective for measles in the beginning stages and so is contraindicated by some for later stages of the disease.

Dosage: 3 - 9 grams

Notes: The major function of Lithospermum root is to Cool and vitalize Blood. It can be taken with herbs such as Cicada (Chan Tui), Schizonepeta (Jing Jie) and Arctium (Niu Bang Zi) to treat and prevent measles. It detoxifies the blood and lubricates the intestines, increasing bowel evacuation. Externally, Lithospermum is very effective as a wash for poison oak or ivy dermatitis for which it can be combined with Sophora (Ku shen) and Lycii Bark (Di Gu Pi).

Cynanchi Baiwei　　　　　　　　**Bai Wei**　　(3)

Common Name: Swallow wort

Part Used: Root (Radix)

Family: Asclepiadaceae

Energy and Flavor: bitter, salty and Cold

Organ Meridians Affected: Stomach, Kidney, Liver and Lung

Actions: 1. Cools the Blood and expels Deficient Heat; 2. Clears Heat in the Blood by encouraging urination; 3. Detoxifies when used either internally or externally.

Indications: 1. For Heat entering the Blood in cases of Yin Deficiency, especially for persistent fever in children or fever in the aftermath of a febrile disease which has injured the Yin and/or the Blood, or after childbirth; 2. For Hot painful urination where there is blood in the urine, acute urinary tract infections; it should be especially remembered when these problems present themselves before or after childbirth; 3. For Hot toxic and swollen sores, sore throat or abscesses, also for snakebite; for this it can be applied either externally or taken internally.

Contraindications: This herb should not be used by those with diarrhea or those with no true Heat signs. It is also antagonistic with Astragalus (Huang Qi), Jujube Date (Da Zao), Dried Ginger (Gan Jiang), Cornus fruit (San Zhu Yu), Rhubarb (Da Huang), Euphorbia (Da Ji).

Dosage: 3 - 9 grams

Notes: Cynanchi is Cool and descending and is able to clear Heat from the Blood. This makes it very important in gynecological problems. It can also be used for Heat that enters the Blood level. Some uses are as follows: for postpartum inflammation, septicemia and/or accompanying restlessness, combine with Angelica sinensis (Dang Gui), Ginseng (Ren Shen) and Licorice (Gan Cao); for urinary tract infections caused by Yin Deficiency combine with Lophatherum (Dan Zhu Ye) and Ginseng (Ren Shen).

Lycii Chinense (Radicis)   Di Gu Pi   (2)
Common Name: Lycium Rootbark, Wolfberry Rootbark
Part Used: Root Bark (Radicis Cortex)
Family: Solanaceae
Energy and Flavor: sweet and Cold
Organ Meridians Affected: Liver, Lung and Kidney

Actions: 1. Clears Yin Deficient Heat; 2. Clears Lung Heat and stops cough; 3. Cools the Blood when there is reckless movement of Blood; 4. Drains Fire when Kidney Water is unable to control Fire.

Indications: 1. For Yin Deficiency with signs of Heat and symptoms of night sweats, chronic low-grade fever, a red tongue and a rapid thin pulse; 2. For Lung Heat with symptoms of cough and wheezing with yellow sputum; also for tuberculosis; 3. For Heat in the Blood which causes bleeding with symptoms of blood in the urine, nosebleed, coughing or vomiting blood; 4. For Fire not being controlled by Water with symptoms of toothache, diabetes mellitus, hypertension and other Deficiency Fire symptoms.

Contraindications: This herb should not be used by those with weakness in the Spleen or Stomach.

Dosage: 6 - 12 grams

Notes: Lycii bark is combined with Mulberry bark (Sang Bai Pi) and Apricot seed (Xing Ren) for dyspnea, cough and bleeding from the Lungs caused by Lung Heat. When Lung Heat is cleared, the Lungs will again be able to generate Qi. It is indicated for various types of recurring afternoon fevers; combined with Moutan peony (Mu Dan Pi), it is effective for vomiting of blood, epistaxis, purpuric rashes, abnormal menstrual bleeding with accompanying Blood Deficiency.

Lycium bark is very effective externally for fungus infections. For genital itch caused by trichomonas and other microorganisms, use as a vaginal douche with Caulis Polygonum Multiflorum (Ye Jiao Teng), Alumen (Ming Fan), Cnidium (She Chuang Zi), Lithospermum (Zi Cao) and Sophora (Ku Shen). The same combination can be used topically as a wash for the treatment of poison oak or ivy dermatitis and other rashes.

Stellaria Dichotomae   Yin Chai Hu (3)

Common Name: Stellaria Root
Part Used: Root (Radix)
Family: Caryophyllaceae
Energy and Flavor: sweet, bitter and slightly Cold
Organ Meridians Affected: Liver, Kidney and Stomach

Actions: 1. Clears Yin Deficient Heat; 2. Clears Heat in the aftermath of febrile diseases; 3. Clears Heat caused by malnutrition in children; 4. Cools the Blood when there is reckless movement of Blood.

Indications: 1. For fever caused by Yin Deficiency; also when there are night sweats; 2. For fever that remains at the end of a febrile disease; 3. For childhood malnutrition which is cause by accumulation of Heat; 4. For bleeding that is caused by Heat with symptoms of Heat and blood in the urine, sputum, nosebleed or abnormal uterine bleeding.

Contraindications: This herb should not be taken by those with the common cold or flu when caused by Wind and Cold nor by those with Blood Deficiency or no true Heat signs.

Dosage: 3 - 9 grams

Notes: Stellaria is used for chronic fevers, muscle Heat fever and Steaming Bone Heat which originates from the bone marrow. It can be used for children with fever caused by parasites with accompanying restlessness, thirst and irritability. This herb is used for Yin Deficient Heat caused by wasting and/or parasites.

For Heat caused by Yin Deficiency, with afternoon fever and night sweats combine with Lycii Bark (Di Gu Pi), Turtle Shell (Bie Jia) and Sweet Wormwood (Qing Hao); for infantile malnutrition with general emaciation and swollen abdomen, combine with Gardenia (Zhi Zi), Codonopsis (Dang Shen) and Scutellaria (Huang Qin).

Discrimination:

All herbs clear Blood Heat as well as:

Rhinoceros Horn (Xi Jiao) and its substitute Water Buffalo horn – the primary substance for Cooling Blood Heat fever, bleeding, spasms, convulsions and coma.

Moutan Peony (Mu Dan Pi) – invigorates the Blood and clears Deficiency Fire without perspiration.

Unprepared Rehmannia (Sheng Di Huang) – moistens the Yin and generates Fluids.

Lycii Bark (Di Gu Pi) – clears Deficiency Heat or Fire with perspiration.

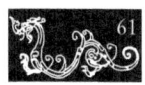

Scrophularia (Xuan Shen) — moistens Dryness, similar to Unprepared Rehmannia (Sheng Di Huang).

Lithospermum Root (Zi Cao) — detoxifies Blood, treats obstinate skin diseases.

Cynanchi (Bai Wei) — clears Deficient Heat, urinary infections and promotes urination.

Stellaria Root (Yin Chai Hu) — clears Deficient Heat with night sweats, Heat and abnormal bleeding associated with childhood malnutrition.

HERBS THAT CLEAR HEAT AND DRY DAMPNESS

This category of herbs are all bitter and Cold. They treat Damp Heat conditions which include hepatitis, Gallbladder disease and any purulent discharges. Some would be classified in Western herbalism as cholagogues (herbs that discharge bile) while others have secondary laxative properties.

Scutellaria Baicalensis   Huang Qin (1)

Common Name: Scute, Chinese Skullcap, Scutellaria

Part Used: Root (Radix)

Family: Labiatae

Energy and Flavor: bitter and Cold

Organ Meridians Affected: Liver, Lung, Heart, Gallbladder and Large Intestine

Actions: 1. Expels Heat and Dampness; 2. Clears Upper Burner Heat, especially of the Lung; 3. Clears Heat and stops reckless movement of Blood; 4. Clears pathogenic Heat which is upsetting the fetus; 5. Cools the Liver, reducing Liver Yang rising syndrome; 6. Externally for Hot sores.

Indications: 1. Expels Damp-Heat especially in the Lower Burner (Stomach and Intestines) with symptoms of diarrhea, jaundice, urinary tract infections, febrile diseases with fever and thirst without wanting to drink; 2. For cough with Heat in the Lung with symptoms of high fever and viscous yellow sputum; 3. For bleeding caused by Heat with symptoms of blood in the urine, stool, sputum or vomiting of blood; 4. For threatened miscarriage or aggravated fetus caused by Heat; 5. For Liver Yang rising with symptoms of hypertension, headache, irritability or painful red eyes; 6. For external application to Hot Damp sores and swellings.

Contraindications: This herb should not be used by those with Deficiency Heat in the Lungs, with Coldness in the Middle Burner with diarrhea, nor by those mothers with restless fetus due to Cold conditions.

Dosage: 3 - 9 grams

Notes: Scutellaria clears Heat, dries Dampness, stops bleeding and secures the fetus. Being both Cold and bitter, it has antibiotic and antiviral properties, making it useful for most types of Heat including coughing with bleeding in the lungs, diarrhea caused by dysentery, gonorrhea, carbuncles and boils caused by fever and Heat, and infectious diseases. For these conditions it is usually combined with Coptis (Huang Lian), Phellodendron (Huang Bai) and Gentiana (Long Dan Cao). If there is constipation, Rhubarb root (Da Huang) may be added, which becomes the representative detoxifying formula known as the "Four Yellows". This combination is also useful as a treatment for different types of cancer.

Scutellaria can be used for various types of bleeding disorders caused by Heat, such as epistaxis, blood in the stool, menorrhagia, spitting of blood. By clearing the Heat, Scutellaria prevents the Blood from going in the wrong direction (for instance, bloody nose) .

For either acute or chronic Lung Heat cough combine with Mulberry Bark (Sang Bai Pi), Lycii bark (Di Gu Pi) and Apricot seed (Xing Ren).

Coptidis Chinensis   Huang Lian   (1)
Common Name: Coptis
Part Used: Rhizome (Rhizoma)
Family: Ranunculaceae
Energy and Flavor: bitter and Cold
Organ Meridians Affected: Heart, Liver, Stomach and Large Intestine
Actions: 1. Expels Damp-Heat especially in the Lower Burner; 2. Eliminates Fire toxicity especially when there is associated Dampness; 3. Acts as a sedative by eliminating Heart Fire; 4. Eliminates Stomach Fire; 5. Applied topically for Damp-Heat sores.

Indications: 1. For Damp-Heat in the Stomach and Intestines, with symptoms of diarrhea, dysentery or vomiting associated with Heat; 2. For patterns of Fire toxicity with symptoms of high fever, conjunctivitis, irritability, a red tongue and a big rapid pulse; 3. For Heart Fire because of poor communication between the Heart and the Kidney with symptoms of insomnia, high fever, irritability and restlessness; 4. For Stomach Fire with symptoms of poor digestion with associated bad breath, sores and inflammation of the mouth and tongue and dental decay; 5. For Damp-Heat sores of the skin such as carbuncles, abscesses, sores of the mouth and tongue and red, swollen and painful eyes.

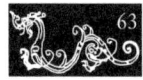

Contraindications: This herb should not be used by those with Stomach or Spleen Qi Deficiency especially when there is diarrhea. It should also not be used by those with Yin Deficiency, or when there is vomiting or nausea due to Cold.

Dosage: 1 - 9 grams

Notes: This is one of a number of herbs together with Phellodendron (Huang Bai), Barberry root (Berberis spp.) and North American Goldenseal (Hydrastis Canadensis) that contain berberine. The biochemical similarity of all of these herbs makes them possible alternatives for each other. For an overabundance of Heart Fire with restlessness, insomnia possibly with delirium, combine Coptis with Phellodendron (Huang Bai) and Gardenia (Zhi Zi). Coptis drains all types of Damp Heat and can be combined with Gardenia (Zhi Zi) for Heat in all the Three Burners (throughout the entire body) with symptoms of irritability, dry mouth and dark urine. When it is combined with Cinnamon Bark (Rou Gui), even though it is a Hot natured, spicy herb, it treats a type of insomnia caused by a lack of communication between the Heart and Kidneys. When combined with Saussurea (Mu Xiang), a Qi regulating herb, it is effective for Hot type dysentery. In fact, this herb is effective either taken alone as a powder for various types of inflammatory conditions, or when combined with any herb, regardless of its energy or flavor to clear Heat in the area relevant to the conducting herb. It can also be used as an eyewash to treat conjunctivitis.

If there is diarrhea with Stomach Heat and an inability to ingest food, combine Coptis with Ginseng (Ren Shen) in a tea and sip throughout the day. If the patient vomits, it will be all right. Even one mouthful retained in the stomach can cure this condition. Commonly Coptis is combined with Scutellaria (Huang Qin) and Phellodendron (Huang Bai) for general detoxification and for the treatment of cancer. This general detoxifying formula is called the "Three Yellows". When Rhubarb (Da Huang) is added if there is constipation, it is called the "Four Yellows". A basic combination to Cool Heat and stop diarrhea is with Saussurea (Mu Xiang). To neutralize acidity and Cool the Liver, combine with Evodia (Wu Zhu Yu).

Phellodendron Amurense   Huang Bai   (1)
Common Name: Phellodendron Bark
Part Used: Bark (Cortex)
Family: Rutaceae
Energy and Flavor: bitter and Cold
Organ Meridians Affected: Kidney, Urinary Bladder and Large Intestine

Actions: 1. Expels Damp-Heat in the Lower Burner; 2. Clears Kidney Yin Deficient Heat; 3. Applied externally for toxic Fire, especially associated with Dampness.

Indications: 1. For Damp-Heat especially in the Lower Burner with symptoms of diarrhea, dysentery, urinary tract infections, Hot vaginal discharge and jaundice; 2. For Kidney Yin Deficiency with Heat signs such as night sweats, afternoon fever, and nocturnal seminal emission; 3. For Damp-Heat skin conditions such as abscesses, boils, carbuncles, furuncles and eczema.

Contraindications: This herb should not be used by those with Spleen or Stomach Deficiency with or without diarrhea.

Dosage: 3 - 9 grams

Notes: Phellodendron cortex is one of the Three Yellows Combination, with Scutellaria (Huang Qin) and Coptis (Huang Lian) for general detoxification. While Scutellaria (Huang Qin) and Coptis (Huang Lian) clear Heat from the Upper and Middle Warmers, Phellodendron (Huang Bai) clears Heat from the Lower Warmer. It is used to clear Kidney Fire with symptoms of wet dreams in men, insatiable urge to masturbate and insatiable sex drive in either men or women. For Yin Deficiency with Heat, it is added along with Anemarrhena (Zhi Mu) to Rehmannia Six Formula (Liu Wei Di Huang Wan). It is used with any formula intending to treat Damp Heat in the Lower Warmer including symptoms of hemorrhoids, jaundice, diarrhea, dysentery and leukorrhea. Because it is Cold, if it is used for a long time, it should be combined with Qi tonic herbs.

Gentiana Scabra   Long Dan Cao   (1)

Common Name: Chinese Gentian, Gentian

Part Used: Root (Radix)

Family: Gentianaceae

Energy and Flavor: bitter and Cold

Organ Meridians Affected: Liver, Gallbladder and Stomach

Actions: 1. Expels Damp-Heat especially in the Liver and Gallbladder meridians; 2. Clears Liver Fire; 3. Clears Liver Wind

Indications: 1. For Damp-Heat in the Liver and Gallbladder with symptoms of jaundice, conjunctivitis, sore throat and ears, putrid vaginal discharge with itching or other Damp-Heat conditions associated with the genitalia or surrounding regions; 2. For Liver Fire with symptoms of headache and swollen, red and painful eyes; 3. For Liver Wind with symptoms of spasms, dizziness, fever, convulsions and pains and sores that move on the Liver meridian.

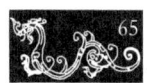

Contraindications: This herb should not be used by those with diarrhea caused by Spleen/Stomach Qi Deficiency or by persons without true Damp-Heat symptoms.

Dosage: 3 - 9 grams

Notes: Gentiana is the primary herb in Gentiana Combination, which is used as the representative formula to detoxify and clear Damp Heat. As such, it is useful for the treatment of hepatitis, jaundice and cholecystitis as well as urinary tract infections such as cystitis and red swollen eyes. Other uses include the treatment of inflammatory pain and swelling of the testicles. For deafness or ringing in the ears caused by Damp Heat combine with Calculus Bovis (Niu Huang) and a small amount (no more than 0.03 to 0.1 grams) Borneol (Bing Pian). When combined with Bupleurum (Chai Hu), Scutellaria (Huang Qin) and Coptis (Huang Lian) it can be taken for a variety of Damp Heat symptoms ranging from eye inflammation, sharp stabbing pains in the chest, herpes zoster to bitter taste in the mouth

Sophora Flavescentis   Ku Shen   (2)

Common Name: Sophora

Part Used: Root (Radix)

Family: Leguminosae

Energy and Flavor: bitter and Cold

Organ Meridians Affected: Heart, Liver, Stomach, Large and Small Intestine, Urinary Bladder

Actions: 1. Expels Damp-Heat; 2. Scatters Wind and relieves itching; 3. Promotes urination and expels Heat; 4. Kills parasites; 5. Applied externally for Damp-Heat.

Indications: 1. For Damp-Heat with symptoms of vaginal discharge, jaundice, dysentery and carbuncles; 2. For Wind itching with symptoms of Damp-Heat sores, vaginitis, eczema and genital itching; 3. For Damp-Heat conditions of the Urinary Bladder and Small Intestine with symptoms of acute urinary tract infection, dysentery and edema associated with Damp-Heat; 4. For ringworm; 5. For external application to Damp-Heat sores.

Contraindications: This herb should not be used by those with weakness and Cold in the Spleen and Stomach. Caution: This herb should not be used with Radix Veratri.

Dosage: 3 - 12 grams

Notes: Sophora is primarily used for Damp Heat dysentery, jaundice, leukorrhea and sores. For trichomonas, genital itch and fungus infections use as an external wash or vaginal douche combined with Alumen (Ming Fan), Cnidium (She Chuang Zi), Lycii Bark (Di Gu Pi), Caulis Polygonum

Multiflorum (Ye Jiao Teng) and Lithospermum (Zi Cao). For urinary infections during pregnancy combine with Angelica (Dang Gui) and Fritillary Bulb (Chuan Bei Mu). For weeping eczema, combine with Cnidium (She Chuang Zi), Salvia Miltiorrhiza (Dan Shen) and Lithospermum (Zi Cao).

Fraxini Rhynchophylla   Qin Pi   (3)
Common Name: Korean Ash Bark, Fraxinus
Part Used: Bark (Cortex)
Family: Oleaceae
Energy and Flavor: bitter and Cold
Organ Meridians Affected: Liver, Gallbladder, Stomach and Large Intestine
Actions: 1. Expels Damp-Heat diarrhea; 2. Eliminates Liver Fire and brightens the eyes; 3. Dispels Wind-Damp painful obstruction (Bi Pain); 4. Relieves cough and wheezing.
Indications: 1. For diarrhea and dysenteric disorders associated with Damp-Heat; 2. For Liver Fire with symptoms of swollen, red and painful eyes and cataracts; 3. For painful obstruction (Bi Pain) associated with Wind-Damp-Heat conditions; 4. For cough and asthma associated with Heat.
Contraindications: This herb should not be used by those with weakness and Cold in the Stomach and Spleen.
Dosage: 3 - 12 grams
Notes: This is specifically useful with Pulsatilla (Bai Tou Weng), Phellodendron (Huang Bai) and Sophora (Ku Shen) for Hot dysentery.

Picrorhiza Scrophulariaflora   Hu Huang Lian   (3)
Common Name: Picrorhiza
Part Used: Rhizome (Rhizoma)
Family: Scrophulariaceae
Energy and Flavor: bitter and Cold
Organ Meridians Affected: Liver, Stomach and Large Intestine
Actions: 1. Expels Damp-Heat in the Lower Burner; 2. Dispels Yin Deficient Heat; 3. Cools Heat associated with childhood malnutrition.
Indications: 1. For Damp-Heat conditions in the Lower Burner such as diarrhea and piles; 2. For Yin Deficiency Heat with symptoms of low grade fever, thirst, red tongue and a thin rapid pulse; 3. For malnutrition in children where there is Heat.
Contraindications: This herb should not be used by those with Deficiency in the Stomach or Spleen.
Dosage: 3 - 9 grams

Notes: Picrorhiza clears Damp Heat and Heat associated with Yin Deficiency. As such it can be combined with Lycium Bark (Di Gu Pi) for afternoon tidal fever, steaming bone disorder (a feeling of heat radiating out from the bones), children's fever caused by starvation and malnutrition. For chronic diarrhea with blood in the stool, it is combined with Dry Ginger (Gan Jiang) to tonify and Warm the Spleen and Stomach.

Discrimination:

All herbs clear Damp Heat as well as:

Scutellaria (Huang Qin) – clears Heat in the Upper Warmer, calms restless fetus.

Coptis (Huang Lian) – strongest herb for clearing Damp Heat, detoxifies Heart Fire for associated irritability and insomnia.

Phellodendron (Huang Bai) – drains Damp Heat especially in the Lower Warmer, clears Kidney Yin Deficiency Heat.

Gentiana (Long Dan Cao) – clears Damp Heat from the Liver and Gallbladder.

Fraxini (Qin Pi) – clears Damp Heat associated with dysentery.

Sophora (Ku Shen) – dysentery, toxic skin conditions as well as genital itching.

Picrorhiza (Hu Huang Lian) – clears Deficient Heat, treats diarrhea and hemorrhoids, Heat associated with childhood malnutrition.

HERBS THAT CLEAR HEAT AND RELIEVE TOXICITY

This is the largest category of Heat clearing herbs; they serve as broad spectrum herbal antibiotics and antivirals. Besides directly inhibiting bacteria and viruses, their complex chemistry serves to support the host resistance to such pathogens.

Lonicera Japonica   Jin Yin Hua   (1)

Common Name: Honeysuckle Flower, Lonicera

Part Used: Flower (Flos)

Family: Caprifoliaceae

Energy and Flavor: sweet and Cold

Organ Meridians Affected: Lung, Heart, Stomach and Large Intestine

Actions: 1. Expels Heat and Fire from toxicity; 2. Dispels Wind-Heat derived from an External pathogen; 3. Expels Damp-Heat from the Lower Burner.

Indications: 1. For most any Hot infection where there is pain and swelling such as boils, sore throat, conjunctivitis, upper respiratory tract infection

and intestinal abscesses; 2. For external Wind-Heat with symptoms of fever, sore throat, common cold, influenza and headache; 3. For dysentery and acute urinary tract infection.

Contraindications: This herb should not be used by those with Deficiency in the Spleen/Stomach when there is Cold or diarrhea. It should be used carefully when there is Qi or Yin Deficiency.

Dosage: 6 - 15 grams; large doses (up to 60g) can be used effectively and safely in severe cases.

Notes: This is a broad spectrum antimicrobial herb used to clear infections and inflammations of various types associated with External Wind Heat. It is commonly paired with Forsythia (Lian Qiao) for many types of inflammatory conditions. It can be combined with other herbs that have a stronger conducting property to direct the anti-inflammatory effects of Lonicera to that area. For instance: for Summer Heat (heat stroke) combine with Elsholtzia (Xiang Ru) and Dolichoris (Bian Dou); for severe high fever combine with Scutellaria (Huang Qin) and Coptis (Huang Lian); for swollen and painful sore throat combine with Platycodon (Jie Geng) and Arctium (Niu Bang Zi); for bloody dysentery combine with Pulsatilla (Bai Tou Weng) and Sophora (Ku Shen). It can be used for many purulent diseases like erysipelas, mastitis, peritonitis and appendicitis. Picking Honeysuckle flowers is a wonderful meditation. The stem and leaves share the properties of the flowers. With the extensive overuse of such Western Heat-clearing herbs as Goldenseal and Echinacea, equally effective Heat-clearing herbs such as Lonicera and Forsythia should be a welcome addition to the world's herbal armamentarium. The tender, young stems of the Honeysuckle (Ren Dong Teng) are picked in autumn or winter and have many of the anti-inflammatory properties of the flowers but in high dosage (16 - 20 grams) are specifically used to treat arthritis and rheumatic inflammations. For this, they can be combined with Mulberry twigs (Sang Zhi) and Chaenomeles (Mu Gua).

Forsythia Suspensa   Lian Qiao   (1)
Common Name: Forsythia Fruit
Part Used: Fruit (Fructus)
Family: Oleaceae
Energy and Flavor: bitter and Cool
Organ Meridians Affected: Heart, Liver, Lung and Gallbladder
Actions: 1. Expels Heat and toxicity from the Blood; 2. Dispels External Wind-Heat; 3. Reduces lumps, swollen lymph nodes and sores of a Heated nature.

Indications: 1. For Heat in the Blood with symptoms of high fever with thirst or infection of any kind; 2. For invasion of External Wind-Heat with symptoms of high fever often accompanied by chills, thirst, sore throat, headache; 3. For abscesses, carbuncles, furuncles and scrofula.

Contraindications: This herb should not be used by those with Deficiency and Cold Spleen/Stomach conditions, nor should it be used for sores that are already open or caused by Yin Deficiency.

Dosage: 3 - 12 grams

Notes: Forsythia is most often combined with Lonicera Flowers for Wind-Heat fevers with sore throat. The two herbs have complementary antimicrobial properties with Forsythia being more effective for *Shigella spp* and *Staphylococcus aureus* while Lonicera is more effective for *Salmonella typhi* and *Streptococcus*.

Taraxacum Mongolicum   Pu Gong Ying (1)

Common Name: Dandelion

Part Used: Aerial portion (Herba) and root (Radix)

Family: Compositae

Energy and Flavor: bitter, sweet and Cold

Organ Meridians Affected: Liver and Stomach

Actions: 1. Expels Heat and Fire toxicity; 2. Dispels Damp-Heat in the Lower Burner; 3. Increases lactation.

Indications: 1. For Heat, especially in the Liver with symptoms of conjunctivitis, boils, furuncles, carbuncles, abscesses and other infections; 2. For Damp-Heat in the Lower Burner with symptoms of jaundice, urinary tract infection and hepatitis; 3. For insufficient lactation due to Heat.

Contraindications: This is a very safe herb but overdoses could cause mild diarrhea.

Dosage: 10 - 30 grams

Notes: Dandelion root is one of the most effective herbs for the treatment of liver disorders such as cirrhosis and hepatitis. The whole herb is strongly diuretic but the leaves even more so. It is a specific for breast diseases of all kinds ranging from mastitis, breast lumps and cancer, to lack of breast milk. The root when ground and roasted makes a delicious warm beverage that one can use as a substitute for coffee. Dandelion root is also good for stomach pains. For hepatitis and/or symptoms of jaundice caused by Damp Heat, combine with Capillaris (Yin Chen Hao).

Isatis Tinctoria   Da Qing Ye   (2)

Common Name: Isatis Leaf, Indigo

Part Used: Foliage (Folium)

Family: Cruciferae

Energy and Flavor: bitter and Cold

Organ Meridians Affected: Heart, Lung and Stomach

Actions: 1. Clears Heat and toxicity from the Blood; 2. Clears Heat associated with contagious febrile diseases.

Indications: 1. For any kind of Heat and toxicity in the Blood associated with infection, skin rashes, fever, or sores; 2. For febrile diseases of the contagious nature such as influenza, pneumonia, viral infections where there are symptoms of Heat.

Contraindications: This herb should not be used by those with weak and Cold Spleen or Stomach.

Dosage: 9 - 15 grams

Notes: Da Qing Ye together with Isatis tinctoria root (Ban Lan Gen) represent two of the most powerful antiviral herbs in all of herbal medicine. Often combined together, they can be used for either bacterial or viral sore throat and for any infectious conditions anywhere on the body. For the common cold, influenza and epidemic fevers of various kinds for individuals regardless of their constitution, these are among the most powerful herbs taken alone or with other herbs such as Lonicera (Jin Yin Hua) and Forsythia (Lian Qiao) for sore throat, sores and mumps. Taken with Gypsum, the properties of these herbs will be focused more on relieving Internal Heat with high fever and mania.

Isatis Tinctoria   Ban Lan Gen   (1)

Common Name: Isatis

Part Used: Root (Radix)

Family: Cruciferae

Energy and Flavor: bitter and Cold

Organ Meridians Affected: Lung, Heart and Stomach

Actions: 1. Expels Heat and Fire toxicity; 2. Cools the Blood; 3. Dispels Damp-Heat in the Lower Burner.

Indications: 1. For febrile diseases, especially infectious diseases such as mumps and others associated with viral infections; 2. For febrile diseases with symptoms of fever, rapid pulse and a red tongue body with a yellow coat; 3. For jaundice and hepatitis.

Contraindications: This herb should not be used by those who are Deficient or are without true Fire toxicity.

Dosage: 10 - 30 grams

Notes: See notes for the previous herb, Isatis leaf (Da Qing Ye). These herbs are good to use to Cool the Blood and relieve blotches and skin eruptions caused by Blood Heat. As such it is very good to use for agent orange disease. A Western herb with similar properties is Baptisia tinctoria.

Pulsatilla Chinensis Bai Tou Weng (3)

Common Name: Pulsatilla, Chinese Anemone

Part Used: Root (Radix)

Family: Ranunculaceae

Energy and Flavor: bitter and Cold

Organ Meridians Affected: Liver, Stomach and Large Intestine

Actions: 1. Expels Heat and toxicity from the Blood; 2. Clears Damp-Heat in the Lower Burner; 3. Treats vaginal parasites and other conditions such as trichomonas.

Indications: 1. For Heat in the Blood with reckless movement of Blood such as nosebleed and blood in the stool; 2. For Damp-Heat in the Lower Burner with symptoms of dysentery, vaginitis or hemorrhoids; 3. For vaginal protozoa with symptoms of inflammation, itchy tissue with frothy and fetid discharge.

Contraindications: This herb should not be used by those with Deficiency in the Spleen/Stomach that causes diarrhea or chronic dysenteric symptoms.

Dosage: 6 - 15 grams

Notes: Pulsatilla is effective against *Entamoeba histolytica, Trichomonas vaginalis,* and *Shigella dysenteriae*. It is used for acute Hot natured dysentery disorders and intestinal parasites including bacteria and amoebas, for which it can be combined with Phellodendron (Huang Bai), Coptis (Huang Lian) and Brucea (Ya Dan Zi). It can be combined with Sophora (Ku Shen) as a douche for vaginal itch including trichomonas.

Viola Yedoensis Zi Hua Di Ding (3)

Common Name: Yedoens Violet, Viola

Part Used: Aerial Portion and Root (Herba cum Radice)

Family: Violaceae

Energy and Flavor: acrid, bitter and Cold

Organ Meridians Affected: Heart and Liver

Actions: 1. Expels Heat and toxicity and reduces swellings; 2. Cools and reduces Hot swellings applied topically.

Indications: 1. For Heat with symptoms of swollen and painful eyes, sore throat, abscesses and boils; 2. Can be applied externally for Hot infections where there is swelling such as abscesses, carbuncles, furuncles and boils.

Contraindications: This herb should not be used by those who have Deficiency with Cold.

Dosage: 9 - 15 grams

Notes: Violet leaves clear Heat and yet are gentle enough to serve as a delicious steamed green vegetable. For medicine, the whole herb is used with the root. It is also used to soften hard lumps and for the treatment of cancer. Violet syrup is an old time over the counter remedy sold as an expectorant and for the treatment of sore throat.

Chrysanthemum Indicum   Ye Ju Hua   (3)

Common Name: Wild Chrysanthemum Flower

Part Used: Flower (Flos)

Family: Compositae

Energy and Flavor: acrid, bitter and slightly Cold

Organ Meridians Affected: Lung and Liver

Actions: 1. Expels Heat and Fire toxins; 2. Clears Liver Wind or Liver Yang rising when associated with Yin Deficiency Heat.

Indications: 1. For Heat and toxicity with symptoms of sore throat, boils, furuncles and carbuncles; 2. For Liver Wind or Liver Yang rising with symptoms of red painful eyes, eczema, itchy skin or scalp and hypertension.

Contraindications: This is a very safe herb although there is a possibility of nausea or vomiting in high dosages in some patients.

Dosage: 9 - 15 grams

Notes: This herb can be used alone or combined with Lonicera (Jin Yin Hua) and Dandelion (Pu Gong Ying) for the treatment of hypertension. It has stronger detoxifying effects than cultivated Chrysanthemum (Ju Hua) and may be very similar to the Western herb known as Feverfew (Chrysanthemum parthenium). It can be taken internally or applied externally for the treatment of all types of inflammations ranging from toxic sores, carbuncles, sore throats to conjunctivitis.

Patrinia Villosa et Scabiosaefolia   Bai Jiang Cao   (3)

Common Name: Patrinia

Part Used: Herb and Root (Herba cum Radice)

Family: Valerianaceae

Energy and Flavor: acrid, bitter and slightly Cold

Organ Meridians Affected: Liver, Stomach and Large Intestine

Actions: 1. Expels Heat and toxicity and drains pus; 2. Moves Blood and relieves pain caused by Blood Stasis; 3. Reduces inflammation.

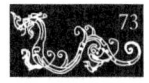

Indications: 1. For both internal and external application to sores, abscesses, carbuncles or any internal toxic condition; 2. For any pain caused by Stagnation of Blood when there is Heat associated, such as postpartum pain, postoperative pain, endometriosis and pain in the chest and abdomen; 3. For any inflammation where there is Heat associated and especially where there is Blood Stagnation.

Contraindications: This herb should be avoided by those with diarrhea, lack of appetite or digestive weakness associated with Spleen and Stomach Deficiency.

Dosage: 6 - 15 grams

Notes: This is specifically useful for the treatment of colitis or other conditions classified as Heat in the Intestines, especially when combined with Coptis (Huang Lian) and Pueraria (Ge Gen).

Houttuynia Cordata   Yu Xing Cao (3)

Common Name: Houttuynia

Part Used: Herb and Root (Herba cum Radice)

Family: Saururaceae

Energy and Flavor: acrid and slightly Cold

Organ Meridians Affected: Liver, Lung and Urinary Bladder

Actions: 1. Expels Heat and toxins; 2. Reduces inflammation and expels pus; 3. Dispels Damp-Heat and stimulates urination.

Indications: 1. For any kind of infections, but is especially useful for Lung infections and abscesses; 2. For boils, carbuncles and other toxic swellings, can be used either internally or externally; 3. For Damp-Heat in the Lower Burner especially when there is inflammation with symptoms of diarrhea, urinary tract infection or colitis.

Contraindications: This herb is contraindicated for those with Cold from Deficiency symptoms.

Dosage: 15 - 40 grams only lightly decocted

Notes: Houttuynia is grown in gardens of the west as an ornamental. The entire herb is used to remove Heat from the Lungs. As such it is very good to give in formulas for treating the adverse effects of tobacco addiction. To aid in the withdrawal from tobacco addiction, combine with Ginseng (Ren Shen), Mulberry root bark (Sang Bai Pi), Trichosanthes Fruit (Gua Lou) and Platycodon (Jie Geng). Make into a fine powder and take two 00 sized capsules every hour or two. Providing the patient is resolved to quit tobacco, frequent use of this formula, hourly if necessary, will significantly lessen the craving and hasten detoxification. One should lessen the frequency of dosage after 3 or 4 days.

Lygodium Japonica   Jin Sha Teng (3)

Common Name: Japanese Fern

Part Used: Aerial portion (Herba)

Family: Lygodiaceae

Energy and Flavor: sweet and Cold

Organ Meridians Affected: Urinary Bladder and Small Intestine

Actions: 1. Drains Damp-Heat and stimulates urination; 2. Expels stones; 3. Expels Heat and toxicity.

Indications: 1. For Damp-Heat in the Lower Burner with symptoms of urinary tract infection or blood in the urine; 2. For stones of any kind especially when there is Heat involved; 3. For swollen and sore throat and mumps.

Contraindications: None noted in the literature.

Dosage: 15 - 50 grams

Notes: The spores of this herb, Spora Lygodium Japonica (Hai Jin Sha), are more specific for stones and are not considered as Cooling as the entire plant. They should not be used if the urinary problems are due to Yin Deficiency. Lygodium can be used with Polygonum Avicularis (Bian Xu) to clear Heat from the urinary tract. When combined with Isatis (Ban Lan Gen) and/or Da Qing Ye, it is effective to treat sore throat, tonsillitis and mumps.

Brucea Javonica   Ya Dan Zi   (3)

Common Name: Brucea, Java Brucea Fruit

Part Used: Fruit (Fructus)

Family: Simarubaceae

Energy and Flavor: bitter, Cold and toxic

Organ Meridians Affected: Liver and Large Intestine

Actions: 1. Reduces fever and clears toxins; 2. Clears chronic dysentery caused by Cold; 3. Treats malaria; 4. Applied externally for warts.

Indications: 1. For fever due to toxic buildup; 2. For chronic dysentery caused by Stagnation, also for dysentery caused by amoebas and protozoas; 3. For malaria where there is alternating chills and fever; 4. Apply as an ointment for warts, corns or for vaginal parasites as a douche or wash.

Contraindications: This herb should not be used by those with Cold weak Spleen and Stomach nor by pregnant women or young children. This herb should not be used for extended periods of time.

Dosage: 10 - 30 fruits

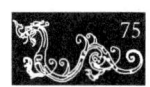

Notes: This herb is specific for amoebic dysentery. The fruits are slightly crushed and each one placed in the center of the sweet tasting Longan Berry (Long Yan Rou) with anywhere from 10 to 30 fruits consumed twice a day. This is continued for seven to 10 days while eating only brown rice that was previously toasted in an open dry pan. Beans may be eaten with the rice but it is extremely important to avoid all sugar and/or fruit and fruit juices.

Portulaca Oleracea   **Ma Chi Xian** (3)

Common Name: Purslane

Part Used: Aerial portion (Herba)

Family: Portulacaceae

Energy and Flavor: sour and Cold

Organ Meridians Affected: Liver, Heart and Large Intestine

Actions: 1. Clears Heat and Cools the Blood; 2. Clears Damp-Heat associated with skin disorders; 3. Treats pain and swelling from insect and snake bites.

Indications: 1. For Heat in the Blood and Lower Burner with symptoms of painful and bloody urine or dysenteric disorders; 2. Applied internally or externally as a wash for Damp-Heat skin disorders such as boils, non-healing sores, carbuncles and vaginitis with discharge; 3. For swelling and pain due to insect or snake bites it can be used both internally and externally but is most effective externally.

Contraindications: This herb should be avoided by those with weak Cold Spleen and Stomach and by women during pregnancy.

Dosage: 15 - 60 grams; it can be juiced and drunk as a green drink and is a delightful vegetable.

Notes: Purslane is prized as a vegetable in many Latin countries and in France. A delicious recipe is to steam the early spring stems, add olive oil and salt to taste. This herb is regarded as an invasive weed because of its ability to produce seeds throughout its growing season and the ability of even a small leaf to sprout into a mature plant; its seeds can remain dormant in the soil for years. At least part of any effort to eradicate it should be to consume it regularly as a healthful Yin nourishing vegetable.

Lasiosphaera seu Calvatiae (Fructificatio)   Ma Bo   (3)

Common Name: Puffball, Lasiosphaera

Part Used: Fruiting Body (Fructificatio)

Family: Lycoperdaceae

Energy and Flavor: acrid and neutral

Organ Meridians Affected: Lung

Actions: 1. Clears Lung Fire and benefits the throat; 2. Stops bleeding when applied externally.

Indications: 1. For Lung Fire with symptoms of swollen painful throat, loss of voice or cough; 2. For bleeding of the mouth, gums or nose; for this it is applied topically.

Contraindications: This herb should not be used by those with loss of voice due to chronic cough when associated with Wind-Cold conditions.

Dosage: 1 - 4 grams

Notes: The puffball mushroom occurs in many parts of the world and is eaten as a food. As it begins to fade, the entire contents of the mushroom develops powdery spores which have been topically applied to wounds and sores to staunch bleeding.

Sophora Tonkinensis et Subprostrata   Shan Dou Gen   (3)

Common Name: Sophora root

Part Used: Root (Radix)

Family: Leguminosae

Energy and Flavor: bitter and Cold

Organ Meridians Affected: Heart, Lung and Large Intestine

Actions: 1. Clears Fire in the Upper Burner and benefits the throat; 2. Stops cough due to Lung Heat.

Indications: 1. For conditions of Fire toxicity in the Upper Burner with symptoms of swollen and painful throat, gum disease or cancer of the respiratory tract, can also be applied topically to gums where there is swelling and pain; 2. For cough due to Heat in the Lung.

Contraindications: This herb should be avoided by pregnant women and by those with diarrhea caused by Spleen Qi Deficiency.

Dosage: 3 - 9 grams

Notes: This herb can be combined with Arctium (Niu Bang Zi) and Platycodon (Jie Geng) for sore throat. For mouth sores and gingivitis it can be combined with Isatis (Ban Lan Gen). For genital itch combine with Lycii Bark (Di Gu Pi), Lithospermum (Zi Cao), and Caulis Polygonum Multiflorum (Ye Jiao Teng).

Achyranthis Aspera et Longumfolia   Tu Niu Xi   (3)

Common Name: Tu Niu Xi Root, Achyranthes

Part Used: Root (Radix)

Family: Amaranthaceae

Energy and Flavor: bitter, sour and neutral

Organ Meridians Affected: Liver and Kidney

Actions: 1. Clears Heat and Fire toxins; 2. Moves Blood and breaks up Stagnation; 3. Antidote to snakebite.

Indications: 1. For Heat and Fire toxins with symptoms of swollen and painful throat, abscesses, sores, and diphtheria; 2. For Stagnant Blood with symptoms of amenorrhea or dysmenorrhea; 3. For poisonous snakebite.

Contraindications: This herb should not be used during pregnancy.

Dosage: 10 - 30 grams

Notes: This herb can be used for the combination of blood detoxifying and diuretic properties. It is used for colds, fevers, malaria, dysentery, tonsillitis, mumps, rheumatic arthritis, traumatic injury, urinary tract stones, nephritic edema, dysmenorrhea, amenorrhea. For mumps the roots can be powdered and mixed with water and topically applied as a poultice.

Scutellaria Barbata   Ban Zhi Lian   (1)

Common Name: Barbat Skullcap

Part Used: Aerial portion (Herba)

Family: Labiatae

Energy and Flavor: acrid, bitter and Cold

Organ Meridians Affected: Liver, Lung and Stomach

Actions: 1. Cools the Blood and moves Stagnation of Blood; 2. Clears Heat and reduces swelling; 3. Clears Liver Heat.

Indications: 1. For abscesses and traumatic injury associated with Blood Heat or Stagnation of Blood; 2. For toxic swellings and snakebite; 3. For Liver Heat with symptoms of hepatitis or cirrhosis.

Contraindications: This herb should not be used by pregnant women or those with Blood Deficiency.

Dosage: 15 - 30 grams

Notes: This herb has been shown to have anticancer properties.

Belamcanda Chinensis   She Gan   (3)

Common Name: Belamcanda

Part Used: Rhizome

Family: Iridaceae

Energy and Flavors: bitter, Cold

Organ Meridians Affected: Lungs

Actions: 1. Clears Heat; 2. Detoxifies Fire poison especially for sore throat, 3. Resolves Phlegm and lowers Lung Qi

Indications: 1. Especially indicated for sore throat, acute tonsillitis, acute laryngitis; 2. Cough with Hot and abundant Phlegm .

Contraindications: Not to be used during pregnancy or for Spleen Deficiency diarrhea.

Dosage: 3 to 6 grams

Notes: Belamcanda has anti-hyaluronidase activity that makes it especially useful to control and eliminate inflammations. It can be used topically for sores and dermatitis or with a little salt and lemon juice in water as a gargle for severe sore throat.

Dictamni Dasycarpi   Bai Xian Pi   (3)

Common Name: Dittany Rootbark

Part Used: Bark (Cortex)

Family: Rutaceae

Energy and Flavor: bitter, salty and Cold

Organ Meridians Affected: Spleen, Stomach and Urinary Bladder

Actions: 1. Expels Heat and toxicity especially when associated with Dampness; 2. Expels Wind and Dampness.

Indications: 1. For Hot sores, boils and carbuncles when there is fetid discharge or yellow pus; 2. For Wind-Damp skin ailments such as rashes and scabies with Dampness of the affected area.

Contraindications: This herb should not be used by those with conditions of Cold nor by those with Deficient Qi where there is Cold in the abdomen.

Dosage: 6 - 12 grams

Notes: Combined with Sophora (Ku Shen), Dictamni is effective in treating Damp Heat diseases such as fungal diseases associated with pruritis and itching. For eczema and hives it can be combined with Ledebouriella (Fang Feng) and Tribulus (Bai Ji Li). It is effective for dermatitis, psoriasis, and itching of the skin.

Smilacis Glabrae   Tu Fu Ling   (2)

Common Name: Smilax Glabra Root

Part Used: Rhizome (Rhizoma)

Family: Liliaceae

Energy and Flavor: sweet, bland and neutral

Organ Meridians Affected: Liver, Stomach and Kidney

Actions: 1. Expels Damp-Heat especially from the skin; 2. Clears Heat and dispels Dampness.

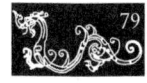

Indications: 1. For Damp-Heat with symptoms of urinary tract infection, boils, carbuncles and jaundice; 2. For Heat and Damp when associated with painful obstruction of the joints.

Contraindications: This herb should not be used by those with Yin Deficiency of the Liver and Kidney.

Dosage: 15 - 60 grams

Notes: Similar blood and lymphatic purifying properties to Western Sarsaparilla (Smilax Officinalis). It is uniquely able to penetrate the blood brain barrier which makes it useful for spirochete type microbes such as syphilis and Lyme's disease as well as herpes. Smilax glabra is used for Damp Heat, urinary infections and for the treatment of spirochete diseases such as syphilis in combination with Lonicera (Jin Yin Hua), Licorice (Gan Cao), Dictamni (Bai Xian Pi), Portulaca (Ma Chi Xian) and Dandelion (Pu Gong Ying). As such it may be a very good combination for the treatment of another bacterial spirochete disease called Lyme's disease.

Rhapontici seu Echinops   Lou Lu (3)

Common Name: Rhaponticum or Echinops

Part Used: Root (Radix)

Family: Compositae

Energy and Flavor: bitter, salty and Cold

Organ Meridians Affected: Stomach and Large Intestine

Actions: 1. Expels Heat and reduces toxic swellings; 2. Increases the flow of mothers' milk.

Indications: 1. For the early stages of Hot sores where there is inflammation; it is especially good when the symptoms arise in the breast area; 2. For decreased flow of mothers' milk when associated with Heat.

Contraindications: This herb should not be used by pregnant women nor by those with Deficient Qi.

Dosage: 3 - 12 grams

Notes: The many uses for Rhapontici include its use as a glandular and lymphatic purifier for Heat Stagnation and to reduce toxic swelling. It is also effective for relieving Heat Stagnation of the mammary glands and to increase the secretion of milk. For swollen glands combine it with Forsythia (Lian Qiao) and Rhubarb root (Da Huang); for mastitis, combine it with Dandelion (Pu Gong Ying) and Trichosanthes fruit (Gua Lou).

Discrimination:

Lonicera (Jin Yin Hua) – clears Heat, detoxifies Fire poison from all three Warmers.

Forsythia Fruit (Lian Qiao) – clears Heat and Poison, dissipates nodules, boils and swollen lymph glands.

Taraxacum (Pu Gong Ying) – clears Liver Heat and poisons, promotes lactation, treats breast problems.

Isatis Foliage (Da Qing Ye) – strong antiviral and antibiotic, treats highly contagious Heat diseases.

Isatis Root (Ban Lan Gen) – similar to Isatis foliage.

Lasiophaerae (Ma Bo) – clears Lung Heat and diseases of the mouth.

Lygodium (Jin Sha Teng) – clears Heat especially from the urinary tract with symptoms of stones and bleeding.

Oldenlandia (Bai Hua She She Cao) – clears Heat, detoxifies Fire Poisons, treats cancer and tumors of the G.I. tract.

Pulsatilla (Bai Tou Weng) – treats dysentery.

Smilax (Tu Fu Ling) – treats urinary tract infections, joint pains and Damp Heat skin diseases including herpes and syphilis.

Belamcanda (She Gan) – relieves sore throat and Phlegm in the lungs and bronchioles, lowers Lung Qi.

Dictamni Bark (Bai Xian Pi) – internally for rashes and measles, externally for scabies and fungus infections.

Sophora Root (Shan Dou Gen) – sore throat, skin diseases, venomous bites, cancer of the lungs, throat or bladder.

Violet (Zi Hua Di Ding) – treats toxicity, reduces swellings, abscesses, boils and carbuncles.

Wild Chrysanthemum Flower (Ye Ju Hua) – clears symptoms of Liver Wind or Liver Yang rising as well as Yin Deficiency Heat with symptoms of hypertension, conjunctivitis, itchy skin and scalp.

Patrinia (Bai Jiang Cao) – drains pus, relieves pain caused by Blood Stagnation.

Houttuynia (Yu Xing Cao) – clears Lung Heat, urinary infection and colitis.

Brucea Fruit (Ya Dan Zi) – amoebic dysentery, malaria, externally for warts.

Portulaca (Ma Chi Xian) – skin conditions caused by Damp Heat, dysentery and urinary infections, venomous bites and stings.

Achyranthes Aspera (Tu Niu Xi) — moves Blood, sore throat, diphtheria, amenorrhea or dysmenorrhea, snakebite poison.

Scutellaria Barbata (Ban Zhi Lian) — inflammations and injuries, swellings, hepatitis and cirrhosis.

Rhapanticum (Lou Lu) — reduces toxic swellings, breast diseases, increases the flow of mothers' milk.

HERBS THAT CLEAR SUMMER HEAT

Summer Heat is a seasonal condition characterized by External Heat caused by hot humid weather and Internal Cold Dampness caused by overeating cold raw foods and cold drinks in hot weather. Because of the Internal Damp symptoms, the condition is associated with Spleen Dampness.

Nelumbinis Nucifera   He Ye   (1)

Common Name: Lotus Leaf

Part Used: Foliage (Folium)

Family: Nymphaeaceae

Energy and Flavor: slightly sweet, bitter, neutral

Organ Meridians Affected: Heart, Liver, Spleen, Stomach

Actions: 1. Relieves Summer Heat; 2. Lifts the Spleen Yang; 3. Halts bleeding caused by Heat or Stagnation.

Indications: 1. For Summer Heat with symptoms of reduced urination, fever, sweating and diarrhea; 2. For diarrhea caused by Deficiency of Spleen Yang; 3. For bleeding in the Lower Burner especially when caused by Heat and Stagnation with symptoms of blood in the urine, stool or vomiting of blood.

Contraindications: This herb should not be used when there is a Cold Deficiency pattern.

Dosage: 3 - 9 grams

Notes: The reverence the Chinese and all Eastern countries have for the Lotus is in its spiritual symbology. Out of the depths of a pond, representing the mud of confusion and negativity, and amidst the abundance of its leaves representing aspirations, arises the pristine beauty of the lotus flower that symbolizes achievement and spiritual enlightenment. All parts of the lotus are used for medicine. The tuber is used for fevers and bleeding (240 grams taken in several doses of the juice extract); the leaves are taken internally for Heat stroke, enteritis, hematemesis, epistaxis and other bleeding disorders (5 - 12 grams, calcine and use the ash for bleeding disorders); the stalks are used for Heat

stroke, fainting and chest fullness (3 - 5 grams); the flowers are used for trauma, bleeding and impetigo (3 - 5 grams); the stamens are used for nocturnal emission, leukorrhea, frequent urination, enuresis (3 - 10 grams); the receptacle is used for massive uterine bleeding, lower abdominal pain from Blood Stagnation; the seeds are used as food for malabsorption, diarrhea, nocturnal emission, leukorrhea (5 - 12 grams); the green center of the seeds are used for febrile conditions, thirst, palpitations, insomnia, hypertension (1.5 to 3 grams).

Phaseolus radiatus   Lu Dou   (1)
Common Name: Mung Bean
Part Used: Seed (Semen)
Family: Leguminosae
Energy and Flavor: sweet and Cool
Organ Meridians Affected: Heart and Stomach
Actions: 1. Treats and used as a preventative for Summer Heat; 2. Antidote for Radix Lateralis Aconiti Carmichaeli Praeparata (Fu Zi) poisoning.
Indications: 1. For Summer Heat with symptoms of thirst and fever; 2. For overdose of Prepared Aconite (Fu Zi).
Contraindications: Because of their Cooling nature Mung beans should be avoided by those with a Cold weak Spleen.
Dosage: 15 - 30 grams; 120 grams are cooked with 60 grams of Licorice for treatment of Aconite (Fu Zi) poisoning

Notes: The mung bean is a very important herb for both its nutritional as well as medicinal properties. It is uniquely a proteinaceous food that is Cooling, lowers cholesterol, triglycerides, hypertension and detoxifies the blood. It figures prominently in South Indian cuisine as "mung dahl". The dish called "Kichari" is a combination of mung beans and rice cooked with the three basic curry herbs - turmeric, coriander seed and cumin - which contributes to the therapeutic properties of the dish. Rock salt and ghee also add to their therapeutic benefits. This is commonly used by Ayurvedic doctors, yogis and sages as a sole, completely balanced healing food. One legend states that eating Kichari for 3 weeks will cure all diseases. I standardly prescribe a 10 day Kichari fast to be repeated periodically. It is especially useful because it detoxifies and neutralizes acids without causing nutritional deficiencies.

A simple method for treating hypertension is to begin each morning by pouring a glass of boiling hot water over 2 tablespoons of uncooked mung beans. Let it stand until it is cool enough to drink. At noon, pour another glass of hot water over the same beans and drink that as well.

Repeat this one more time in the evening and then eat the beans. This is very good for lowering or regulating blood pressure. It is also a simple but effective treatment for heat stroke.

Citrullus Vulgaris   Xi Gua   (2)

Common Name: Watermelon

Part Used: Fruit (Fructus)

Family: Curcurbitaceae

Energy and Flavor: sweet and Cold

Organ Meridians Affected: Heart, Stomach, Urinary Bladder

Actions: 1. Treats Summer Heat and thirst; 2. Brings on urination.

Indications: 1. For Summer Heat with symptoms of thirst and diminished urination; 2. For urinary difficulties with symptoms of dark scanty urination and jaundice.

Contraindications: Watermelon should be avoided by those who have either Damp or Cold conditions or a combination of both.

Dosage: 9 - 30 grams; a cup or two of the fresh juice is the best

Notes: Watermelon, and indeed all melons, are cooling and useful for treating heat stroke and promoting urination. Crushed watermelon seeds are commonly used by herbalists around the world as a diuretic and treatment for urinary infections.

Artemisia Annua   Qing Hao   (1)

Common Name: Sweet Annie

Part Used: Aerial portion (Herba)

Family: Compositae

Energy and Flavor: acrid, bitter and Cold

Organ Meridians Affected: Liver, Kidney and Gallbladder

Actions: 1. Treats malaria; 2. Treats Summer Heat; 3. Clears symptoms of Deficient Heat; 4. Clears Blood Heat and stops bleeding.

Indications: 1. For malaria with symptoms of alternating chills and fever; 2. For Summer Heat with symptoms of heat stroke, low grade fever, headache and distention in the chest; 3. For Yin or Blood Deficiency with Heat signs, such as fever in the night without sweating; 4. For Blood Heat with symptoms of rashes and nosebleed.

Contraindications: This herb should be used with caution by those with diarrhea due to weak, Cold Spleen and Stomach and by those without Heat signs due to Yin Deficiency.

Dosage: 3 - 9 grams

Notes: Modern research has shown that Artemisia annua is an effective herb for malaria. During the Ming dynasty (1368 - 1644), Li Shi Shen described it as important for the treatment of "malaria with chills and fever". It is important because of all the herbs that clear Heat, it is the only aromatic herb, that has a bitter flavor and Cold energy. This means that it is versatile for a wide range of patterns that involve both Heat and Dampness, and yet because of its aromatic properties will not injure the Spleen with its bitterness or Coldness. Further, even though it is bitter, it will not injure the Yin; while Cold, it will not aggravate Dampness. Because it has a fragrant or spicy Qi, it is able to decongest turbidity. Finally, being light and clear, it is able to rise upward and release Evil through the surface. It is useful for treating all four stages of Heat Evils: Wei, Qi, Ying and Xue, as either the primary or secondary herb in a formula. It is generally useful for clearing all types of Heat. Being weaker than either Scutellaria (Huang Qin) or Coptis (Huang Lian), because of its more neutral energy, it has less side effects. This is why it is ideal for treating Warm diseases.

It is recognized by the United States government as an effective herb to take in place of the standard pharmaceutical drug for the prevention of malaria while traveling to foreign countries. Research has revealed that one of its constituents destroys various malarial parasites and an extract is capable of inhibiting the proliferation of spirochetes.

Artemisia annua is also an important herb to clear External conditions of Summer Heat especially in combination with Dolichoris lablab (Bian Dou) and/or Herba Elsholtziae splendens (Xiang Ru).

Glycines Germinatum   Dou Juan (2)

Common Name: Soybean Sprout

Part Used: Seed (Semen)

Family: Leguminosae

Energy and Flavor: sweet and neutral

Organ Meridians Affected: Spleen and Stomach

Actions: 1. Treats Summer Heat; 2. Clears Damp-Heat.

Indications: 1. For Summer Heat especially when there are symptoms of Dampness; 2. For Damp-Heat with symptoms of joint pain, diarrhea and a thick greasy tongue coating.

Contraindications: According to some texts, this herb should not be used with Chinese Gentian (Long Dan Cao).

Dosage: 6 - 18 grams

Notes: Soya bean sprouts are a part of the traditional Chinese diet where they are added to stir fry recipes. They are cooling and a tea of soya sprouts is an effective treatment for heat stroke. They are highly nutritious and contain genistein, an important estrogen precursor. Genistein is taken up by the estrogen receptor sites in the body and either converts to estrogen if needed or inhibits its uptake and conversion if it is not needed. As a result, it is believed that the regular consumption of soya beans and soya products in Eastern countries is at least partially responsible for the lower incidence of estrogen sensitive cancers such as breast or uterine cancer in women.

Dolichoris lablab — Bian Dou (2)

Common Name: Hyacinth Bean

Part Used: Seed (Semen)

Family: Leguminosae

Energy and Flavor: sweet and slightly Warm

Organ Meridians Affected: Spleen and Stomach

Actions: 1. Treats Summer Heat; 2. Strengthens the Spleen and clears Damp-Heat; 3. Relieves diarrhea and vomiting.

Indications: 1. For Summer Heat, especially when there are symptoms of Dampness; 2. For Damp-Heat with symptoms of vomiting.

Preparation: Presoak at least 4 hours in warm water and 3 hours (or at least 1 hour) before adding any other herbs in formula. The cooked herb is edible. When dry-fried it can be used for chronic Deficiency diarrhea and borborygmus as well as leukorrhea caused by Spleen Deficiency.

Contraindications: Avoid with alternating fever and chills and Cold disorders.

Dosage: 6 - 18 grams

Notes: Dolichoris, also known as hyacinth beans, are used as a food medicine. They must, however, be cooked, since uncooked hyacinth beans can inhibit the enzymes trypsin and amylase. These undesirable side-effects are significantly lessened, though not entirely so, when they are cooked. For gastroenteritis, boil 50 grams of hyacinth beans in water and eat throughout the day. Another method is to bake them until dry and grind into a powder. Fifteen grams of the powder can be taken twice a day with warm water.

Discrimination:
Artemisia Annua (Qing Hao) — Summer Heat with no sweating, low fever, treats and prevents malaria.

Lotus Leaf (He Ye) – Summer Heat with less urination and bleeding.

Mung Bean (Lu Dou) – treats and prevents Summer Heat, neutralizes acidity in the blood, antidotes aconite poisoning.

Watermelon (Xi Gua) – promotes urination, relieves thirst.

Soybean Sprout (Dou Juan) – clears Dampness and Heat.

Dolichoris (Bian Dou) – Summer Heat with Dampness, diarrhea and vomiting, slightly Warm energy making it more useful for associated Spleen Deficiency.

HERBS THAT DRAIN DOWNWARD: PURGATIVES

The herbs in this category are those that treat constipation. They do this by either stimulating peristalsis or by lubricating the Intestines. There are three subcategories: purgatives, moist laxatives and cathartics.

Purgatives treat Excess conditions by clearing Internal Heat in the Intestines and/or Stomach and treat constipation caused by either Excess Internal Heat or External Wind-Heat that has moved to the Interior and caused Dryness. These herbs increase peristalsis, clear Heat and drain Fire.

Demulcent laxatives are generally seeds, nuts and oils. Having a high oil content, they are used for Deficient rather than Excess conditions. Deficiency of Yin, Blood and Qi can cause Dryness. In order to assist in the passage of waste, an important function of the Intestines is the reabsorption of fluid and water. By definition, the nature of such Deficiencies implies Dryness, and when this occurs the stool becomes hard and is unable to descend. The moist oily nature of these herbs lubricates the Intestines and assists the function of the Intestines to move the stool from the body.

Cathartics or hydrogogues strongly eliminate both solid and fluid waste and should be used with caution and only for severe intestinal blockage or gastrointestinal swelling. They can be used for a limited number of times for such conditions to relieve Fluid Stagnation in the Middle and Lower Warmers.

Rheum Palmatum (Rhei)   Da Huang   (1)
Common Name: Rhubarb Root
Part Used: Root and Rhizome (Radix et Rhizoma)
Family: Polygonaceae
Energy and Flavor: bitter and Cold

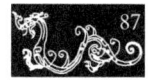

Organ Meridians Affected: Liver, Spleen, Large Intestine, Stomach and Pericardium

Actions: 1. Drains Excess Heat and eliminates Dampness, especially when in the Sunlight Yang stage; 2. Cools the Blood and stops bleeding; 3. Invigorates Blood, breaks up Stasis and relieves pain; 4. Clears Heat and toxins from Excess; 5. Applied topically for Hot sores and Blood Stasis.

Indications: 1. For Damp-Heat conditions of Excess with symptoms of constipation, high fever, jaundice, painful urination and fullness of the abdomen; 2. For Heat in the Blood with reckless movement of Blood, with symptoms of blood in the stool, vomiting of blood or nosebleed; 3. For amenorrhea, dysmenorrhea, sharp pain, pain due to injury and abscesses, it can be applied externally or taken internally to break up Stasis and relieve pain; 4. For Heat at the Blood level accompanied by toxic build-up with symptoms of fever, jaundice, acute appendicitis, swollen eyes and abscesses; 5. Applied topically for burns, abscesses, carbuncles and Blood Stasis.

Contraindications: This herb should only be used where there is a definite condition of Heat and Dampness; Rhubarb should be used by nursing mothers with extreme caution.

Dosage: 3 - 12 grams

Notes: The active purging constituents in Rhubarb are anthraquinone glycosides including chrysophanol, emodin, aloe-emodin, rhein and physcion. It also contains astringent elements such as rheum tannic acids. It purges in from 6 to 8 hours. This herb is widely used by Western herbalists as a laxative. In large doses it is laxative while in smaller doses of less than 0.3 grams it is an astringent. As such it has opposing functions of treating both constipation as well as diarrhea and dysentery. Rhubarb, characteristic of most potent herbs, has seemingly opposite and paradoxical effects, combining laxative, Cooling alterative or detoxifying, Blood moving and astringent properties. For fibroids, abdominal cysts and blocked menstruation combine Rhubarb (Da Huang) with Poria (Fu Ling) and Red Peony (Chi Shao); combine with Mirabilitum (Mang Xiao) and Immature Citrus peel (Zhi Shi) for constipation and Dryness; with Mirabilitum (Mang Xiao) and Persica seed (Tao Ren) for intestinal inflammation and acute stage of appendicitis.

Like many Chinese herbs, different properties of Rhubarb are amplified as a result of processing. For burns soak Rhubarb in vinegar for 1 - 3 days and apply directly. This is not intended for use on open sores. For Blood Stagnation, wine-soaked Rhubarb is most effective. For diarrhea and bleeding, carbonize Rhubarb root in an open pan. Take 5 - 15 grams internally or applied externally to stop bleeding.

Mirabilitum   Mang Xiao   (1)

Common Name: Glauber's Salt

Part Used: The rock powder

Energy and Flavor: bitter, acrid, salty and very Cold

Organ Meridians Affected: Stomach and Large Intestine

Actions: 1. Purges Stagnation in the Intestines caused by Heat and Dryness; 2. Cools Heat and abates swelling.

Indications: 1. For constipation caused by Heat and Dryness; 2. For Heat accompanied by swelling with symptoms of red swollen eyes, breast lumps, inflammation of the throat and mouth and appendicitis.

Contraindications: As this substance has a strong descending action, it should not be used during pregnancy, menstruation or post-partum; it should also be avoided by those with Spleen Deficiency and by the elderly.

Dosage: 3 - 12 grams

Notes: Mirabilitum or Sodium sulfate is commonly sold as a laxative in pharmacies throughout the Western world. It is used as a stool softener and in Chinese herbalism it is commonly used with Rhubarb (Da Huang) for a smooth evacuation. Mirabilitum, like Rhubarb and other purging herbs, has a strong downward Qi and is contraindicated during pregnancy.

Cassia Angustifolia   Fan Xie Ye   (2)

Common Name: Senna Leaf

Part Used: Foliage (Folium)

Family: Leguminosae

Energy and Flavor: sweet, bitter and Cold

Organ Meridians Affected: Large Intestine

Actions: 1. Purges Internal Heat

Indications: 1. For constipation and abdominal fullness caused by Heat.

Contraindications: This herb should not be used by those with chronic constipation with weakness nor by pregnant, menstruating or post-partum women.

Dosage: 3 - 9 grams

Notes: Because Senna, like all Cold natured purging herbs has a Cold energy, it can cause severe abdominal cramps called 'griping'. To counteract this, it is important to combine a smaller amount of a Warming spice or Qi regulating herb. Typically, a Western herbalist might add Ginger as an assistant to a well formulated laxative combination. Chinese herbalists often use Citrus peel for a similar reason, which is explained in traditional Chinese medical theory as 'adding a

small amount of Warm, circulating herbs to protect the righteous Qi of the Spleen-Stomach'. A small amount of Senna (3 grams) will only loosen the stool; more than this will cause a purge in 2-3 hours.

Aloe Vera   Lu Hui   (2)

Common Name: Aloe

Part Used: Aerial portion (Herba)

Family: Liliaceae

Energy and Flavor: bitter and Cold

Organ Meridians Affected: Liver, Stomach and Large Intestine

Actions: 1. Clears Heat; 2. Cools the Liver and clears Heat in the Liver channel; 3. Dispels parasites.

Indications: 1. For acute and chronic constipation caused by Heat in the Intestines; 2. For Heat in the Liver and its channel with symptoms of fever, headache, red eyes, dizziness and abdominal distention; 3. Kills roundworm and ringworm; 4. For childhood malnutrition caused by digestive weakness associated with intestinal parasites.

Contraindications: This herb should not be used by pregnant or menstruating women nor should it be used by those with Cold weak Spleen and Stomach.

Dosage: .5 - 2 grams

Notes: This is the same Aloe Vera that is topically applied as a first aid treatment for burns and scalds. The watery juice is called "Kumari" meaning 'goddess' because Ayurvedic medicine teaches that a woman can prevent wrinkles and maintain feminine beauty if it is taken daily. Aloe juice is rich in enzymes and is justifiably promoted as a powerfully rejuvenative health aid with extensive research to support and back up the claims of the distributors. Some of that research coincides with the Chinese who have discovered it to have potent anti-carcinogenic properties, including the inhibition of liver cancers.

Aloe as a laxative is made from the dried concentrated leaf juice. The sap or juice is decocted and concentrated. This is then evaporated and powdered. It drains Heat from the Liver and is effectively combined with other Heat draining herbs such as Gentiana (Long Dan Cao) and Scutellaria (Huang Qin). As with all Cold laxatives, a small amount of a Warm Qi regulating herb such as Anise, Ginger or Citrus peel will prevent possible gastrointestinal discomfort.

Discrimination:

Rhubarb (Da Huang) – standard herb used for constipation, moves Blood.

Mirabilitum (Mang Xiao) — softens stool.

Aloe (Lu Hui) — mild laxative, useful for children and conditions associated with intestinal parasites.

Senna (Fan Xie Ye) — used occasionally for Food Stagnation.

LUBRICATING LAXATIVES

Cannabis Sativa   Huo Ma Ren   (1)
Common Name: Cannabis Seed
Part Used: Seed (Semen)
Family: Cannabiaceae
Energy and Flavor: sweet and neutral
Organ Meridians Affected: Large Intestine, Spleen, Stomach

Actions: 1. Moistens the Intestines and unblocks Food Stagnation caused by Dryness; 2. Nourishes the Yin and relieves constipation caused by Yin Deficiency; 3. Cools Heat and aids healing of sores.

Indications: 1. For constipation caused by Dry Intestines, especially for the elderly and following a febrile disease; 2. Mildly tonifies Yin and relieves constipation caused by Yin Deficiency; 3. For Hot sores, speeds healing used internally and externally.

Contraindications: Although it is considered safe, it should not be taken for extended periods of time. Substitute Psyllium.

Dosage: 9 - 30 grams

Notes: Traditionally, none of the ancient Herbal Classics mention the intoxicating effects of marijuana. Its effects when used in that way are considered toxic. The seeds, however, are considered a nutritionally dense source of oils with essential fatty acids. They contain barely a trace amount of the intoxicating principle (cannabinol) of the plant and to prevent them from germinating, they are processed by roasting. They lubricate the Intestines and relieve chronic constipation, especially in the debilitated and elderly. The seeds must always be ground before use. For Yin and Blood Deficiency with constipation caused by a lack of fluids, combine with Angelica sinensis (Dang Gui) and Prepared Rehmannia (Shu Di Huang); for constipation caused by Dryness and Heat, combine with Peach seed (Tao Ren), White Peony (Bai Shao Yao) and Immature Citrus (Zhi Shi).

Prunus Japonica   Yu Li Ren   (2)
Common Name: Bush Cherry Pit
Part Used: Seed (Semen)

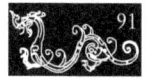

Family: Rosaceae

Energy and Flavor: acrid, sweet, bitter and neutral

Organ Meridians Affected: Spleen, Small and Large Intestine, Urinary Bladder

Actions: 1. Moistens the Intestines and invigorates Qi; 2. Increases the flow of urine.

Indications: 1. For constipation caused by Dryness and Stagnation of Qi; 2. For edema with lack of urination and Stagnant Qi.

Contraindications: This herb should be avoided by pregnant women and those with Yin Deficiency.

Dosage: 3 - 9 grams

Notes: The herb contains up to 60 to 75% oils which gives it the property of lubricating the intestines to relieve constipation. Because is also has a spicy or acrid flavor, it helps to break through congestion to further circulate the Qi downward. At the same time it is diuretic and relieves edema. It can be combined with either Peach seed (Tao Ren) or Apricot seed (Xing Ren) and Cannabis seed (Huo Ma Ren) for chronic constipation.

Discrimination:

Cannabis Seed (Huo Ma Ren) — softens the stool, lubricates the Intestines, nourishes Yin.

Prunus Japonica (Yu Li Ren) — invigorates the Qi, increases urine flow.

STRONG PURGATIVES

CATHARTICS AND HYDROGOGUES

Pharbitidis Nil   Qian Niu Zi   (2)

Common Name: Morning Glory Seeds

Part Used: Seed (Semen)

Family: Convolvulaceae

Energy and Flavor: acrid, bitter, Cold and toxic

Organ Meridians Affected: Kidney, Lung and Large Intestine

Actions: 1. Clears Heat and drains Dampness through the urine and the stool; 2. Relieves Food Stagnation and constipation; 3. Kills and expels parasites.

Indications: 1. For Heat and accumulation of water with symptoms of edema and urinary difficulty; 2. For Damp-Heat with symptoms of constipation; 3. For intestinal parasites accompanied with Food Stagnation.

Contraindications: This herb should not be used by pregnant women and should be avoided by those with Deficiency of the Spleen or Stomach.

Dosage: 3 - 9 grams in decoction, 1.5 - 3 grams used alone as a powder

Notes: Morning glory seeds can be ground into a powder with Peach seeds (Tao Ren) and mixed with honey to form a pill. They are used for constipation and strongly lower the Qi, clear leg edema and promote urination. They are usually harvested in the Fall and powdered and taken as a tea. While Pharbitidis is the mildest herb in this category and can be taken longer for Food Stagnation and parasites, in general all strong purgatives are only indicated for short term (from one or two days to a week or so) or occasional use. In large doses, morning glory seeds are hallucinogenic.

Euphorbiae Kansui   Gan Sui   (1)

Common Name: Kansui Root

Part Used: Root (Radix)

Family: Euphorbiaceae

Energy and Flavor: bitter, Cold and toxic

Organ Meridians Affected: Lung, Spleen, Kidney and Large Intestine

Actions: 1. Relieves water retention and congestion of Fluids; 2. Cools swellings and reduces inflammation when applied topically; 3. Strong purgative, driving water and Food Stagnation out though the stool.

Indications: 1. For accumulation of water and Fluids in the chest and abdomen with symptoms of ascites, edema and distention in the chest and abdomen; 2. Apply topically for painful sores and abscesses associated with Damp-Heat; 3. For constipation with Damp-Heat Fluid Stagnation.

Contraindications: This herb should not be used by pregnant women nor by those that are Deficient.

Dosage: 1 - 3 grams in decoction, .5 - 1 grams as a powder; when taken in this form it should be roasted so as to reduce its toxicity that causes vomiting. This herb is traditionally considered incompatible with Glycyrrhizae Uralensis (Gan cao).

Notes: Combine with Pharbitidis (Qian Niu Zi) for edema and ascites; with roasted, dry Ginger for stopped urination, constipation, abdominal swelling and ascites. The juice can be applied topically as a counterirritant to clear warts and other skin nodules. It is in the spurge family of which another member, popularly called "Gopher spurge" (E. Lathyris) can be planted and allowed to freely proliferate throughout the garden to eliminate gophers and moles. It is believed that the root has the same drastic purgative action it has on humans. Perhaps when they deliberately

or accidentally nibble on the roots of the plant, they experience severe gastrointestinal irritation, a violent cathartic reaction and possibly death.

Another member of the spurge family, Euphorbiae seu Knoxiae (Da Ji) has very similar properties to Euphorbiae Gan Sui and they are usually combined together.

Daphne Genkwa   Yuan Hua   (1)

Common Name: Genkwa Flower

Part Used: Flower (Flos)

Family: Thymelaeceae

Energy and Flavor: acrid, Warm and toxic

Organ Meridians Affected: Lung, Kidney and Large Intestine

Actions: 1. Relieves chronic congestion of Fluids in the chest and stops cough; 2. Drains congested Fluids through the urine and the stool; 3. Expels parasites.

Indications: 1. For Stagnation of Fluids with symptoms of fluid congestion, edema, ascites and severe congestion in the abdomen and chest; 2. Used topically for scabies and ringworm; 3. As an expectorant, diuretic and harsh cathartic it clears chronic congestion in the chest for such ailments as chronic bronchitis.

Contraindications: This herb should not be used by pregnant women nor by those with weak constitutions. It should also not be used with Licorice root (Gan Cao) because it counteracts it.

Dosage: 1.5 - 3 grams used in a powder; it can be fried with vinegar to reduce its toxicity.

Notes: For sudden cough with Cold-Damp chronic bronchitis, combine Genkwa flower with Jujube dates (Da Zao); for facial edema combine 20 grams each of Genkwa flower (Yuan Hua), Euphorbia seu Knoxiae (Da Ji), Euphorbia Gan Sui (Gan Sui) and Jujube Dates (Da Zao). This is called Ten Jujubes Decoction (Shi Zao Tang) and is used for different types of edema and water accumulation in the chest, hypochondrium, stomach and intestines. It might be considered for ascites, pleurisy, liver cirrhosis and chronic nephritis.

Phytolacca Acinosa   Shang Lu   (3)

Common Name: Poke Root

Part Used: Root (Radix)

Family: Phytolaccaceae

Energy and Flavor: bitter, Cold and toxic

Organ Meridians Affected: Spleen, Kidney, Lung and Urinary Bladder

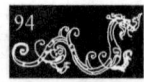

Actions: 1. Drains water retention associated with Excess; 2. Abates swellings, tumors and sores associated with Damp-Heat and Stagnation.

Indications: 1. For Excess conditions with symptoms of scanty urination, edema and constipation; 2. Internally for tumors and swellings and applied topically for sores and tumors; when used externally it should be used fresh.

Contraindications: This herb should be reserved for those with Excess conditions and not used by pregnant women.

Dosage: 3 - 9 grams

Notes: Phytolacca, commonly known as Poke root in Western herbalism, is used for much the same reasons as it is used in Chinese medicine. Western herbalism uses it as an alterative, blood and lymphatic purifier or for conditions the Chinese describe as Excess Damp Heat. Again, in both systems, it is specifically used for glandular affections including inflammation of the mammary glands, lymph glands and glands of the reproductive organs. It is also very important in both systems for the treatment of cancer. In its fresh form it may cause gastrointestinal distress. Aging the dried root for at least 3 months and combining it in formula with other herbs and/or prolonged cooking for at least an hour will neutralize its toxic elements. Chinese herbalism lessens the toxicity associated with the drastic purging action of Phytolacca by stir frying it with rice vinegar.

Croton Tiglii   Ba Dou   (3)

Common Name: Croton Seed

Part Used: Seed (Semen)

Family: Euphorbiaceae

Energy and Flavor: acrid, Hot and toxic

Organ Meridians Affected: Stomach and Large Intestine

Actions: 1. Strongly purges Stagnation and accumulation due to Cold; 2. Drains water; 3. Dissolves Phlegm; 4. Clears warts and speeds healing of abscesses, carbuncles and furuncles; 5. Can be used as an insecticide.

Indications: 1. For Stagnation due to Cold with symptoms of constipation, pain and abdominal distention; 2. For edema and ascites due to Cold; 3. For Phlegm obstructing the throat, Lungs or the Heart with symptoms of difficulty breathing, wheezing; 4. Topically applied to promote the resolution and healing of ulcers and abscesses; 5. Used environmentally to kill insects.

Contraindications: This herb should not be used by pregnant women nor by those with a weak constitution; one should not ingest hot liquids while taking this herb. If diarrhea persists, a Cold bowl of rice cereal or a tea with Cold herbs such as Phellodendron and Coptis should be taken. This herb should not be used with Semen Pharbitidis. This is a very strong and penetrating herb and only used internally or externally in prescribed dose and with caution.

Dosage: 0.1 - 0.5 grams

Toxicity: Twenty drops of Croton oil is a lethal dose for humans.

Notes: This herb is used to drive out excess water from the Stomach and Intestines and reduce ascites. It is very strong and potentially toxic in even a comparatively small dose. Combine with Rhubarb (Da Huang) and Dried Ginger (Gan Jiang) to purge and remove Internal Coldness. The seeds contain 40 - 60 percent fat, both saturated and unsaturated, 18 percent protein and 4 - 6 percent ash. The toxic element is the crotin which is found in the protein. The Chinese also use defatted Croton (Ba Dou Shuang) which eliminates the toxic oil from the seeds and moderates its drastic purging action.

Discrimination:

Pharbitidis (Qian Niu Zi) — Clears Heat, drains Dampness and promotes urine flow.

Euphorbiae Kansui (Gan Sui) — reduces inflammation.

Daphne Genkwa (Yuan Hua) — expels parasites.

Phytolaccae (Shang Lu) — treats tumors, cancers and sores.

Croton Tiglii (Ba Dou) — dissolves Phlegm, clears warts, heals abscesses and boils.

HERBS THAT DRAIN DAMPNESS

Herbs that drain Dampness are diuretics. There are many forms and causes of Dampness, with the Spleen, Kidneys and Lungs being variously involved in the regulation of Fluids. Damp accumulates first in the lower limbs, causing edema and impaired movement. From there it can move upward and invade the deeper organic levels involving the functions of the Kidney and Spleen. The resulting Stagnation of Fluids congests and impairs digestion, Fluid metabolism and eventually the respiratory system. As with any Stagnation, Fluid Stagnation, if it is unresolved, can eventually transform into Heat, giving way to a new and more complex condition, Damp-Heat. This can manifest as urinary tract infections, diarrhea, jaundice and moist skin diseases such as eczema. These conditions are treated not only with the herbs in this category but

also with Heat clearing herbs, specifically those that Drain Damp and Clear Heat, a subcategory within the Heat clearing category. Damp-Cold is a condition where the Dampness has accumulated due to Internal Cold. This condition is most often a Phlegm issue and another category of herbs are used to treat it; they are called Herbs that Transform Phlegm.

Dampness can be differentiated into extra-cellular fluid and intra-cellular fluid. Being a part of Yin, one can have an Excess in either area. Thus one can appear Damp and obese and still have intracellular Fluid or Yin Deficiency, as in the case of some diabetics. In this case, there is a profound disturbance of electrolyte balance of potassium and sodium ions between the fluid in and out of the cells. This involves the Spleen and Kidney function. Because mushrooms generally, and specifically the Chinese medicinal mushrooms Poria (Fu Ling) and Polyporus (Zhu Ling), are used to regulate intra- and extra-cellular fluid, they may be considered to have more nutritive and tonic properties as well. In contrast, herbs such as Plantaginis (Che Qian Zi) and Dianthus (Qu Mai) are more discharging, pure diuretics.

Another group of herbs in this category enter the Heart and Small Intestine and, having a Cool nature, are used for draining Heat and Dampness invading the Heart through the Small intestine. These are useful for the treatment of high blood lipids and congestive heart conditions.

Most herbs that drain Dampness have a bland or mild flavor and a neutral to Cold or Cool atmospheric energy. Those that have a Cool or Cold energy are used to drain Heat. In general, salt, which causes fluid retention, should be avoided when taking diuretics.

Alisma Orientalis   Ze Xie   (1)
Common Name: Alisma, Water Plantain Rhizome
Part Used: Rhizome (Rhizoma)
Family: Alismataceae
Energy and Flavor: sweet and Cold
Organ Meridians Affected: Kidney and Urinary Bladder

Actions: 1. Encourages urination and regulates water in the body; 2. Clears Damp-Heat in the Lower Burner especially when caused by Kidney Yin Deficiency.

Indications: 1. For Damp conditions that are causing Stagnation with symptoms of edema, urinary difficulty, nephritis and acute diarrhea; 2. For Damp-Heat conditions associated with Kidney Yin Deficiency with symptoms of Heat such as dark scanty urination, rapid pulse and a thick, greasy and yellow tongue coating, dizziness and tinnitus.

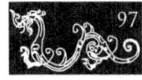

Contraindications: This herb should not be used when there are excretions caused by Kidney Yang Deficiency, such as seminal emission or vaginal discharge, as well as Damp-Cold conditions.

Dosage: 6 - 12 grams

Notes: Alisma is a diuretic that Cools Damp Heat flowing into the Bladder. For painful or frequent urge to urinate, combine with Plantain seeds (Che Qian Zi), Akebia (Mu Tong), Gardenia (Zhi Zi) and Talc (Hua Shi). Alisma Congee is taken for inhibited urination, edema, leukorrhea, obesity, high cholesterol, high blood pressure, chronic liver disease. It is made by stir frying 10 grams of alisma and grinding it to a fine powder. Cook 50 grams of polished rice in 4 cups of water and then stir in the Alisma powder (Ze Xie) and cook a little longer. It can be taken warm twice daily. Three days constitutes one course of treatment.

Poria Cocos **Fu Ling** (1)

Common Name: Poria, Hoelen

Part Used: Sclerotium

Family: Polyporaceae

Energy and Flavor: sweet, bland and neutral

Organ Meridians Affected: Spleen, Heart, Lung, Urinary Bladder

Actions: 1. Encourages urination and drains Dampness; 2. Tonic to the Spleen/Stomach; 3. Assists the Heart and calms the Spirit.

Indications: 1. For Dampness with symptoms of edema, difficult urination and Damp-Heat conditions with scanty urination; 2. For weakness in the Spleen/Stomach with symptoms of Dampness, lack of appetite, abdominal distention, diarrhea and conditions of Phlegm in the Upper Burner with a thick greasy tongue coating; 3. Calms the Heart when there are insomnia and palpitations.

Contraindications: This herb should not be used when there is frequent and copious urination when associated with a Cold Deficiency.

Dosage: 6 - 15 grams

Notes: Fu ling is a member of the polyporaceae family and there is at least one species that was used by the Native Americans and early settlers of the Southeast U.S. There it was known as "Indian Bread" or "Tuckahoe". It is usually found adhering to the roots of pine trees. The part that attaches to the tree is more specifically used for calming the mind.

Poria is high in potassium salts which may account for its unique fluid regulating properties. Instead of directly increasing the flow of urine, it frees up interstitial fluid for excretion and also regulates

intercellular fluid. This is the reason that Poria, unlike most diuretics, does not cause thirst.

For Dampness and edema combine with Polyporus (Zhu Ling), Alisma (Ze Xie), Atractylodes (Bai Zhu) and Cinnamon twigs (Gui Zhi) in Hoelen Five Herb Combination (Wu Ling San); to strengthen the Spleen and remove Dampness combine with Codonopsis (Dang Shen), Atractylodes (Bai Zhu) and Licorice (Gan Cao) in Four Major Herbs (Si Jun Zi Tang); to calm the spirit use the part of Poria that attaches itself to the host tree or root. This is called Fu Shen. It can be combined with Zizyphus Seeds (Suan Zao Ren) and Polygala (Yuan Zhi). Poria skin (Fu Ling Pi) is better for reducing edema while Red Poria (Chi Fu Ling) is used for removing Damp Heat.

Polyporus Umbellatus   Zhu Ling   (1)

Common Name: Polyporus, Grifola

Part Used: Sclerotium

Family: Polyporaceae

Energy and Flavor: sweet, bland, neutral

Organ Meridians Affected: Urinary Bladder, Kidney and Spleen

Actions: 1. Drains Dampness and encourages urination; 2. Grifola, which is often used as Zhu Ling, has been used recently for tumors and cancer.

Indications: 1. For Stagnant Dampness with symptoms of edema, urinary difficulty, scanty urination, jaundice and diarrhea; 2. Grifola has the same properties of polyporus but is used for tumors and cancer.

Contraindications: This herb should not be used when there is an absence of Dampness.

Dosage: 6 - 15 grams

Notes: Polyporus is very similar to Poria except that it is more purely diuretic. It is used for difficult or painful urination associated with urinary inflammations such as cystitis. It is often combined with Poria (Fu Ling) to augment its diuretic action. For painful urination it can be combined with Akebia (Mu tong) and Talcum (Hua Shi).

Talcum   Hua Shi   (1)

Common Name: Talcum

Part Used: The rock powder

Energy and Flavor: sweet and Cold

Organ Meridians Affected: Stomach and Urinary Bladder

Actions: 1. Encourages urination; 2. Expels Damp-Heat from the Urinary Bladder; 3. Dispels Summer Heat; 4. Dries Dampness when applied topically.

Indications: 1. For urinary dysfunction with symptoms of scanty urine, painful urination and diarrhea; 2. For Damp-Heat in the Urinary Bladder with symptoms of painful and dark urine, scanty urination, eczema, diarrhea, fever and a sensation of feeling heavy; 3. For Summer Heat with symptoms of thirst, fever, difficult urination and irritability; 4. Applied topically for Damp skin sores.

Contraindications: This substance should not be used when there are no signs of a Damp-Heat condition and should be avoided during pregnancy.

Dosage: 9 - 12 grams in decoction and should be placed in a cheese cloth to separate from the rest of the herbs.

Notes: Talcum is a mineral that has a similar use to Gypsum in relieving Summer Heat (heat stroke) but also a more particular use as a cooling demulcent to relieve urinary irritations and painful urination. Because of this, it is usually added to formulas for dissolving and passing urinary stones. For urinary infections combine Talc (Hua Shi) with Akebia (Mu Tong), Plantain seed (Che Qian Zi), Polygonum (Bian Xu) and Gardenia (Zhi Zi). For heat stroke combine Talc (Hua Shi) with Licorice root (Gan Cao). Externally for boils, eczema, itch and other skin irritations mix it with Gypsum (Shi Gao) and Calamine lotion available from a drug pharmacy and apply externally.

Coix Lachryma-jobi   Yi Yi Ren   (1)

Common Name: Job's Tears, Coix

Part Used: Seed (Semen)

Family: Gramineae

Energy and Flavor: sweet, bland and slightly Cold

Organ Meridians Affected: Spleen, Stomach, Kidney, Lung and Large Intestine

Actions: 1. Regulates water and encourages urination; 2. Tonic to the Spleen and stops diarrhea caused by Spleen Deficiency; 3. Reduces inflammation and eliminates pus; 4. Dispels Wind-Damp Bi Pain; 5. Expels Damp-Heat.

Indications: 1. For improper water metabolism with symptoms of edema, urinary difficulty, ascites and Damp leg Qi; 2. For Spleen Deficiency with diarrhea; 3. For abscesses of the Lung and Intestines as well as pus filled inflammations of the Exterior; 4. For painful obstruction associated with Wind and Damp with symptoms of lack of mobility, inflammation and spasms; 5. For any kind of Damp-Heat with symptoms of digestive difficulty with a thick greasy tongue coating and a slippery rapid pulse.

Contraindications: This herb should not be used by pregnant women.

Dosage: 9 - 30 grams

Notes: Coix is used primarily to regulate fluid metabolism. It drains Dampness while moistening the skin at the same time. It can be taken as a Coix congee. First dry-fry the Coix until is light brown. Then grind it to a flour and cook in enough water to make it into a porridge. This can be taken sweetened with raw, unrefined sugar to taste. Alternatively, Coix may be cooked with rice and eaten as a grain. It is good for Spleen and Stomach Deficiency, rheumatic arthritis, edema, warts and fatty tumors. For rheumatic and arthritic conditions, combine it with Ephedra (Ma Huang), Apricot seed (Xing Ren) and Licorice (Gan Cao); for colitis combine it with Patrinia (Bai Jiang Cao), Pueraria (Ge Gen), Moutan (Mu Dan Pi); for diarrhea caused by Spleen Deficiency combine roasted Coix with Atractylodes (Bai Zhu) and Poria (Fu Ling). Research has shown Coix to be an effective anti-cancer herb.

Dianthus Superbus (Dianthi)   Qu Mai   (2)

Common Name: Dianthus, Chinese Pink Flower

Part Used: Aerial portion (Herba)

Family: Caryophyllaceae

Energy and Flavor: bitter and Cold

Organ Meridians Affected: Heart, Small Intestine and Urinary Bladder

Actions: 1. Encourages urination and expels Damp-Heat; 2. Dissolves Blood Stasis and assists blocked menstruation.

Indications: 1. For urinary difficulty associated with Damp-Heat with symptoms of dark or bloody and scanty urine, acute urinary tract infection, lack of urine or dribbling; 2. For amenorrhea due to Blood Stasis.

Contraindications: This herb should not be used by pregnant women nor by those with Deficiency of Qi of the Kidneys or Spleen.

Dosage: 6 - 12 grams

Notes: This herb is a strong diuretic that also promotes intestinal peristalsis. It is used for urinary infections and other urinary dysfunctions caused by Damp-Heat in the Bladder. For this it can be combined with Akebia (Mu Tong), Talc (Hua Shi) and Polygonum avicularis (Bian Xu) as found in Dianthus Formula (Ba Zheng San). This is a member of the Carnation family and is easily cultivated in Western herb gardens.

Desmodium Styracifolium   Jin Qian Cao   (3)

This is an interesting example where many diverse herbs used for the same purpose have the same Chinese name. Besides the species listed, Ground Ivy (Glechoma longumtuba), Lysimachia christinae, Dichondra repens and Hydrocotyle sibthorpiodes are all used for a similar purpose. The translation of the Chinese describes the primary herb used which is "gold coin herb".

Family: varies with the species

Energy and Flavor: The species listed is sweet, bland and neutral, Glechoma is bitter, spicy and Cool, both dichondra and hydrocotyle are slightly salty and neutral.

Organ Meridians Affected: Heart, Small Intestine and Urinary Bladder

Actions: 1. Expels urinary stones and gallstones; 2. Clears Damp Heat of the Liver; 3. Detoxifies Fire poison, venomous bites, abscesses, injuries and burns.

Indications: 1. A major group of herbs for urinary and gallstones; 2. They can be externally applied to speed the healing of burns.

Contraindications: No known toxicity

Dosage: 15 to 30 grams

Notes: This herb is a common easily grown ground cover available as Lysimachia at most nurseries. The leaves vary from greenish in the shade to bright gold in full sun.

Juncus Effusi   **Deng Xin Cao** (2)

Common Name: Juncus

Part Used: Inner pith or medulla

Family: Junceae

Energy and Flavor: Cold and sweet

Organ Meridians Affected: Lung, Heart, Small Intestine

Actions: 1. Diuretic, promotes urination; 2. Clears urinary tract infections.

Indications: This herb is specific for urinary tract infections, sore throat, Damp Heat, incessant crying of babies.

Contraindications: Not for individuals with Spleen and Stomach Coldness and Deficiency

Dosage: 2 to 3 grams

Notes: Juncus is a common grass-like herb found in many parts of the world. The Chinese variety is sold in neatly tied bunches with the pith stripped out and wrapped around the outer, hollow stem. Like Dianthus, it is used for Damp Heat conditions or infections of the Bladder or Kidneys.

Akebia Trifoliata   **Mu Tong**   (3)

Common Name: Akebia

Part Used: Stem (Caulis)

Family: Lardizabalaceae

Energy and Flavor: bitter and Cold

Organ Meridians Affected: Heart, Small Intestine and Urinary Bladder

Actions: 1. Encourages urination and clears Heat; 2. Clears Heat and inflammation of the Heart; 3. Promotes lactation; 4. Moves and smoothes the flow of Blood; 5. Used for painful obstruction associated with either Dampness, Blood Stagnation, Wind or Heat.

Indications: 1. For urinary difficulty with symptoms of acute urinary tract infection, painful urination and edema; 2. For Heart Fire with symptoms of irritability, scanty urination, mouth sores and restlessness; 3. For the lack of proper milk by a nursing mother; 4. For amenorrhea associated with Blood Stagnation; 5. For Bi syndrome (painful obstruction) with symptoms of pain, stiffness and inflammation of the joints.

Contraindications: This herb should not be used during pregnancy and should be used with caution with patients who have Yin Deficiency.

Dosage: 3 - 9 grams

Notes: Akebia helps the communication between the Heart and Small Intestine with the Bladder. It is indicated for urinary dysfunctions associated or caused by irritability and emotional stress. For edema and urinary tract infections combine with Plantain seeds (Che Qian Zi); for edema combine with Poria (Fu Ling) and Polyporus (Zhu Ling).

Kochia Scoparia   Di Fu Zi   (3)

Common Name: Kochia Fruit, Broom Cypress Fruit

Part Used: Fruit (Fructus)

Family: Chenopodiaceae

Energy and Flavor: sweet, bitter and Cold

Organ Meridians Affected: Kidney and Urinary Bladder

Actions: 1. Encourages urination and dispels Damp-Heat; 2. Drains Dampness and arrests itching.

Indications: 1. For Damp-Heat in the Urinary Bladder with symptoms of acute urinary tract infection, dark and scanty urination and painful urination; 2. For Damp skin diseases where itching is the major complaint as in eczema, scabies and poison oak or ivy; for this it can be used either internally or externally.

Contraindications: This herb should only be used when there is presence of Dampness and Heat.

Dosage: 6 - 15 grams

Notes: For urinary inflammation and pain, combine with Polyporus (Zhu Ling), Dianthus (Qu Mai), Plantain Seed (Che Qian Zi) and Talc (Hua Shi).

Polygonum Avicularis **Bian Xu** (3)

Common Name: Knotweed, Polygonum

Part Used: Aerial portion (Herba)

Family: Polygonaceae

Energy and Flavor: sweet, bitter and Cool

Organ Meridians Affected: Urinary Bladder

Actions: 1. Expels Damp-Heat and encourages urination; 2. Drains Dampness and stops itching; 3. Kills parasites.

Indications: 1. For Damp-Heat in the Lower Burner with symptoms of painful urination, acute urinary tract infection and jaundice; 2. For Damp skin ailments accompanied by infection and itching; 3. For intestinal parasites as well as vaginal trichomonas.

Contraindications: This herb should be used with caution by those with Deficient Qi.

Dosage: 9 - 15 grams

Notes: This is a common wayside weed known as Polygonum or Knotgrass. It is found throughout the world and herbalists use it for urinary tract inflammations.

Plantaginis Asiatica **Che Qian Zi** (2)

Common Name: Plantain Seed

Part Used: Seed (Semen)

Family: Plantaginaceae

Energy and Flavor: sweet and slightly Cold

Organ Meridians Affected: Kidney, Lung, Liver, Urinary Bladder and Small Intestine

Actions: 1. Encourages urination and clears Heat; 2. Stops diarrhea by expelling water through urination; 3. Brightens the eyes, used in combination either for Deficiency or Heat; 4. Reduces inflammation of infections; 5. Arrests cough and expectorates Phlegm.

Indications: 1. For Damp-Heat in the Lower Burner with symptoms of edema, urinary dysfunction and urinary tract infection; 2. For diarrhea caused by either Damp-Heat or Damp-Summer Heat; 3. For red eyes caused by either Deficiency of the Kidneys or Liver or Heat in the Liver depending on the other herbs in the formula; 4. For infections accompanied by inflammation; 5. For cough and Phlegm associated with Lung Heat where there is abundant copious Phlegm.

Contraindications: This herb should not be used during pregnancy, constipation, Deficiency of Qi or with signs of Damp Heat.

Dosage: 3 - 9 grams

Notes: There is hardly a more common wayside weed than Plantain. Generally two varieties are used by Western herbalists: broadleaf (Plantago major) and narrow or lanceleaf (Plantago minor). It contains aucubin which is both an anti-inflammatory and acts as a mild pain reliever especially when topically applied on injuries and wounds. The leaves can be chewed or lightly steamed to more quickly release their healing benefits. Used in this way, the leaves can be topically applied to relieve bee stings and other venomous bites and stings.

Zea Mays   **Yu Mi Xu**   (3)

Common Name: Cornsilk

Part Used: Stylus

Family: Gramineae

Energy and Flavor: sweet, bland and neutral

Organ Meridians Affected: Liver, Urinary Bladder and Small Intestine

Actions: 1. Encourages urination; 2. Stimulates the Gallbladder and eliminates jaundice; 3. Regulates blood sugar for wasting and thirsting disorders such as diabetes mellitus; 4. Stops bleeding.

Indications: 1. For lack of urination with symptoms of acute or chronic edema, cirrhosis of the Liver or urinary dysfunction with painful urination caused by urinary tract infection or stones; 2. Stimulates the flow of bile from the Gallbladder for Stagnation which has led to jaundice of either a Yin or Yang nature; 3. For wasting and thirsting disorders such as diabetes mellitus where the blood sugar is not regulated properly in the body; 4. For bleeding of the nose or gums.

Contraindications: None noted

Dosage: 6 - 20 grams

Notes: Corn silk consists of the tassels that grow at the top of an ear of corn. Ideally these should be used fresh. Corn silk is a standard Western herbal diuretic useful for urinary tract infections and to help dispel and expel stones.

Lobelia Chinensis   **Ban Bian Lian** (3)

Common Name: Chinese Lobelia

Part Used: Herb and Root (Herba cum Radice)

Family: Campanulaceae

Energy and Flavor: sweet and neutral

Organ Meridians Affected: Liver, Kidney, Heart, Lung, Small intestine

Actions: 1. Diuretic, reduces edema; 2. Detoxifying, and anti-inflammatory; 3. Anti-cancer.

Indications: It is used for edema, snake bites, enteritis, dysentery, eczema, Liver cirrhosis, cancer, inflamed sores, abscesses and venomous snake bites.

Contraindications: Use with caution for individuals with all types of Deficiencies.

Dosage: 15-30 gms

Notes: Chinese Lobelia is one of the primary herbs used by the Chinese to treat cancer. It has a combination of alkaloids very similar to Western Lobelia inflata, the latter being used as an antispasmodic, stimulant, emetic and expectorant by Western herbalists. Lobelin is similar to nicotine, so that an extract of Lobelia inflata has been used commercially as a drug for the treatment of tobacco addiction. Chinese Lobelia, unlike Lobelia inflata, is classified and used as a diuretic. There is no mention of Chinese Lobelia being employed for its emetic properties. However, since there are several different North American species of Lobelia including L. syphilitica and L. cardinalis for instance, one of these may be even more similar to the Chinese species. This may be especially important in view of the fact that at least one of these may have similar therapeutically anti-neoplastic properties to the Chinese species.

Stephania Tetrandra   **Han Fang Ji**   (2)

Common Name: Stephania

Part Used: Root (Radix)

Family: Menispermaceae

Energy and Flavor: acrid, bitter and Cold

Organ Meridians Affected: Spleen, Kidney, Lung and Urinary Bladder

Actions: 1. Encourages urination; 2. Allays pain and dispels Wind-Damp painful obstruction (Bi Pain).

Indications: 1. For Dampness accumulation with symptoms of edema, rumbling intestines, ascites and abdominal distention; 2. For Wind-Damp painful obstruction with symptoms of Heat, pain and swollen joints.

Contraindications: This herb should not be used by those with chronic Dampness nor by those with Yin Deficiency.

Dosage: 3 - 9 grams

Notes: Stephania is specifically useful for leg edema. For edema with Heat combine Stephania (Fang Ji) with Lepidium seeds (Ting Li Zi); for edema with weakness combine it with Astragalus (Huang Qi) and Atractylodes (Bai Zhu) as used in the formula Stephania and Astragalus Combination (Fang Ji Huang Qi Tang).

Aristolochia Fangchi   Guang Fang Ji   (3)

Common Name: Aristolochia

Part Used: Root (Radix)

Family: Aristolochiaceae

Energy and Flavor: acrid, bitter and Cold

Organ Meridians Affected: Bladder, Spleen and Kidney

Actions: 1. Dispels Wind-Damp-Heat painful obstruction (Bi Pain); 2 Encourages urination.

Indications: 1. For Wind-Damp-Heat painful obstruction (Bi Pain) with symptoms of aches and pains accompanied by thirst, a rapid and slippery pulse and a thick, yellow and greasy tongue coating; 2. For edema, especially of the face, and wheezing.

Contraindications: This herb should be used with caution by those with Yin Deficiency.

Dosage: 3 - 9 grams

Notes: Combine with Astragalus (Huang Qi) and Clematis (Wei Ling Xian) for swollen, painful joints; with Coix (Yi Yi Ren) for pain in the extremities caused by Damp Heat.

Artemisia Capillaris   Yin Chen Hao   (1)

Common Name: Capillaris, Oriental Wormwood

Part Used: Aerial portion (Herba)

Family: Compositae

Energy and Flavor: bitter, acrid and Cool

Organ Meridians Affected: Spleen, Liver, Gallbladder, Stomach and Urinary Bladder

Actions: 1. Drains Damp and clears Heat, especially from the Liver and Gallbladder; 2. Eliminates Heat and relieves the Exterior.

Indications: 1. For Damp-Heat in the Liver and Gallbladder, also for jaundice caused by either Damp-Heat or Damp-Cold; 2. For symptoms of Heat accompanied by fever and chills, bitter taste in the mouth, dizziness, nausea and loss of appetite.

Contraindications: This herb should not be used where there is jaundice caused by Qi Deficiency with no signs of Damp-Heat.

Dosage: 9 - 15 grams

Notes: Commonly known as Capillaris, this herb is specific for hepatitis and jaundice, for which it can be combined with Gardenia (Zhi Zi) and Rhubarb (Da Huang). We have found it effective for the treatment of acute hepatitis B. It can also be taken with Talc (Hua Shi) as an alternative to Artemisia annua (Qing Hao) for heat stroke. For Damp-Cold jaundice

it can be combined with Dried Ginger (Gan Jiang), Prepared Aconite (Fu Zi) and Poria (Fu Ling).

Abutili seu Malvae   Dong Kui Zi   (3)

Common Name: Abutilon Seeds, Malva Seeds
Part Used: Seed (Semen)
Family: Malvaceae
Energy and Flavor: sweet and Cold
Organ Meridians Affected: Urinary Bladder, Large and Small Intestine
Actions: 1. Encourages urination; 2. Promotes lactation; 3. Moistening and soothing to the urinary tract and Intestines.
Indications: 1. For urinary difficulty with Hot and painful urination, also useful for urinary stones; this herb is especially useful when there is constipation accompanied by the above mentioned symptoms; 2. For difficulty in lactation as well as painful breasts and the beginnings of breast abscesses; 3. For urinary tract infections or stones in the urinary tract as well as constipation.
Contraindications: This herb should not be used by those with diarrhea due to Spleen Deficiency nor by pregnant women.
Dosage: 6 - 15 grams

Notes: Abutilon seeds are used similarly to that of the Western Althea officinalis (Marshmallow root) to relieve irritation accompanying urination, as a result of Dryness. Both Althea and Abutilon also increase lactation and the richness of mother's milk. This herb can be tried as a milder demulcent substitute for Talc (Hua Shi) in relieving urinary irritation and pain.

For dysuria and edema, combine with Poria (Fu Ling) and Atractylodes (Bai Zhu); for scanty, painful urination with blood, combine with Plantain seeds (Che Qian Zi), Lygodium Spores (Hai Jin Sha) and Talc (Hua Shi).

Dioscorea Hypoglauca   Bei Xie   (3)

Common Name: Hypoglauca Yam, Fish-Poison Yam
Part Used: Rhizome (Rhizoma)
Family: Dioscoreaceae
Energy and Flavor: bitter and neutral
Organ Meridians Affected: Liver, Stomach and Urinary Bladder
Properties: antibacterial, antifungal, antirheumatic, antiinflammatory, antitussive, antiparasitic

Actions: 1. Encourages urination and eliminates cloudy urine; 2. Eliminates Wind-Damp; 3. Relieves Damp-Heat from the skin.

Indications: 1. For cloudy urine caused by either Damp-Heat or Deficiency; 2. For Wind-Damp with symptoms of lower back pain and muscle aches and rheumatic arthritis; 3. For Damp-Heat skin ailments such as eczema and sores.

Contraindications: This herb should not be used by those with Kidney Yin Deficiency.

Dosage: 9 - 15 grams

Notes: This Dioscorea is similar to the one used by Western herbalists (D. villosa), also used for Damp Heat conditions associated with jaundice, hepatitis, Gallbladder and rheumatic diseases. For urinary bladder infections combine with Phellodendron (Huang Bai) and Plantain Seed (Che Qian Zi); for Cold Dampness rheumatic conditions, combine with Cinnamon twigs (Gui Zhi) and Prepared Aconite (Fu Zi).

Discrimination:

Sclerotium Poria Cocos (Fu Ling) — Spleen tonic, calms the mind.

Sclerotium Polyporus Umbellatus (Zhu Ling) — a more pure diuretic than Fu ling, used for cancer.

Talcum (Hua Shi) — lubricates and moistens Dryness and relieves urinary pain.

Semen Coix lachryma-jobi (Yi Yi Ren) — used for diarrhea and to relieve Wind-Damp Bi pain (rheumatic pains).

Dianthus (Qu Mai) — relieves Damp Heat and Blood Stagnation.

Akebia (Mu Tong) — clears Heat from the Heart, promotes circulation.

Kochia Scoparia (Di Fu Zi) — clears Damp Heat, stops itching.

Polygonum Avicularis (Bian Xu) — clears Damp Heat, stops itching, kills parasites.

HERBS THAT DISPEL WIND AND DAMPNESS

Wind-Damp is a pathogenic factor that settles in the bones, joints, muscles and sinews, causing pain, stiffness and numbness as a result of the obstruction of Blood and Qi. When this happens, it is called *bi*, or painful obstruction, and corresponds to arthritic and rheumatic conditions. Wind-Damp painful obstruction is usually accompanied by Heat or Cold. In the different patterns one of the Pathogenic Factors - Wind, Damp, Heat or Cold - is always most predominant. Wind Damp Heat can be caused by Liver Deficiency especially when it affects the

sinews and tendons, or the Kidneys when it affects the joints and bones. Most of the herbs in this category are aromatic, Warm and drying in nature and may injure Blood or Yin. Thus they should be used with caution for those with deficiencies of Blood and Yin.

Wind Damp Cold can be caused by a Deficiency of Yang or Qi and is treated with Warming and circulating herbs. These should be accompanied with the use of Qi or Yang tonics.

Because these patterns are often chronic and difficult to treat, other methods of more localized treatment should be used when treating them. This should include the local application of medicated oils, plasters, fomentations, moxibustion, acupuncture and magnets, all of which are highly complementary and effective in relieving Bi pain.

When Wind is the predominant factor the symptoms are soreness, pain and limited movement in the joints and muscles. More importantly, the pain moves from place to place in the body. In an acute case of Wind predominant painful obstruction, the pulse would be floating and slightly rapid.

When Damp is the predominant factor, the symptoms are pain, swelling, feeling of heaviness and numbness, and the condition is fixed because Damp does not easily move around the body. The condition will be aggravated by Damp weather. In an acute case of Damp predominant painful obstruction, the pulse would be slow and slippery.

When Cold is the predominant factor the symptoms are severe pain which is fixed and with a limitation of motion. The condition is aggravated by cold weather. In an acute case of Cold predominant painful obstruction, the pulse would be tight.

When Heat is the predominant factor, there will be symptoms of swelling and severe pain with joints that are hot to the touch, and redness of the affected area with limitation of movement. Other Heat signs will be present such as fever, thirst, a red tongue body with a yellow coat and a rapid pulse.

Angelica Pubescentis   Du Huo   (1)

Common Name: Pubescent Angelica, Angelica Du Huo

Part Used: Root (Radix)

Family: Umbelliferae

Energy and Flavor: acrid, bitter and Warm

Organ Meridians Affected: Kidney and Urinary Bladder

Actions: 1. Disperses Wind, Cold, Dampness; 2. Relieves pain; 3. Relieves Lesser Yang (Shao Yang) headache.

Indications: 1. Treats both acute and chronic rheumatic pains, especially in the lower back and legs; 2. Releases Exterior Cold conditions such as the common cold with fever, headache and muscle pain; 3. Relieves Gallbladder and Liver caused headaches and toothaches.

Contraindications: Do not use when there is Yin Deficiency with Heat signs.

Dosage: 3 - 9 grams

Notes: Like all the Angelica species, Du Huo Warms and promotes Blood and Qi circulation. It may be combined with other herbs as is appropriate for treatment. It counteracts Dampness and Wind (spasms) associated with Bi (blockage) Stagnation. Western Angelica Archangelica, commonly used in digestive liqueurs, is also used for arthritic complaints and as an emmenagogue to promote menstruation. Du Huo can be combined with Loranthes (Sang Ji Sheng), Gentiana (Qin Jiao) and Ledebouriella (Fang Feng) for Wind-Cold Dampness with rheumatic aches and pains; for External Wind-Cold, combine it with Notopterygium root (Qiang Huo).

Gentiana Macrophylla   Qin Jiao   (1)

Common Name: Gentian

Part Used: Root (Radix)

Family: Gentianaceae

Energy and Flavor: acrid, bitter and Cool

Organ Meridians Affected: Liver, Gallbladder and Stomach

Actions: 1. Clears either acute or chronic, Cold or Hot Wind-Damp conditions; 2. Clears Heat from Yin Deficiency; 3. Lubricates the Intestines and promotes bowel movements.

Indications: 1. Relieves acute or chronic pains, spasms caused by Wind-Damp conditions that are either Hot or Cold; 2. Reduces fever, including steaming bone fever caused by Yin Deficiency; 3. Treats hepatitis, jaundice and other Damp-Heat conditions; 4. Relieves constipation caused by Dryness.

Contraindications: Not for conditions of frequent urination and pain in weak and Deficient individuals, especially when there is Spleen Deficient diarrhea.

Dosage: 3 - 9 grams

Notes: This herb counteracts the inflammation associated with arthritic conditions and as such is often combined with other more circulating herbs such as Angelica Du Huo, Cinnamon twigs (Gui Zhi) and Aconite root (Fu Zi). Its Damp Heat clearing properties are synergistically aided with the addition of Honeysuckle stems (Ren Dong Teng), Gardenia (Zhi Zi) and Artemisia annua (Qing Hao). It possesses similar anti-

inflammatory properties as all Gentians except it must be more circulating.

Acanthopanax Gracilistylus   Wu Jia Pi   (2)
(includes Eleuthrococcus Senticosus-Si Wu Jia)

Common Name: Acanthopanax Rootbark, Thorny Ginseng, Chinese Siberian Ginseng

Part Used: Root Bark (Cortex and Radix)

Family: Araliaceae

Energy and Flavor: acrid and Warm

Organ Meridians Affected: Liver and Kidney

Actions: 1. Relieves Wind-Damp and strengthens the bones and sinews; 2. Drains Damp.

Indications: 1. For painful obstruction (Bi Pain) caused by chronic Wind-Cold-Damp with a Deficiency of the Liver and Kidneys and obstruction of Qi and Blood; 2. For edema and urinary difficulty.

Contraindications: This herb should not be used when there is Yin Deficiency with Heat signs.

Dosage: 3 - 12 grams

Notes: China's most honored herbalist, Li Shih Shen, told of six Chinese politicians and scholars who lived 300 years as a result of their regular consumption of Acanthopanax root (Wu Jia Pi). It is commonly sold as a Chinese wine for which it is listed as good for neurasthenia, insomnia, many dreams, forgetfulness, dizziness, poor appetite, palpitations, coronary heart disease, and angina pectoris. Prolonged consumption is necessary to treat leukopenia caused by physiotherapy and chemotherapy. A similar plant that grows in Russia known as Eleutherococcus senticosus has been extensively researched for its ability to counteract stress and improve work and athletic performance.

For rheumatic pain with motor impairment of the joints and limbs combine with Chaenomeles (Mu Gua), Achyranthes (Niu Xi) and Prepared Rehmannia (Shu Di Huang).

Morus Alba (twig)   Sang Zhi   (2)

Common Name: Mulberry Twig

Part Used: Branches (Ramulus)

Family: Moraceae

Energy and Flavor: bitter and Cool

Organ Meridians Affected: Liver

Actions: 1. Relieves Wind-Damp painful obstruction (Bi Pain) and assists the joints; 2. Encourages urination.

Indications: 1. For Wind-Damp painful obstruction (Bi Pain) especially affecting the joints of the upper extremities; 2. For edema and high blood pressure caused by retention of water.

Contraindications: None noted.

Dosage: 9 - 15 grams (up to 30 grams)

Notes: Used for rheumatic and arthritic conditions with accompanying spasm of the limbs. It can be used alone or combined with Stephania (Fang Ji), Chaenomeles (Mu Gua) and Clematis (Wei Ling Xian).

Clematis Chinensis   Wei Ling Xian(1)

Common Name: Clematis

Part Used: Root (Radix)

Family: Ranunculaceae

Energy and Flavor: acrid, salty and Warm

Organ Meridians Affected: Urinary Bladder

Actions: 1. Relieves Wind-Damp, circulates Qi and alleviates pain; 2. Softens and releases fish bones lodged in the throat.

Indications: 1. For Wind-Damp Bi Pain in any part of the body; 2. Mixed with vinegar and brown sugar it is taken for fish bones lodged in the throat.

Contraindications: This herb should not be used by those with Deficiency of either Qi or Blood.

Dosage: 3 - 12 grams

Notes: The translation of the Chinese is "Temple's Sacred Root" which refers to an ancient story of an old nun who lived in a temple called "the temple of powerful spirits," atop a high mountain. She regularly prescribed this herb for many conditions with great success. Herbs like Clematis that promote circulation, of all properties, are the most likely to be of benefit for more conditions. This is certainly true for conditions associated with Cold and Damp, likely to be found at such a high mountainous location. As with any other Qi or Blood circulating herbs, they may further exhaust Yin or Blood, especially if there is any tendency towards Deficiency of these qualities.

For Wind-Damp obstruction or rheumatic aches and pains combine with Angelica Du Huo (Du Huo), Loranthes (Sang Ji Sheng) and Angelica sinensis (Dang Gui).

Clematis is specifically indicated to help soften and dislodge fishbones stuck in the throat. This property is probably due to its ability to remove spasmodic pain of the larynx.

Chaenomelis Lagenaria — Mu Gua (1)

Common Name: Chinese Quince, Chaenomeles Fruit

Part Used: Fruit (Fructus)

Family: Rosaceae

Energy and Flavor: sour and Warm

Organ Meridians Affected: Liver and Spleen

Actions: 1. Relaxes the sinews by increasing the flow of both Blood and Qi; 2. Assists the function of the Stomach and expels Dampness.

Indications: 1. For pain caused by Wind-Damp painful obstruction, it is especially useful for the lower back and lower extremities and when there is cramping; 2. For excessive Dampness in the Stomach with symptoms of abdominal pain and spasms and cramping pain in the legs.

Contraindications: This herb should not be used by those with Yin Deficiency. It should also be avoided in Exterior conditions.

Dosage: 3 - 9 grams

Notes: Because of its antispasmodic properties, Chaenomeles (Mu Gua) can be used to increase flexibility by relaxing the ligaments and sinews. For Wind-Damp obstruction, stiffness, pain of the limbs and joints combine with Stephania (Fang Ji), Clematis (Wei Ling Xian), Angelica (Dang Gui). Chinese martial arts and Qi Gong or Taoist Yoga are ancient traditions associated with the use of such herbs to treat injuries, strengthen and/or harden various bodily parts and increase flexibility.

Xanthium Sibiricum — Cang Er Zi (2)

Common Name: Xanthium, Cocklebur Fruit

Part Used: Fruit (Fructus)

Family: Compositae

Energy and Flavor: sweet, bitter, pungent, Warm and toxic

Organ Meridians Affected: Lung

Actions: 1. Expels Wind-Damp; 2. Relieves nasal congestion; 3. Drives away Exterior Wind.

Indications: 1. For Wind-Damp which causes either painful obstruction or itching skin; 2. For nasal congestion with thick running discharge that is either chronic or acute and is associated with headache; 3. For invasion of Exterior Wind that causes headache.

Contraindications: This herb should not be used by those with Blood or Yin Deficiency as it is very drying. Overdosing can cause toxic reactions of vomiting, abdominal pain and diarrhea.

Dosage: 3 - 9 grams

Notes: This herb is often included in the External Surface Relieving category since its main function is treating sinus congestion and upper respiratory allergies. For these conditions it represents an alternative to Ma Huang, which is the herb most commonly used. For sinus congestion and allergies combine with Magnolia flower (Xin Yi), and Angelica dahurica (Bai Zhi) as found in the formula Xanthium combination (Cang Er San). It is also used for spasms and joint pain caused by Cold-Damp-Wind Stagnation, for which Clematis (Wei Ling Xian), Cinnamon Bark (Rou Gui), Black Atractylodes (Cang Zhu) and Ligusticum (Chuan Xiong) are added.

Lignum Pini Nodi   Song Jie

Common Name: Pine nodular branch, knotty pine

Part Used: the branch with the node or bend

Family: Pinaceae

Energy and Flavor: bitter and Warm

Organ Meridians Affected: Liver

Actions: 1. Dispels Wind-Damp; 2. Stops pain

Indications: 1. It can be used in teas or soaked in rice wine to treat acute arthritis with severe inflammation and pain; 2. It is used with other Blood moving herbs such as Peach seed (Tao Ren), Safflower (Hong Hua), Frankincense (Ru Xiang) and Myrrh (Mo Yao) for external injury and pain.

Contraindications: This herb should not be used by those with Blood or Yin Deficiency.

Dosage: 9- 15 grams

Notes: This herb is mentioned because it is so commonly available throughout various parts of the world. The nodular pine branch can be soaked in wine and taken for arthritic and rheumatic conditions.

Discrimination:

Angelica Pubescentis (Du Huo) — Cold conditions of the lower back and legs, colds, headaches, toothaches.

Gentiana Macrophylla (Qin Jiao) — with Yin Deficiency Heat, lubricates the Intestines.

Acanthopanax Gracilistyli Radicis (Wu Jia Pi) – Warm, strengthens bones and sinews, edema, tonifies Liver and Kidneys.

Morus Alba (Sang Zhi) – Cool, treats upper extremities pain, edema and high blood pressure.

Clematis Chinensis (Wei Ling Xian) – Cool, circulates Qi, softens fish bones in the throat.

Chaenomelis Lagenaria (Mu Gua) – Warm, spasms and cramps of the lower back and extremities, leg cramps.

Xanthium Sibiricum (Cang Er Zi) – relieves respiratory allergies, itching skin.

Lignum Pini Nodi (Song Jie) – commonly available, counteracts inflammation of the joints.

HERBS THAT TRANSFORM PHLEGM AND STOP COUGH

Phlegm is a condition of Stagnation of Fluids which are thick and viscous. This pattern usually affects the Lungs and Spleen and causes symptoms of coughing, wheezing, stuffiness in the chest when affecting the Lungs, and nausea, vomiting, loss of appetite and distention when affecting the Spleen or Stomach. Phlegm is a further condensation of Fluid or Dampness and originates as a by-product of mal-absorbed food and fluids from a Deficient Spleen. There is always a natural amount of lubrication that is needed by various Organs and parts of the body. Of these, the Lungs, because they are continually exposed to the passage of air, require a certain amount of mucus for normal function. This is perhaps one reason why the Five Elements describe the Earth-Spleen as being the mother of Metal-Lungs. Any excess of Fluid from the Spleen first goes to the Lungs, and if this overly accumulates it thickens and becomes pathological Phlegm.

The herbs in this category act on the Lungs and are considered expectorant, because they eliminate Phlegm and stop coughing. Phlegm, being a form of Stagnation, may start as being Cool and transform to Hot; as a result, herbs in this category are correspondingly Cool or Warm natured.

Phlegm can arise as a result of Deficiency caused by lower metabolism and weak digestion. In such cases, one must employ tonics either as a single therapeutic principle or in combination with herbs from this category as assistants.

Many Phlegm transforming herbs act through the Stomach and Spleen. In TCM theory, Phlegm can also block the channels and obstruct

the Heart, causing conditions such as coma, delirium, lockjaw and seizure. Disorders such as these must be treated with herbs that transform Phlegm and disperse Wind as well as herbs that calm the Spirit (Shen).

There are four subcategorizes within this category: (1) herbs that transform Hot-Phlegm, (2) herbs that transform Cold-Phlegm, (3) herbs that stop coughing and wheezing and (4) herbs that expel Phlegm by inducing vomiting.

Herbs that transform Hot-Phlegm are Cool or Cold in nature and treat conditions of Hot and Dry-Phlegm. They treat cough, goiter, scrofula and Phlegm-Heat convulsions. They have expectorant, antitussive, anti-inflammatory and sedative properties.

Herbs that transform Cold-Phlegm are Warm or Hot in nature and treat conditions of Cold-Phlegm and Wet-Phlegm. They treat cough, wheezing, vomiting and nausea. Many of the herbs in this subcategory are very strong and can be toxic when used improperly; for this reason, care should be used when administering them.

Herbs that stop coughing and wheezing can be either Warm or Cooling in nature and treat branch symptoms. They should be used as assistants to other herbs; for instance, those that treat the Exterior. These herbs have properties such as antitussive, expectorant, diuretic and laxative.

Herbs that expel Phlegm by inducing vomiting are very strong and should only be used for more serious conditions. Because of their strong nature, they should only be used for those with a strong constitution and not for children or pregnant women. This method, although once very popular in China, was employed by famous Western doctors such as Samuel Thompson with his famous Lobelia emetic, but is not now commonly used in TCM and should be done with extreme care, as improper use of these herbs could cause serious injury to the patient.

Since I have found Thompson's Lobelia Emetic treatment extremely effective, especially for asthma, I would like to offer it here. For maximum benefit, it should be only undergone at the height of an acute asthma attack. The patient is instructed to drink one or two quarts of peppermint tea. After this is accomplished, one teaspoon (60 drops) of Lobelia seed extract is taken in ten minute intervals, three times in succession. Before or at this point, the patient should experience strong emesis and the asthma will be relieved.

COOL HERBS THAT TRANSFORM HOT PHLEGM

Fritillaria Cirrhosa   Chuan Bei Mu   (1)

Common Name: Fritillaria

Part Used: Bulb (Bulbus)

Family: Liliaceae

Energy and Flavor: sweet, bitter and Cold

Organ Meridians Affected: Heart and Lung

Actions: 1. Clears Hot Phlegm and stops cough; 2. Clears Lung Heat caused by Yin Deficiency; 3. Clears Heat and reduces hard lumps and swellings.

Indications: 1. For thick yellow sputum with or without blood streaks that is difficult to expectorate; 2. For Lung Yin Deficiency with Fire where there is dry cough and little sputum; 3. For conditions of Phlegm-Fire where there are hard swellings, scrofula, or Lung or breast abscesses.

Contraindications: This herb should not be used by those with Cold-Damp Phlegm conditions.

Dosage: 3 - 9 grams

Notes: For cough caused by Lung Deficiency with dry throat combine with Ophiopogon (Mai Men Dong) and Glehnia (Sha Shen); for cough with thick yellow phlegm combine with Anemarrhena (Zhi Mu), Scutellaria (Huang Qin) and Trichosanthes fruit (Gua Lou); for Wind-Heat cough combine with Mulberry leaf (Sang Ye), Peucedanum (Qian Hu), and Apricot seed (Xing Ren); for swollen glands combine with Scrophularia (Xuan Shen) and Laminaria (Kun Bu); for mastitis combine with Dandelion (Pu Gong Ying) and Forsythia (Lian Qiao); for Lung abscess and tobacco toxicity, combine with Tendrilled Fritillary (Chuan Bei Mu), Houttuynia (Yu Xing Cao) and Coix (Yi Yi Ren).

Fritillaria Thunbergii   Zhe Bei Mu (2)

Common Name: Fritillaria

Part Used: Bulb (Bulbus)

Family: Liliaceae

Energy and Flavor: bitter and Cold

Organ Meridians Affected: Lung and Heart

Actions: 1. Clears Phlegm-Heat and stops cough; 2. Reduces swellings caused by Phlegm-Fire.

Indications: 1. For acute Lung Heat with symptoms of productive cough with thick yellow sputum; 2. For swelling and abscesses of the neck and Lung where there is a pattern of Phlegm-Fire.

Contraindications: This herb should not be used when there is Cold and Damp Phlegm. Notes: The fresh herb is toxic and should never be used without being processed first.

Dosage: 3 - 9 grams

Notes: Similar effect as Tendrilled Fritillary (Chuan Bei Mu) but stronger in its Heat clearing properties. The former is more lubricating but it is considerably more expensive. They are often used interchangeably.

Peucedanum Praeruptorum (Peucedani)   Qian Hu   (1)
Common Name: Hogfennel, Peucedanum
Part Used: Root (Radix)
Family: Umbelliferae
Energy and Flavor: acrid, bitter and Cold
Organ Meridians Affected: Lung and Spleen
Actions: 1. Directs the ascending flow of Lung Qi downward to stop cough; 2. Expels Phlegm; 3. Expels Wind and relieves the Exterior for either Wind-Heat or Wind-Cold, although most frequently used for Wind-Heat patterns because of its Cold nature.
Indications: 1. For coughing and wheezing with thick sputum; 2. For thick, difficult to expectorate sputum; 3. For Externally contracted Wind with thick copious sputum with symptoms of upper respiratory tract infections and acute asthma attack.
Contraindications: This herb should be used with caution by those without true Heat signs.
Dosage: 3 - 9 grams

Notes: For Phlegm Heat in the Lungs with cough, yellow and sticky mucus, combine with Mulberry bark (Sang Bai Pi), Trichosanthes fruit (Gua Lou) and Tendrilled Fritillary (Chuan Bei Mu); for cough caused by Wind-Heat combine with Mentha (Bo He), Arctium (Niu Bang Zi) and Platycodon (Jie Geng).

Trichosanthes Kirilowii (Fructus)   Gua Lou   (1)
Common Name: Trichosanthes Fruit
Part Used: Fruit (Fructus)
Family: Cucurbitaceae
Energy and Flavor: sweet and Cold
Organ Meridians Affected: Lung, Stomach and Large Intestine
Actions: 1. Clears Phlegm-Heat conditions with thick difficult to expectorate sputum; 2. Regulates the Qi of the chest and relieves constriction and swellings of the chest and Lungs.
Indications: 1. For cough associated with patterns of Heat in the Lungs with sputum that is difficult to expectorate; 2. For Stagnation of Qi in the chest with symptoms of stifling sensation, constriction, pain caused by obstruction of Qi, and Lung and breast abscesses.

Contraindications: This herb should not be used by those with Cold and Damp especially when there is Spleen Deficiency.

Dosage: 6 - 18 grams

Notes: The peel of the fruit, Pericarpium Trichosanthes (Gua Lou Pi), has the same energetics as the fruit and is similarly used. It is, however, especially good for dry throat and cough or conditions caused by Wind-Heat Phlegm that is difficult to expectorate.

Trichosanthes Kirilowii (Semen)   Gua Lou Ren (1)

Common Name: Trichosanthes Seed

Part Used: Seed (Semen)

Family: Cucurbitaceae

Energy and Flavor: sweet and Cold

Organ Meridians Affected: Lung, Stomach and Large Intestine

Actions: 1. Cools and nourishes the Lungs; 2. Regulates the Qi in the chest; 3. Used externally, it assists the healing of Phlegm-Heat induced sores and abscesses; 4. Moistens the Intestines.

Indications: 1. For cough associated with Heat injuring the Yin of the Lung with symptoms of thick yellow sputum that is difficult to expectorate; 2. For Stagnation of Qi in the chest with symptoms of Phlegm, constriction and pain; 3. For Phlegm-Heat induced breast abscesses and sores, also good for sores that have Heat but no Phlegm; 4. For constipation associated with Lung Heat.

Contraindications: This herb should not be used when there is diarrhea or when there is no Heat.

Dosage: 9 - 15 grams

Notes: This has a similar use to Trichosanthes Fruit (Gua Lou) but the seeds are demulcent and treat dry constipation associated with thirst; this is in contrast with Cannabis (Huo Ma Ren) that treats dry constipation associated with Qi Deficiency or Peach seeds (Tao Ren) that treat dry constipation associated with Blood Stagnation.

Trichosanthes Kirilowii (Radix)   Tian Hua Fen (1)

Common Name: Trichosanthes Root

Part Used: Root (Radix)

Family: Cucurbitaceae

Energy and Flavor: bitter, slightly sweet, sour and Cold

Organ Meridians Affected: Lung and Stomach

Actions: 1. Clears Heat in the Lungs and moistens Dryness, especially when there is Phlegm that is aggravating the condition; 2. Brings down inflammation and reduces pus.

Indications: 1. For Heat or Phlegm-Heat where the condition is injuring the Fluids of the Lungs with symptoms such as thirst, dry cough or cough with blood streaked sputum; 2. For inflammation of any type, especially of the Lung and Stomach and where there is pus.

Contraindications: This herb should not be used by pregnant women, by those without Heat or by those with diarrhea.

Dosage: 9 - 15 grams

Notes: Trichosanthes Root (Gua Lou Ren) has similar properties to the other parts of the plant but is more specific for reducing Heat and toxicity.

Succus Bambusae   Zhu Li   (2)

(Phyllostachys Nigra)

Common Name: Dried Bamboo Sap

Part Used: Sap (Succus)

Family: Gramineae

Energy and Flavor: sweet and very Cold

Organ Meridians Affected: Heart, Lung and Stomach

Properties: antipyretic, expectorant

Actions: 1. For Phlegm that is associated with Heat in the Lungs; 2. For Phlegm blocking the Heart channel especially when there is Heat.

Indications: 1. For Phlegm-Heat in the Lungs with symptoms of cough with yellow sputum; 2. For Phlegm and Heat that are blocking the Heart orifices with symptoms such as convulsions, fainting, or other loss of sensory control.

Contraindications: This herb should not be used for coughs that are associated with Cold and by those with Spleen Deficiency with symptoms such as diarrhea.

Dosage: 30 - 60 grams generally, while one third of that dosage is usually effective to relieve coughs.

Notes: It is extracted from the freshly cut stalk of the bamboo which is then heated in order to encourage the sap to flow for collection. It is important in Ayurvedic medicine for the preparation of a well known cold and cough remedy known as Sito Paladi Churna. This is an herbal powder made by grinding eight parts dried bamboo sap, sixteen parts raw brown sugar, one part Cinnamon, four parts Black Pepper and two parts Cardamon. It is strongly Warming, anti-mucus and digestive. One teaspoon of the powder can be taken each time with warm water or warm milk. To offset its Cold energy, Chinese herbalists prescribe it with raw Ginger (Sheng Jiang) tea or Ginger juice to help offset its Coldness.

Bambusae in Taeniis   **Zhu Ru**   (2)

(Phyllostachys Nigra)

Common Name: Bamboo Shavings

Part Used: Stem (Caulis)

Family: Gramineae

Energy and Flavor: sweet and slightly Cold

Organ Meridians Affected: Stomach, Gallbladder and Lung

Actions: 1. Clears Phlegm-Heat in the Lungs; 2. Clears Heat in the Stomach and stops vomiting; 3. Cools the Blood and stops bleeding.

Indications: 1. For Phlegm-Heat in the Lungs with symptoms such as infections, cough with thick yellow sputum or with blood in the sputum, and a stifling sensation in the chest; 2. For Heat in the Stomach with vomiting, bad breath, and a yellow, greasy tongue coating; 3. For bleeding of the nose and vomiting blood.

Contraindications: This herb should not be used in cases of Spleen Deficiency or cough caused by Cold.

Dosage: 4.5 - 9 grams

Notes: Bamboo is revered and widely depicted in Chinese Taoist paintings because it symbolizes the essence of spontaneity, simplicity, beauty and usefulness. The Black Bamboo is favored because of the correspondence of the color to the Water Element and the Kidneys as source Qi.

Pumice   **Fu Hai Shi**   (3)

Common Name: Pumice

Part Used: The powdered stone

Energy and Flavor: salty and Cold

Organ Meridians Affected: Lung

Actions: 1. Clears Heat and expels Phlegm from the Lungs; 2. Softens lumps and hardenings associated with Phlegm-Fire and the lymph; 3. Increases urine output and clears Heat in the urinary tract.

Indications: 1. For Heat in the Lung with difficult to expectorate sputum that is either yellow or blood streaked; 2. For scrofula and goiter and other conditions that are related to Phlegm-Fire; 3. For urinary tract infection with hot and painful urination.

Contraindications: This herb should not be used when a person has a cough and is cold and weak.

Dosage: 6 - 15 grams

Notes: For Phlegm Heat with thick, yellow phlegm combine with Trichosanthes seeds (Gua Lou Ren), Scutellaria (Huang Qin), Lonicera (Jin Yin Hua); for swollen glands or goiter combine with Scrophularia

(Xuan Shen), Forsythia (Lian Qiao), Laminaria (Kun Bu) and Sargassum (Hai Zao).

Thallus Algae (Laminaria)   Kun Bu or Hai Dai
Common Name: Kelp thallus, Kombu
Part Used: Leaves
Family: Laminariaceae
Energy and Flavor: salty and Cold
Organ Meridians Affected: Kidneys, Liver and Stomach
Actions: 1. Softens hardness, Cools Hot phlegm; 2. Encourages urination and lessens edema.
Indications: 1. For swollen lymph glands, inflammation of the lymph glands, goiter; 2. For edema.
Contraindications: This herb should not be used by those with Coldness due to Spleen and Stomach Deficiency.
Dosage: 9 - 15 grams

Notes: Kun Bu or Kelp contains alginic acid, laminarin, mannitol, protein, amino acid, Vit. C, iodine, potassium, calcium, cobalt and other trace minerals. It has a wide tradition of nutritional use by Western herbalists to regulate thyroid function and for weight reduction. This is probably due at least in part to its naturally high iodine content. Chinese herbalists often combine it with Sargassum (Hai Zao) for treating goiter, swollen and inflamed lymph glands and to soften hard nodules and tumors for the treatment of cancer. Laminaria (Kun Bu) is also useful for binding with toxins to help their excretion from the body.

Sargassii Pallidum   Hai Zao   (2)
Common Name: Sargassum, Seaweed
Part Used: Aerial portion (Herba)
Family: Sargassum
Energy and Flavor: bitter, salty and Cold
Organ Meridians Affected: Lung, Kidney, Liver, Spleen and Stomach
Actions: 1. Clears Heat and reduces hardening associated with Phlegm-Fire; 2. Encourages urination and lessens edema; 3. Expels phlegm from the lungs.
Indications: 1. For Phlegm-Fire with symptoms of goiter, scrofula and tuberculosis of the lymph nodes; 2. This herb can be used in combination with other herbs for edema; 3. For phlegm in the lungs due to chronic bronchitis or other similar chronic conditions.

Contraindications: This herb should not be used by those with Coldness due to Spleen and Stomach Deficiency.

Dosage: 6 - 15 grams

Notes: Often combined with Laminaria to soften and dissipate swollen glands (especially of the thyroid) and tumors.

Discrimination:

Fritillaria Cirrhosa (Chuan Bei Mu) – Yin Deficiency, Hot Phlegm, reduces lumps and swollen glands.

Fritillaria Thunbergii (Zhe Bei Mu) – clears yellow Phlegm caused by Heat, reduces goiter.

Peucedani (Qian Hu) – Lowers Lung Qi, treats either External Cold or Hot conditions.

Trichosanthes Fructus (Gua Lou) – regulates Lung Qi, relieves constriction in the chest.

Trichosanthes Semen (Gua Lou Ren) – Cools and nourishes the Lungs, moistens the Intestines.

Trichosanthes Radix (Tian Hua Fen) – clears Phlegm and Lung Heat, reduces inflammation and pus.

Pumice (Fu Hai Shi) – clears Hot Phlegm, softens lumps and lymphatic nodules.

Sargassii (Hai Zao) – reduces hard lumps, swelling and goiter, promotes urination, expels Phlegm.

Succus Bambusae (Zhu Li) – Hot Phlegm blocking the Heart's openings.

Bambusae in Taeniis (Zhu Ru) – clears Stomach Heat, stops vomiting, Cools Blood, stops bleeding.

WARM HERBS THAT TRANSFORM COLD PHLEGM

Pinellia Ternata   Ban Xia   (1)

Common Name: Pinellia

Part Used: Rhizome (Rhizoma)

Family: Araceae

Energy and Flavor: Warm, acrid and toxic

Organ Meridians Affected: Lung, Spleen and Stomach

Actions: 1. Drains Dampness and reduces Phlegm; 2. Reverses the flow of Rebellious Qi; 3. Reduces hardenings and relieves distention.

Indications: 1. For cough with abundant Phlegm, especially when associated with Dampness in the Spleen; 2. For most kinds of Rebellious Qi, especially where there is Dampness involved such as vomiting, nausea and morning sickness; 3. For focal distention of the chest or abdomen, lumps, globus hystericus or any Stagnation caused by Phlegm in the body.

Contraindications: This herb should not be used by pregnant women or those with any blood disorders, especially bleeding. It should be used with caution by those with Heat and Dryness. This herb should not be used with Aconite (Fu Zi).

Dosage: 3 - 12 grams

Notes: Because the raw unprocessed herb is toxic, it is only reserved for external use to soften hard swollen lumps, disperse nodules, reduce swelling and stop pain. There is no danger of toxicity when using it externally. Internally, the herb is available in its processed form which is fried with Ginger juice (Sheng Jiang) and Alumen (Bai Fan), sometimes with the addition of Licorice (Gan Cao) and Gleditschiae (Zao Jiao). It is best to use only Ginger-treated Pinellia since long term use of Alumen can have a mildly cumulative toxicity.

Pinellia is one of the strongest antitussives and can be used for either Hot or Cold type coughs with phlegm. It dries Spleen Dampness, stops post-nasal drip and excessive saliva. Having a downward energy, it is frequently combined with Ginger (Gan Jiang) to resolve phlegm, counteract nausea and vomiting. It is most commonly used in Citrus and Pinellia Combination (Er Chen Tang).

Inula Japonica   Xuan Fu Hua   (3)

Common Name: Elecampane Flower

Part Used: Flower (Flos)

Family: Compositae

Energy and Flavor: acrid, bitter and Warm

Organ Meridians Affected: Lung, Spleen, Stomach, Liver, and Large Intestine

Actions: 1. Moves Stagnant Phlegm in the Lungs; 2. Reverses the flow of Rebellious Qi of the Lungs and Stomach.

Indications: 1. For Stagnation of Phlegm in the Lungs with symptoms such as wheezing, bronchitis with excessive Phlegm; 2. For belching and vomiting due to Cold and/or Damp of the Stomach and Spleen or excessive coughing or wheezing.

Contraindications: This herb should be avoided by those with tuberculosis or cough due to Wind-Heat or Deficiency.

Dosage: 3 - 9 grams

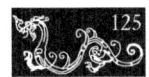

Notes: Elecampane has been used for centuries in the West for chronic coughs and digestive weakness. Western herbalists almost exclusively use the root while the Chinese primarily specify the flower. In any case they are both similarly used for chronic Cold Phlegm disorders, except the root probably has more Qi tonic properties. Interestingly, it contains quercetin and isoquercetin which are used as a natural supplement for upper respiratory allergies.

For asthma and cough with abundant phlegm, combine with Pinellia (Ban Xia) and Asarum (Xi Xin). To Lower the Qi and stop vomiting, combine with Hematite (Dai Zhe Shi).

Arisaema Consanguineum (Arisaematis)   Tian Nan Xing   (2)
Common Name: Jack In The Pulpit
Part Used: Rhizome (Rhizoma)
Family: Araceae
Energy and Flavor: bitter, acrid, Warm and toxic
Organ Meridians Affected: Lung, Liver and Spleen

Actions: 1. Dries and expels Phlegm in the Lung; 2. Clears Wind and Phlegm in the channels and stops convulsions and spasms; 3. Used topically it reduces inflammation and pain.

Indications: 1. For cough and stifling sensation in the chest with excessive Phlegm; 2. For Phlegm and Wind in the channels with symptoms of high fever, convulsions, paralysis, stroke and lockjaw; 3. For topical application on abscesses, traumatic injuries and tumors.

Contraindications: This herb should not be used during pregnancy or by those with Yin Deficient cough with Dry Phlegm.

Dosage: 4 - 9 grams

Notes: Jack in the Pulpit (A. triphyllum, A. dracontium, A. maculatum) naturally occurs in the Southeastern forests of North America. Like the Chinese species, it is also considered toxic in its raw, untreated form. Called "Indian turnip", dried and roasted, the Native Americans ate it as a food. A. triphyllum was official in the USP, 1820-73, and contains a volatile acrid principle, probably an alkaloid, mucilage and calcium oxalate. Chinese Arisaema is regarded as even stronger and more toxic than Pinellia (Ban Xia). Both the North American and the Chinese species are classified stimulant, expectorant, irritant and diaphoretic. Because of toxicity, untreated Arisaema (Tian Nan Xing) is practically never sold but is usually available in the Ginger treated version (Zhi Nan Xing). For Damp, Cold phlegm combine with Pinellia (Ban Xia), Citrus peel (Chen Pi) and Immature Bitter Orange (Zhi Shi).

Platycodum Grandiflorum   Jie Geng   (1)
Common Name: Platycodon, Balloon Flower Root
Part Used: Root (Radix)
Family: Campanulaceae
Energy and Flavor: acrid, bitter and neutral
Organ Meridians Affected: Lung

Actions: 1. Opens the Lungs and smoothes the flow of Lung Qi; 2. Expels Phlegm and pus from the Lungs and throat, can be used for either Wind-Cold or Wind-Heat according to the other herbs in the formula; 3. Directs the actions of other herbs to the Upper Warmer.

Indications: 1. For cough associated with infection in the respiratory tract and abundant Phlegm; 2. For Phlegm and pus associated with infections such as abscesses in the Lung and throat; 3. Can be used, even when there is not a direct call for the herb, to direct the action of the formula to the Upper Warmer.

Contraindications: This herb should not be used if there is blood in the expectoration and so is often not appropriate for tuberculosis.

Dosage: 3 - 9 grams

Notes: Platycodon or Balloon Flower is commonly available in garden stores as an ornamental. Having a neutral energy, it can be used for either Hot or Cold conditions depending on the other herbs with which it is combined. For Wind-Cold cough combine with Apricot seed (Xing Ren), Perilla leaf (Zi Su Ye) and Citrus peel (Chen Pi); for Wind-Heat cough combine with Mulberry leaf (Sang Ye), Apricot seed (Xing Ren) and Trichosanthes fruit (Gua Lou); for sore throat and hoarse voice combine with Scrophularia (Xuan Shen), Licorice (Gan Cao) and Arctium fruit (Niu Bang Zi). For toxic Heat in the Lungs combine with Houttuynia (Yu Xing Cao), Trichosanthes seeds (Gua Lou Ren) and fruit (Gua Lou).

Adenophora trachelioidis or "sweet" Jie Geng is Cold and used to lubricate the Lungs, clear Heat and relieve Fire toxicity. The species described here is known as "Bitter" Jie Geng and is the one most commonly used.

Typhonium Giganteum   Bai Fu Zi   (3)
Common Name: Typhonium
Part Used: Rhizome (Rhizoma)
Family: Araceae
Energy and flavors: acrid, sweet, Warm, toxic
Organ Meridians Affected: Liver, Spleen, Stomach

Actions: 1. Dries Dampness, transforms Phlegm; 2. Dispels Wind and relieves spasms; 3. Disperses hard lumps and nodules; 4. Detoxifies.

Indications: 1. For Wind and Dampness that especially affects the facial nerves, as in Wind-Stroke, Bell's palsy, facial paralysis, hemiplegia or migraine headaches; 2. Epilepsy and tetanus; 3. Swollen glands; 4. Snake and other venomous bites and stings.

Contraindications: Not for pregnant women.

Dosage: 1.5 to 6 grams

Notes: For Wind-Phlegm with convulsions combine with Arisaematis (Tian Nan Xing), Pinellia (Ban Xia) and Gastrodia (Tian Ma); for facial paralysis combine with Bombyx batryticatus (Jiang Can) and Buthus martensi (Quan Xie).

Discrimination:

All herbs transform Cold Phlegm as well as:

Pinellia (Ban Xia) — drains Dampness from the Stomach and Spleen, reduces Phlegm, stops cough, regulates Qi.

Inulae (Xuan Fu Hua) — expectorates Phlegm from the Lungs, lowers Lung and Stomach Qi.

Arisaematis (Tian Nan Xing) — dries Lung Phlegm, antispasmodic, topically reduces pain.

Platycodum (Jie Geng) — opens the Lungs, treats both Hot or Cold symptoms, reduces pus.

Typhonium Giganteum (Bai Fu Zi) — dispels Wind, relieves spasms, especially of the face, resolves swollen glands, detoxifies poisonous bites.

HERBS THAT RELIEVE COUGHING AND WHEEZING

Prunus Armeniaca   Xing Ren   (1)

Common Name: Apricot seed

Part Used: Seed (Semen)

Family: Rosaceae

Energy and Flavor: bitter, slightly Warm, slightly toxic

Organ Meridians Affected: Lung and Large Intestine

Actions: 1. Stops cough and wheezing caused by either Heat or Cold; 2. Lubricates the Intestines and relieves constipation.

Indications: 1. For cough, asthma and either chronic or acute bronchitis; it is especially good for Dry cough; 2. Can be used for constipation.

Contraindications: This herb should be used with caution when there is Yin Deficiency and with infants. It should not be used when there is diarrhea.

Dosage: 3 - 9 grams

Notes: Apricot seed, Loquat leaf and Western Wild Cherry bark all contain hydrocyanic glycosides which can be toxic in large dosage, but in smaller doses they mildly inhibit the cough reflex. Of the three, Apricot has the most tonic properties so that it is favored by the Chinese in most formulas. For Dry cough caused by External Wind-Heat, combine with Mulberry leaves (Sang Ye) and Chrysanthemum flowers (Ju Hua); for Dry cough caused by Wind-Cold combine with Perilla leaves (Zi Su Ye); for cough and asthma caused by Lung Heat combine with Gypsum (Shi Gao), Ephedra (Ma Huang) and Licorice (Gan Cao) in the formula called Ephedra, Apricot and Gypsum Combination (Ma Xing Shi Gan Tang); for constipation caused by Dryness of the Intestines combine with Angelica sinensis (Dang Gui) and Cannabis seeds (Huo Ma Ren). A basic combination to stop cough and dissolve phlegm is with Fritillary (Chuan Bei Mu).

Tussilago Farfarae   **Kuan Dong Hua** (3)

Common Name: Coltsfoot Flower

Part Used: Flower (Flos)

Family: Compositae

Energy and Flavor: acrid and Warm

Organ Meridians Affected: Lung

Actions: 1. Redirects Rebellious Lung Qi and stops coughing.

Indications: 1. For cough with abundant Phlegm caused by a Cold condition, also used for expectoration of blood in the Phlegm.

Contraindications: This herb should not be used for conditions that are of a Hot nature.

Dosage: 3 - 9 grams

Notes: Coltsfoot is an ancient cough remedy used for centuries throughout the world. Western herbalists use the leaves while Chinese herbalism employ the flowers that bloom just before winter. It is excellent for most types of coughs, including whooping coughs, except those that are caused by Yin Deficiency. For cough, combine with Aster Root (Zi Wan).

Asteris Tatarici   **Zi Wan**

Common Name: Aster root

Part Used: root

Family: Compositae

Energy and Flavor: bitter, sweet, slightly Warm

Organ Meridians Affected: Lungs

Actions: Relieves phlegm and stops cough

Indications: For Cold induced cough with copious phlegm or with blood streaked sputum.

Contraindications: Avoid or use cautiously for Yin Deficiency, long term use is not recommended.

Dosage: 3 - 9 grams

Notes: Aster has both expectorant and antibiotic properties against *Shigella sonnei, E. coli, Vibrio proteus,* and *Pseudomonas aeruginosa*. For cough with excessive sputum combine with Schizonepeta (Jing Jie) and Tussilago (Kuan Dong Hua).

Eriobotrya Japonica   Pi Pa Ye   (1)

Common Name: Loquat Leaf

Part Used: Foliage (Folium)

Family: Rosaceae

Energy and Flavor: bitter and Cool

Organ Meridians Affected: Lung and Stomach

Actions: 1. Expels Hot Phlegm in the Lungs and redirects Rebellious Lung Qi; 2. Cools Stomach Heat and redirects Rebellious Stomach Qi.

Indications: 1. For cough associated with Wind-Heat, also for acute and chronic bronchitis; 2. For Stomach Heat with symptoms of nausea, vomiting and belching.

Contraindications: This herb should not be used for cases where there is Cold.

Dosage: 6 - 15 grams

Notes: The Loquat tree is easily grown in many parts of the world. For Lung Heat it can be combined with Mulberry leaf (Sang Ye) and Platycodon (Jie Geng); for nausea and vomiting it can be combined with Bamboo shavings (Zhu Ru) and Phragmites (Lu Gen). As an expectorant it is very mild and probably not very effective as a primary herb for asthma and emphysema.

Perilla Frutescens   Zi Su Zi   (1)

Common Name: Perilla seed

Part Used: Fruit (Fructus)

Family: Labiatae

Energy and Flavor: acrid and Warm

Organ Meridians Affected: Lung and Large Intestine

Actions: 1. Stops coughing and wheezing, expels Phlegm and redirects Rebellious Lung Qi; 2. Lubricates the Intestines.

Indications: 1. For both acute and chronic respiratory conditions such as asthma and emphysema associated with copious thin white sputum and a full, stifling feeling in the chest; 2. For constipation due to Dryness in the Intestines.

Contraindications: This herb should not be used when there is diarrhea.

Dosage: 3 - 9 grams

Notes: For asthma with excessive phlegm, combine with Pinellia (Ban Xia), Ephedra (Ma Huang) and Apricot seed (Xing Ren); for constipation caused by Dry Intestines combine with Trichosanthes seed (Gua Lou Ren) and Cannabis seed (Huo Ma Ren).

Stemona Sessifolia (Stemonae)   Bai Bu   (3)

Common Name: Stemona Root

Part Used: Root (Radix)

Family: Stemonaceae

Energy and Flavor: sweet, bitter, acrid and slightly Warm

Organ Meridians Affected: Lung

Actions: 1. Lubricates the Lungs and stops cough; 2. Kills parasites externally.

Indications: 1. For both acute and chronic cough, especially good for cough due to Deficiency, bronchitis and tuberculosis; 2. For lice and fleas used either as a tincture or a decoction, can also be used as an enema for pinworms.

Contraindications: This herb should not be used when there is Spleen and Stomach Deficiency with diarrhea.

Dosage: 3 - 9 grams

Notes: For Lung Deficiency with Dryness combine with American Ginseng (Xi Yang Shen), Ophiopogon (Mai Men Dong), Unprepared Rehmannia (Sheng Di Huang); for pinworms, use a decoction as an enema; for lice, topically apply either a 20% alcoholic extract or a strong decoction. The herb can also be used as a wash to treat fleas on animals.

Aristolochia Debilis (Aristolochia)   Ma Dou Ling   (3)

Common Name: Aristolochia Fruit, Birthwort Fruit

Part Used: Fruit (Fructus)

Family: Aristolochiaceae

Energy and Flavor: bitter, slightly acrid and Cold

Organ Meridians Affected: Lung and Large Intestine

Actions: 1. Opens the Lungs and transforms Phlegm; 2. Clears Heat in the Lungs, with cough caused by Heat or Deficiency; 3. Lowers blood pressure for hypertension.

Indications: 1. For coughing and wheezing with excessive phlegm, also for asthmatic conditions that present with abundant phlegm; 2. For conditions of Heat in the Lungs with yellow phlegm; 3. For symptoms of Liver Yang rising causing high blood pressure with hypertension.

Contraindications: This herb should not be used in cases of Spleen Deficiency with diarrhea or conditions of Cold and Deficiency with cough and wheezing.

Dosage: 3 - 9 grams

Notes: For Lung Heat asthma with yellow sputum, combine with Loquat leaf (Pi Pa Ye), Peucedanum (Qian Hu) and Scutellaria (Huang Qin); for Lung Deficiency with Dryness, combine with Ophiopogon (Mai Men Dong), Aster root (Zi Wan) and Donkey Skin Gelatin (E Jiao).

Discrimination:

Prunus Armeniaca (Xing Ren) — treats either Hot or Cold coughs and wheezing, lubricates the Intestines.

Tussilago Farfarae (Kuan Dong Hua) — moves Lung Qi down, treats blood in the sputum, treats Dry cough.

Aster Tartaricus (Zi Wan) — dries and expels Cold phlegm.

Eriobotrya Japonica (Pi Pa Ye) — expels Hot Phlegm, moves Lung and Stomach Qi down, Cools Stomach Heat.

Perilla Frutescens (Zi Su Zi) — stops cough and wheezing, moves Lung Qi down, lubricates the Intestines.

Stemona (Bai Bu) — lubricates Dry cough, treats internal or external parasites.

Aristolochia (Ma Dou Ling) — opens the Lungs, removes phlegm and reduces inflammation.

AROMATIC HERBS THAT TRANSFORM DAMPNESS

This category of herbs resolves Cold Damp Stagnation especially as it affects the Stomach and Spleen. Because of their having carminative (Qi regulating) and Food dispersing properties, they are all spicy and either Warm or Hot in nature. Dampness does not represent as congested a state as Phlegm.

Agastache Rugosa Huo Xiang (1)
(Agastaches seu Pogostemi)

Common Name: Agastache; Patchouli
Part Used: Aerial portion (Herba)
Family: Labiatae
Energy and Flavor: acrid and slightly Warm
Organ Meridians Affected: Lung, Spleen and Stomach

Actions: 1. Transforms Dampness that is obstructing the Stomach and Spleen; 2. Harmonizes the Middle Warmer, for nausea and vomiting; 3. Relieves the Exterior for invasion of Cold and Damp.

Indications: 1. For Dampness obstructing the Spleen and Stomach with symptoms such as distended chest and abdomen, lack of appetite, nausea, vomiting and a white and wet tongue coating; 2. For nausea and vomiting associated with Dampness in the Middle Warmer, can also be used for morning sickness; 3. For Externally contracted Wind-Cold with signs of Dampness with symptoms such as stomach ache, nausea and distention in the abdominal region.

Contraindications: This herb should not be used for conditions of Yin Deficiency or Heat.

Dosage: 3 - 9 grams

Notes: To Cool Heat and dissolve Phlegm, combine with Eupatorium fortunei (Pei Lan). For injury caused by overeating cold, raw food as well as invasion of External Wind and Cold in summer with chills, fever, headache, nausea, vomiting and diarrhea combine with Perilla leaf (Zi Su Ye), Pinellia (Ban Xia), Magnolia bark (Hou Po), Citrus peel (Chen Pi) in Huo Xiang Zheng Qi San formula. For morning sickness, combine with Cardamon (Sha Ren) and Fresh Ginger (Sheng Jiang); for vomiting caused by turbid Dampness of the Spleen and Stomach combine with Pinellia (Ban Xia) and Fresh Ginger (Sheng Jiang); for vomiting caused by Damp Heat of the Spleen and Stomach, combine with Coptis (Huang Lian) and Bamboo shavings (Zhu Ru); for vomiting caused by Spleen and Stomach Deficiency combine with Codonopsis (Dang Shen) and Licorice (Gan Cao).

Eupatorium Fortunei   Pei Lan (3)
Common Name: Eupatorium
Part Used: The aerial portions
Family: Compositae
Energy and Flavor: acrid and neutral
Organ Meridians Affected: Spleen, Stomach

Actions: 1. Transforms Dampness that obstructs the Stomach (Middle Warmer), 2. Relieves Summer Heat.

Indications: 1. For Damp conditions with symptoms of chest fullness, lack of appetite, nausea and vomiting with the tongue presenting a white, moist coat. 2. Being neutral, it can also be used for Damp Heat of the Spleen with bad breath, sweet, sticky mouth taste and excessive saliva. 3. For External Summer Heat conditions with Dampness and nausea.

Contraindications: Even though the neutral energy of this herb will also not lead to Dryness it should not be used with Yin Deficiency.

Dosage: 4 - 9 grams

Notes: For Dampness obstructing the Middle Warmer with abdominal and chest fullness and lack of appetite, combine with Amomum (Bai Dou Kou); for indigestion caused by Heat or overindulgence in greasy foods with acid indigestion, combine with Coptis (Huang Lian); for Summer Heat with Dampness combine with Agastache (Huo Xiang) and Artemisia annua (Qing Hao).

Magnolia Officinalis   Hou Po   (1)

Common Name: Magnolia Bark

Part Used: Bark (Cortex)

Family: Magnoliaceae

Energy and Flavor: acrid, bitter, aromatic and Warm

Organ Meridians Affected: Spleen, Lung, Stomach and Large Intestine

Actions: 1. Moves Rebellious Qi downward, dries Dampness and relieves Food Stagnation. 2. Transforms Phlegm and redirects Rebellious Qi of the Lung.

Indications: 1. For Damp conditions with symptoms of nausea, vomiting, abdominal distention, loss of appetite and diarrhea; 2. For cough, wheezing and asthma due to abundant Phlegm obstructing the Lungs; also for the condition called peach-pit or plum-pit throat, where it feels as if there is something lodged in the throat.

Contraindications: This herb should not be used by pregnant women or by those with Stomach or Spleen Deficiency.

Dosage: 3 - 9 grams

Notes: Magnolia bark gently stimulates intestinal peristalsis and can be used for Damp Stagnation that is associated with either constipation or diarrhea. It is antimicrobial against *Streptococcus pneumoniae, hemolytic Streptococcus, Shigella sonnei, Staphylococcus aureus* but in this regard considerably weaker than berberine compounds such as Coptis (Huang Lian). For acid regurgitation with Stagnation of Food combine with Black Atractylodes (Cang Zhu) and Citrus peel (Chen Pi) in Magnolia and Ginger combination (Ping Wei San Formula); for cough and asthma combine with Apricot seed (Xing Ren); for constipation with abdominal

discomfort combine with Rhubarb (Da Huang) and Immature Bitter Orange (Zhi Shi). Magnolia is very effective with herbs such as Coptis (Huang Lian), Pulsatilla (Bai Tou Weng), Rhubarb (Da Huang), Fresh Ginger (Sheng Jiang) and Citrus (Chen Pi) for dysentery.

Atractylodes Lancea   Cang Zhu   (1)
Common Name: Black Atractylodes
Part Used: Rhizome (Rhizoma)
Family: Compositae
Energy and Flavor: aromatic, bitter, acrid and Warm
Organ Meridians Affected: Spleen and Stomach
Actions: 1. Dries Damp and tonifies the Spleen; 2. Relieves the Exterior for invasion of Wind-Cold-Damp; 3. Relieves Wind-Damp painful obstruction; 4. Dries Damp for either Damp-Cold or Damp-Heat when combined with the correct herbs; 5. Clears the eyes and improves sight.

Indications: 1. For weakness in the Spleen and Stomach with Damp obstructing the function of the Organ system of Earth with symptoms of loss of appetite, diarrhea, nausea and vomiting with a thick greasy tongue coating; 2. Releases the Exterior for conditions where Damp is prevalent with symptoms such as body aches, distention and pain in the abdomen, nausea, headache and absence of sweating; 3. For painful obstruction where Damp is prevalent with symptoms of swollen and painful joints; can be used for either Hot or Cold conditions when combined with the correct herbs; 4. For conditions of Dampness with symptoms such as body aches, vaginal discharge, Phlegm and localized fluid retention; 5. For poor night vision or loss of vision.

Contraindications: This herb should not be used by those with Qi Deficiency or Yin Deficiency with Heat.

Dosage: 3 - 9 grams

Notes: This is a strong Drying herb for Spleen and Stomach Dampness. It has no significant diuretic properties but increases the excretion of urinary salts. For certain kinds of diabetes mellitus, it can have a dramatic effect in lowering blood sugar. For Spleen and Stomach Dampness with bloating, poor appetite, nausea or vomiting combine with Magnolia bark (Hou Po) and Citrus peel (Chen Pi) in Magnolia and Ginger combination (Ping Wei San); For Wind-Damp-Cold obstruction of the lower back and limbs combine with Chaenomeles (Mu Gua), Loranthes (Sang Ji Sheng) and Angelica Du Huo (Du Huo); for Exterior invasion of Wind-Damp-Cold combine with Ledebouriella (Fang Feng) and Asarum (Xi Xin); for pain of the lower limbs caused by Damp Heat combine with Phellodendron (Huang Bai) and Achyranthes (Niu Xi).

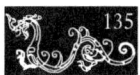

Amomum Villosum   Sha Ren   (1)
also Cardamon cluster (Bai Dou Kou)
(A. Kravanh)
Common Name: Cardamon
Part Used: Fruit (Fructus)
Family: Zingiberaceae
Energy and Flavor: acrid, Warm and aromatic
Organ Meridians Affected: Spleen, Stomach, Kidney, Lung

Actions: 1. Warms the Spleen and transforms Dampness; 2. Promotes the movement of Qi for Damp and Stagnant conditions of the Stomach and Spleen; 3. Settles a restless fetus and stops morning sickness; 4. Prevents cloying and Stagnation sometimes caused by tonifying herbs.

Indications: 1. For Damp conditions of the Spleen with symptoms such as nausea, distention and pain in the abdominal region and diarrhea; 2. For Damp Stagnant conditions with symptoms such as loss of appetite, pain in the abdomen, diarrhea and nausea; 3. For threatened abortion, restless fetus and morning sickness; 4. Used with tonifying herbs to prevent cloying and Stagnation.

Contraindications: This herb should not be used by those with Yin Deficiency when there are Heat signs.

Dosage: 2 - 5 grams

Notes: There are two main types of Cardamon used in Chinese herbalism: the seeds (Sha Ren) and the fruit cluster containing the seeds (Bai Dou Kou). They both have very similar properties for the treatment of bloating, nausea, vomiting and diarrhea and are used singly or interchangeably. However, the seeds (Sha Ren) are better for the Middle and Lower Warmer (Stomach and Intestines) while the fruit cluster (Bai Dou Kou) are more for the Middle and Upper Warmer with symptoms of nausea and vomiting. For bloating, nausea and vomiting caused by blocked Qi of the Spleen and Stomach combine both types of Cardamon together with Magnolia bark (Hou Po) and Citrus peel (Chen Pi); for infantile vomiting combine the two with Licorice (Gan Cao); for vomiting caused by Coldness of the Spleen and Stomach combine either type with Agastache (Huo Xiang), Pinellia (Ban Xia) and Ginger (Gan Jiang); for Excess Damp Heat with lack of appetite, chest fullness and greasy, sticky tongue coat, combine Sha Ren with Talc (Hua Shi) and Coix (Yi Yi Ren); for Excess Heat combine Bai Dou Kou with Scutellaria (Huang Qin), Coptis (Huang Lian) and Talc (Hua Shi).

As with all seeds, the pods and/or seeds should be crushed before using.

Discrimination:

Agastache Rugosa (Huo Xiang) – relieves Dampness in the Middle Warmer, stops nausea and vomiting.

Magnolia Officinalis Bark (Hou Po) – regulates Qi downward, relieves Food Stagnation, transforms Phlegm.

Atractylodes Lancea (Cang Zhu) – dries Damp, treats Wind-Cold-Damp (rheumatic) conditions.

Amomum Kravanh (Sha Ren and Bai Dou Kou) – Warms and dries the Spleen and Stomach, removes digestive Stagnation, calms the fetus.

HERBS THAT RELIEVE FOOD STAGNATION

Herbs that relieve Food Stagnation share some common qualities and attributes with Aromatic Herbs for Transforming Dampness and Herbs to Relieve Qi Stagnation. The major difference is that Food Stagnation necessitates the use of specific herbs that possess digestive and Food moving properties as they relate to the Stomach and Spleen. To facilitate this, some of these herbs are high in digestive enzymes, and have varying specific abilities to promote the digestion of fats, carbohydrates and proteins.

Crataegus Pinnatifida   Shan Zha   (1)

Common Name: Hawthorn Berry, Crataegus

Part Used: Fruit (Fructus)

Family: Rosaceae

Energy and Flavor: sour, sweet and slightly Warm

Organ Meridians Affected: Heart, Liver, Spleen and Stomach

Actions: 1. Improves digestion and reduces Food Stagnation; 2. Invigorates the Blood and breaks Stasis; 3. Treats hypertension and heart disease.

Indications: 1. For digestive conditions caused by Stagnation of fatty and greasy foods with symptoms of abdominal distention especially after eating, loss of appetite, nausea, digestive pains and diarrhea; 2. For pain due to Blood Stasis with symptoms such as amenorrhea, postpartum abdominal pain, retention of placenta; also used for hernial disorders; 3. Used in Western herbalism and more recently by Chinese herbalists for the treatment of hypertension and coronary heart disease.

Contraindications: This herb should be avoided by those with Spleen and Stomach Deficiency.

Dosage: 9 - 15 grams

Notes: Hawthorn berries are traditionally used in Chinese herbalism to help digest protein and fats. Following the Five Elements cycle, sour is the flavor of the Wood element and sweet of the Earth element. Protein, especially meat protein, and fat are classified as sweet so that the sour flavor of substances such as hawthorn, lemons and vinegar are considered an antidote for oily and fatty foods (i.e. lemon or vinegar and oil dressing for vegetables). Hawthorn is also made into a confection with sugar and given to young children to stimulate their appetite and aid digestion.

Western herbalists use this as a primary herb for the heart. It has the ability to increase the uptake of oxygen by the heart, increase enzyme metabolism in the heart muscle and mildly dilate both the coronary and peripheral vessels. By so doing, it helps lower blood pressure and ease the burden on the heart.

It can generally be used to reduce cholesterol and blood lipids as well as for the treatment of cardiac weakness, angina pectoris, heart valve murmurs and an enlarged heart. It will relieve heart strain and improve coronary circulation. Western research has established that the active principles of hawthorn are in the flavonoids, and that these components are also abundantly present in the leaves and flowers of the hawthorn tree.

Hordeum Vulgaris Germinatus   Mai Ya   (2)

Common Name: Barley Sprout, Malt

Part Used: Fruit (Fructus)

Family: Gramineae

Energy and Flavor: sweet and neutral

Organ Meridians Affected: Spleen and Stomach

Actions: 1. Assists the Stomach to move Food Stagnation; 2. Strengthens the Spleen; 3. Stops the flow of mother's milk; 4. Assists in the smooth flow of Liver Qi.

Indications: 1. For accumulation of starchy foods and poorly digested milk by infants which causes poor digestion and poor appetite from Stagnation; 2. For digestive weakness with lack of appetite; 3. For mothers who wish to stop nursing, also for distended breasts; 4. For pain in the abdomen and epigastric region with a sensation of fullness, belching and loss of appetite.

Contraindications: This herb should not be used during pregnancy, by nursing mothers or those without Food Stagnation.

Dosage: 9 - 15 grams; a dose up to 60 grams can be used to stop lactation.

Notes: For Food Stagnation with bloating and no appetite, combine with Hawthorn (Shan Zha), Massa fermentata (Shen Qu) and Chicken Gizzard skin (Ji Nei Jin); for blocked lactation with breast distention make a decoction of half raw and half fried barley sprouts, about 50 grams twice daily. For severe Food Stagnation with indigestion take calcined Hordeum (Mai Ya), Massa Fermentata (Shen Qu) and Crataegus (Shan Zha).

Oryza Sativa Germinatus   Gu Ya   (2)
Common Name: Rice Sprout, Oryza
Part Used: Fruit (Fructus)
Family: Graminae
Energy and Flavor: sweet and neutral
Organ Meridians Affected: Spleen and Stomach
Actions: 1. Strengthens the Spleen and improves the appetite; 2. Harmonizes the Stomach and removes Food Stagnation.
Indications: 1. For poor appetite with digestive weakness; 2. For symptoms of Food Stagnation caused by over-eating of starchy foods.
Contraindications: Sprouted rice should not be used by nursing mothers or by those without Stagnation of Food, nor should it be used for an extended period of time.
Dosage: 9 - 15 grams
Notes: For Food Stagnation take with Medicated Leaven (Shen Qu) and Hawthorn (Shan Zha).

Massa Fermentata   Shen Qu   (1)
Common Name: Medicated Leaven
Energy and Flavor: sweet, acrid and Warm
Organ Meridians Affected: Spleen and Stomach
Actions: 1. Assists the Stomach in removing Food Stagnation; 2. Harmonizes the Earth element and improves digestion.
Indications: 1. For symptoms of Food Stagnation such as distention, fullness, loss of appetite and diarrhea; 2. For poor digestion, painful digestion and lack of appetite.
Contraindications: This product should not be used by pregnant women nor by those with Stomach Fire.
Dosage: 9 - 15 grams
Notes: This is a fermented combination of wheat flour, Artemisia annua, Xanthium, Polygonum hydropiper and other herbs. It is rich in digestive enzymes, for which it is facetiously called "Chinese yogurt". For Food

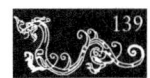

Stagnation it can be taken singly or in combination with any of the other herbs in the category. It is also good for stomach flu.

Raphanus Sativus   Lai Fu Zi   (1)

Common Name: Radish seed
Part Used: Seed (Semen)
Family: Cruciferae
Energy and Flavor: acrid, sweet and neutral
Organ Meridians Affected: Lung, Spleen and Stomach

Actions: 1. Warms the digestion and unblocks Food Stagnation; 2. Reverses Rebellious Lung Qi and transforms Phlegm.

Indications: 1. For Food Stagnation associated with Cold, with symptoms of fullness, pain, distention, belching with a rotten smell, acid regurgitation and diarrhea; 2. For chronic cough and wheezing with copious Phlegm.

Contraindications: This herb should not be used by those who are weak with Deficient Qi.

Dosage: 6 - 12 grams

Notes: For Food Stagnation, bloating, acid regurgitation combine with Hawthorn (Shan Zha) and Medicated Leaven (Shen Qu); for Cold cough with white phlegm combine with White Mustard seed (Bai Jie Zi) and Perilla seed (Zi Su Zi).

Chicken Gizzard's Skin   Ji Nei Jin   (1)

Part Used: Lining of the chicken gizzard
Family: Phasianidae
Energy and Flavor: sweet and neutral
Organ Meridians Affected: Small Intestine, Bladder, Spleen and Stomach

Actions: 1. Strongly unblocks Food Stagnation; 2. Dissolves stones in either the biliary or urinary tract.

Indications: 1. For all kinds of Food Stagnation, especially associated with Cold, improves the Spleen's transportive function; 2. For frequent and nighttime urination and bed wetting; 3. Gall stones and urinary stones; 4. For childhood malnutrition.

Contraindications: none

Dosage: It is generally taken as a powder of 1.5 to 3 grams two or three times daily (considered more effective). For treating stones, dry fry it first.

Notes: Combine with any of the herbs in this category for Food Stagnation; if there is accompanying Spleen Qi Deficiency with diarrhea add Atractylodes (Bai Zhu), Codonopsis (Dang Shen) and Dioscorea (Shan Yao); for childhood malnutrition combine with Atractylodes (Bai Zhu), Codonopsis (Dang Shen), Poria (Fu Ling) and Dioscorea (Shan

Yao); for biliary and urinary tract stones combine with Lysimachia (Jin Qian Cao).

Discrimination:
Crataegus Pinnatifida (Shan Zha) – digests fatty and greasy foods, removes Blood Stagnation.

Hordeum Vulgaris Germinatus (Mai Ya) – digests starchy foods, strengthens the Spleen, stops the flow of mother's milk.

Oryza Sativa Germinatus (Gu Ya) – digests starchy foods, stimulates appetite.

Massa Fermentata (Shen Qu) – abdominal fullness and distention, diarrhea, lack of appetite.

Raphanus Sativus (Lai Fu Zi) – Cold digestion with Stagnation, directs Lung Qi downward, resolves Phlegm.

Chicken Gizzard (Ji Nei Jin) – digestive, dissolves biliary and urinary stone, good for childhood malnutrition.

HERBS THAT REGULATE QI

One of the Five Stagnations, along with Blood, Cold, Food and Phlegm, Qi Stagnation, considered the mother of all Stagnations, especially relates to conditions associated with the Stomach, Liver, and to a lesser extent, the Lungs. Stagnation of the Stomach Qi requires herbal carminatives with a spicy flavor that promote the circulation of Qi in the Stomach.

Since the Liver is responsible for the smooth flow of Qi, Stagnant Qi of the Liver involves some impairment of the Liver's ability to store and release glycogen to help maintain a steady level of energy and the transformation of stress hormones. Stagnation of Liver Qi is frequently associated with psychological symptoms of depression and mood swings. Since these can be hormonally influenced, Stagnant Liver Qi can be associated with premenstrual syndrome (PMS), menopausal symptoms, the development of breast and lower pelvic fibroid cysts and swellings as well as inappropriate or inordinate symptoms of anger, irritability and hypertension.

Stagnant Liver Qi symptoms can coexist with digestive disorders, giving rise to a variety of food related disorders such as food allergies and other conditions of food susceptibility. These are described as Liver and Stomach Qi Stagnation or Liver attacking the Spleen conditions. Because herbs in this category tend to have spicy or bitter flavors with Drying properties, they are contraindicated or should be used cautiously for conditions of Deficient Qi, Blood or Yin.

Citri Reticulatae   **Chen Pi**   (1)

Common Name: Tangerine Peel, Citrus Peel

Part Used: Peel (Pericarpium)

Family: Rutaceae

Energy and Flavor: acrid, bitter, Warm and aromatic

Organ Meridians Affected: Spleen and Lung

Actions: 1. Warms the Spleen and regulates the Middle Burner Qi; 2. Dries Dampness and disperses Phlegm from the Lungs and Middle Burner; 3. Reduces the potential for Stagnation caused by tonifying herbs.

Indications: 1. For regulating the function of the Spleen, with symptoms of fullness and distention in the Middle Burner, bloating after eating and belching; also for Rebellious Qi of the Stomach, with symptoms of nausea and vomiting; 2. For Qi Stagnation with Phlegm or Dampness affecting either the chest or abdomen; it is especially good when both the Lungs and Spleen are involved, with symptoms of distention, stifling sensation, copious watery phlegm, loss of appetite, loose stool with a thick greasy tongue coating and a slippery Excess pulse; 3. Often used with tonifying herbs to reduce the chance of them causing Stagnation.

Contraindications: This herb should not be used when there is cough with Yin or Qi Deficiency; this could manifest as Dry cough or coughing blood. It should also be avoided when there is sticky yellow phlegm.

Dosage: 3 - 9 grams

Notes: Chinese Citrus peel is derived from the tangerine. However, tree ripened orange peels can also be used if no other type is available. They can be made into a delicious confection by candying them in sugar syrup, grinding them fresh or dried and mixed into an electuary (honey pill mass) with honey. The best quality Chen Pi is that which is aged the longest. One pharmacy proudly showed me expensive Chen Pi that was aged since the 1940's. So much for the theory that only the freshest of every herb is the best. All substances, fresh or old, have their own unique energy which can be used therapeutically, depending on the indications and needs.

For Spleen and Stomach Qi Stagnation with symptoms of bloating, belching, nausea, vomiting, poor appetite, combine withImmature Bitter Orange (Zhi Shi) and Saussurea (Mu Xiang); if there is Qi Deficiency add Atractylodes (Bai Zhu) and Codonopsis (Dang Shen); if there is nausea and vomiting add Pinellia (Ban Xia) and Fresh Ginger (Sheng Jiang). For Dampness obstructing the Spleen and Stomach combine with Black Atractylodes (Cang Zhu) and Magnolia Bark (Hou Po); for phlegm and mucus caused by Spleen Dampness combine with Pinellia

(Ban Xia), Poria (Fu Ling) and Licorice (Gan Cao) in Citrus and Pinellia Combination (Er Chen Tang).

Citri Reticulatae Viride   Qing Pi   (1)
Common Name: Green Tangerine Peel, Blue Citrus Peel
Part Used: Peel (Pericarpium)
Family: Rutaceae
Energy and Flavor: bitter, acrid and Warm
Organ Meridians Affected: Liver, Gallbladder and Stomach
Actions: 1. Smooths the flow of Liver Qi and releases Stagnation; 2. Reduces Food Stagnation; 3. Dries Damp and reduces Phlegm.
Indications: 1. For Stagnation of Liver Qi with symptoms of pain in the chest, hypochondrium and breasts; 2. For Food Stagnation with symptoms of pain and distention in the Middle Burner and a stifling sensation in the Middle Burner; 3. For conditions of Phlegm-Damp with symptoms of cirrhosis of the liver, chills, fever and sweating, in that order, and breast abscesses.
Contraindications: This herb should be used with caution by those who are weak with low energy due to Spleen Qi Deficiency.
Dosage: 3 - 9 grams

Notes: For Stagnant Liver Qi combine with Bupleurum (Chai Hu), Cyperus (Xiang Fu) and Curcuma root (Yu Jin); for abdominal pain caused by Food Stagnation combine with Massa Fermentata (Shen Qu), Hordeum Germinatus (Mai Ya) and Crataegus (Shan Zha); for hernia pains, testicular pains caused by Cold invading the Liver Channel add Lindera (Wu Yao), Fennel seeds (Xiao Hui Xiang) and Saussurea (Mu Xiang); for mastitis add Trichosanthes fruit (Gua Lou), Honeysuckle flower (Jin Yin Hua), Dandelion (Pu Gong Ying) and Forsythia (Lian Qiao).

Immaturus Citri Aurantii   Zhi Shi   (1)
Common Name: Immature Bitter Orange, Chih-Shih
Part Used: Fruit (Fructus)
Family: Rutaceae
Energy and Flavor: bitter, sour, acrid and slightly Cold
Organ Meridians Affected: Spleen, Stomach and Large Intestine
Actions: 1. Regulates the flow of Qi in the Middle Burner and reduces Food Stagnation; 2. Moves Qi downward and helps constipation; 3. Reduces Stagnant Phlegm and lessens distention and pain; 4. For prolapse of organs when used with the appropriate herbs.

Indications: 1. For pain and distention in the abdominal region, indigestion and gas; 2. For constipation caused by Stagnation of Qi; 3. For stifling sensation with fullness in the chest and epigastrium with a thick, sticky, yellow coat on the tongue caused by Phlegm; 4. For prolapse of the Stomach, rectum or uterus, only when in combination with the appropriate herbs.

Contraindications: This herb should be used with caution during pregnancy, when there is Qi Deficiency or when there is Cold in the Stomach.

Dosage: 3 - 9 grams

Notes: For Food Stagnation with bloating and foul smelling belching, combine with Hawthorn (Shan Zha), Hordeum (Mai Ya) and Massa Fermentata (Shen Qu); for Food Stagnation with constipation combine with Rhubarb (Da Huang); for dysentery with diarrhea caused by Food Stagnation and Damp Heat combine with Rhubarb (Da Huang), Coptis (Huang Lian) and Scutellaria (Huang Qin).

Areca Catechu   Da Fu Pi   (3)

Common Name: Areca Peel, Betel Husk

Part Used: Peel (Pericarpium)

Family: Palmae

Energy and Flavor: acrid and Warm

Organ Meridians Affected: Spleen, Stomach, Large and Small Intestine

Actions: 1. Assists in the downward movement of Qi and relieves Food Stagnation; 2. Removes Stagnation of Water by draining downward.

Indications: 1. For Stagnation of Food with symptoms such as regurgitation, belching, pain in the epigastric region and bloating, also when constipation is associated with these symptoms; 2. For Stagnant Water in the Intestines, Stomach and general edema with symptoms of distention in the abdominal region and edema; 3. Leg edema.

Contraindications: This herb should not be used by those who are weak with Qi Deficiency.

Dosage: 3 - 9 grams

Notes: For abdominal bloating, tendency towards difficult bowel movements with Dampness and Qi Stagnation combine with Citrus (Chen Pi) and Magnolia Bark (Hou Po).

Cyperus Rotundus   Xiang Fu   (2)

Common Name: Cyperus, Nutgrass

Part Used: Rhizome (Rhizoma)

Family: Cyperaceae

Energy and Flavor: acrid, bitter, sweet and neutral

Organ Meridians Affected: Liver, Triple Burner and Stomach

Actions: 1. Unblocks Stagnant Liver Qi and relieves pain; 2. Regulates the Liver and Spleen; 3. Assists the regulation of menses and relieves pain.

Indications: 1. For Stagnant Liver Qi causing pain and distention in the epigastic region; 2. For aggressive Liver Qi that attacks the Spleen with symptoms of abdominal distention and acid and food regurgitation; 3. For painful menstruation as well as lack of menstrual flow and irregular menstruation; 4. Breast masses, swollen breasts, especially around the time of menstruation.

Contraindications: Because of its Drying nature, this herb should not be used when there is Yin or Qi Deficiency, especially when there is Heat associated with the condition.

Dosage: 4 - 12 grams

Notes: Because of the neutral property of this herb it is very widely used. The natives of Northern California roasted the rhizomes and ate them as food, thus the popular name 'Nutgrass'. The Indians of the Peruvian Amazon use them for gynecological problems as do the Chinese. Certain Amazon tribes use Cyperus for birth control. This may be partially explained by the presence of an ergot-like fungus with oxytocic properties that seems to grow on the fine root hairs, especially in a humid jungle environment. For Liver Qi Stagnation combine with Bupleurum (Chai Hu) and Curcuma root (Yu Jin); for bloating, abdominal distention, lack of appetite, nausea, diarrhea, caused by Food and Qi Stagnation add Cardamon (Sha Ren); for dysenteric diarrhea add Coptis (Huang Lian).

Saussurea Lappa   Mu Xiang   (1)

(Aucklandia Lappa)

Common Name: Saussurea, Costus Root Auklandia

Part Used: Root (Radix)

Family: Compositae

Energy and Flavor: acrid, bitter and Warm

Organ Meridians Affected: Spleen, Liver, Lung, Gallbladder, Large Intestine and Stomach

Actions: 1. Relieves the Stagnation of Qi of the digestion in the Spleen, Stomach and Intestines; 2. Relieves Qi Stagnation of the Liver and Gallbladder; 3. Strengthens the Spleen and is used with tonifying herbs to prevent their potential cloying effects.

Indications: 1. For digestive Stagnation with symptoms of pain and distention in the abdominal region, nausea, loss of appetite and vomiting; 2. For Stagnant Qi of the Liver and Gallbladder with symptoms of flank pain and abdominal distention; 3. Is typically used with tonifying herbs to

prevent the potential cloying effect they can have on the Spleen.

Contraindications: This herb should not be used by those with Yin and Blood Deficiency.

Dosage: 3 - 9 grams

Notes: Next to Citrus peel, this is the most commonly indicated herb for Stomach and Spleen Qi Stagnation which would involve digestion. As with many of the Qi regulating herbs, its properties are closely related to its volatile oils. Therefore, it is always added during the last 5 minutes or so of decoction. For Qi Stagnation of the Spleen and Stomach combine with Amomum (Sha Ren) and Atractylodes (Bai Zhu). In most cases, when treating constipation with purgatives such as Rhubarb (Da Huang), a small amount of a Qi regulating herb such as Saussurea (Mu Xiang) or Citrus (Chen Pi) is added to prevent griping abdominal spasms. Western herbalists commonly use Ginger (Sheng Jiang) which is very effective for counterbalancing any negative reactions to Cold natured laxatives such as Rhubarb (Da Huang). It can be combined with either Warm or Cool herbs such as Coptis (Huang Lian), Green Citrus (Zhi Shi or Qing Pi), Bupleurum (Chai Hu) or Artemisia (Yin Chen Hao) when there are symptoms of Qi Stagnation.

Lindera Strychnifolia   Wu Yao   (3)

Common Name: Lindera Root

Part Used: Root (Radix)

Family: Lauraceae

Energy and Flavor: acrid and Warm

Organ Meridians Affected: Spleen, Lung, Kidney, Urinary Bladder, Stomach

Actions: 1. Warms and stimulates the flow of Qi and relieves pain; 2. Disperses Cold and Warms the Kidneys.

Indications: 1. For Stagnation of Qi caused by Cold with symptoms of pain and distention of the abdominal and epigastric region, menstrual pain and Bi Pain associated with Cold; 2. For Cold in the Kidneys with symptoms of inability to hold urine and frequent urination.

Contraindications: This herb should not be used by those with Qi Deficiency or Interior Heat.

Dosage: 3 - 9 grams

Notes: Lindera contains borneol, a camphoraceous constituent which is very penetrating and pain relieving. As an isolated chemical it is not suitable in its pure form for long term internal use. As part of the biochemistry of the plant, however, it is very useful in relieving pain. It can be combined with Saussurea (Mu Xiang) for hernia and testicular

pains; for nausea, vomiting and morning sickness it can be taken with Amomum (Sha Ren) and/or Perilla leaf (Zi Su Ye) or Fresh Ginger (Sheng Jiang); for painful menstruation combine with Angelica sinensis (Dang Gui) and Ligusticum (Chuan Xiong).

Diospyri Kaki   Shi Di   (3)

Common Name: Persimmon Calyx, Kaki Calyx

Part Used: Calyx

Family: Ebenaceae

Energy and Flavor: bitter and neutral

Organ Meridians Affected: Lung and Stomach

Actions: 1. Directs the flow of Qi downward.

Indications: 1. For upward flow of Qi of the Stomach with symptoms of hiccups and belching; because of its neutral energy can be used for both Hot or Cold conditions.

Contraindications: This herb should be used with caution by those with prolapsed organs due to Deficient Qi as it has a descending energy on the Qi.

Dosage: 3 - 9 grams

Notes: Practically exclusively used to treat hiccups, for which it can be combined with Cloves (Ding Xiang).

Aquilaria Agallocha   Chen Xiang   (3)

Common Name: Aquilaria, Aloewood

Part Used: Wood shavings (Lignum)

Family: Thymelaeaceae

Energy and Flavor: acrid, bitter, Warm and aromatic

Organ Meridians Affected: Spleen, Kidney, Lung and Stomach

Actions: 1. Assists in the flow of Qi and relieves pain; 2. Assists the Kidneys in grasping the Qi of the Lungs; 3. Directs the flow of Qi downward and dispels Cold from the Spleen and Stomach.

Indications: 1. For pain caused by Stagnation associated with Cold from Deficiency or Stagnant Blood with symptoms such as pain and distention in the abdominal region; 2. For the lack of the Kidneys' ability to grasp the Qi of the Lungs with symptoms of asthma and wheezing; 3. For Cold in the Spleen and Stomach with symptoms of vomiting, belching, hiccups and acid regurgitation.

Contraindications: This herb should not be used by those with prolapsed organs caused by Qi Deficiency or by those with Yin Deficiency with Heat signs.

Dosage: 1 - 3 grams

Notes: For Cold Qi Stagnation with symptoms of bloating and abdominal pain combine with Lindera (Wu Yao) and Saussurea (Mu Xiang); for asthma caused by Kidneys unable to receive the Qi, combine with Prepared Rehmannia (Shu Di Huang), Prepared Aconite (Fu Zi) and Cinnamon Bark (Rou Gui).

Melia Toosendan   **Chuan Lian Zi** (3)

Common Name: Chinaberry

Part Used: Fruit (Fructus)

Family: Meliaceae

Energy and Flavor: bitter, Cold, slightly toxic

Organ Meridians Affected: Liver, Spleen and Small Intestine

Actions: 1. Clears Damp Heat; 2. Circulates Qi; 3. Relieves chest, epigastric and abdominal pains; 4. Expels parasites.

Indications: Relieves epigastric, abdominal, chest or hernial pain with Damp-Heat and Stagnant Qi; 2. Kills parasites and relieves associated abdominal pains especially in combination with other herbs that are stronger to kill parasites; 3. It can be powdered and applied topically to relieve athletes' foot, scalp and body itch caused by tinea.

Toxicity: An overdose can cause nausea, vomiting, diarrhea, dyspnea and heart irregularities.

Contraindications: Not for Cold Deficiency of the Stomach and Spleen.

Dosage: 3 - 9 grams

Notes: This herb is good to add when there is Qi Stagnation associated with parasites. To regulate Qi and Blood and stop pain, combine with Corydalis (Yan Hu Suo).

Santali Albi   **Tan Xiang**   (3)

Common Name: Sandalwood

Part Used: Wood Shavings (Lignum)

Family: Santalaceae

Energy and Flavor: spicy, fragrant, Warm

Organ Meridians Affected: Spleen, Stomach, Lung and Heart

Actions: 1. Clears Stagnant Qi of the chest and abdomen.

Indications: 1. Can be used for angina and coronary artery disease; 2. For chest and abdominal pains.

Contraindications: Not for Heart Yin Deficiency.

Dosage: 1 - 6 grams

Notes: For heart angina pains, combine with Red Sage root (Dan Shen) and Corydalis (Yan Hu Suo); for chest and abdominal discomfort combine with Amomum (Sha Ren) and Lindera (Wu Yao).

Rosa Rugosa — Mei Gui Hua

Common Name: Rose flowers
Part Used: the flower
Family: Rosaceae
Energy and Flavor: sweet, slightly bitter, Warm
Organ Meridians Affected: Spleen and Liver
Actions: 1. Regulates Qi and reduces Stagnation of the chest and Liver; 2. Removes Blood Stagnation.
Indications: 1. For Liver and Spleen disharmony with Qi Stagnation of the chest and abdomen with stifling feelings in the chest, pain, epigastric distention, belching, poor appetite; 2. Moves Qi and Blood and is used for Premenstrual Syndrome with depression and menstrual irregularities; 3. Depression.
Contraindications: none
Dosage: 1 - 6 grams

Notes: Rosa Rugosa is also used in Ayurvedic Medicine for depression. A delicious spread is made by picking fresh red rose petals, chopping them as fine as possible and mixing with honey. This can also be combined with fresh tangerine or orange peel both for flavor and to add to the Qi regulating properties of the spread. This can be freely spread on bread, pancakes or crackers and eaten as often as desired.

Discrimination:

All herbs regulate Qi as well as:

Citri Reticulatae (Chen Pi) — Warms digestion, dries Dampness, disperses Phlegm, used with tonics to reduce Stagnation.

Citri Reticulatae Viride (Qing Pi) — stronger for regulating Liver Qi than Chen Pi, removes chest fullness.

Immaturus Citri Aurantii (Zhi Shi) — moves Qi downward, helps constipation.

Areca Catechu (Da Fu Pi) — moves Qi downward, treats stomach acidity and abdominal distention.

Cyperus Rotundus (Xiang Fu) — adjusts Liver and Spleen Qi, regulates menses, relieves pain.

Saussurea Lappa (Mu Xiang) — regulates digestion, treats abdominal distention, used to help digest tonic herbs.

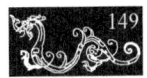

Lindera Strychnifolia (Wu Yao) – Cold Qi Stagnation, Qi pains caused by Coldness, frequent urination.

Diospyri Kaki (Shi Di) – hiccups, belching.

Aquilaria (Chen Xiang) – Cold Qi Stagnation, directs Qi downwards, helps the Lungs grasp Kidney Qi for asthma and wheezing, stomach acidity, hiccups, belching and nausea.

Melia Toosendan (Chuan Lian Zi) –clears Damp Heat, relieves parasites.

Santali Albi (Tan Xiang) – relieves Stagnant Qi of the chest and abdomen.

Rosa Rugosa (Mei Gui Hua) – relieves Stagnant Qi and Blood, can be used as a food and to relieve depression.

HERBS THAT REGULATE BLOOD

Herbs that regulate Blood are further subdivided into herbs that stop bleeding and those that invigorate blood circulation. While these may appear to be opposite properties, in general, some herbs that promote Blood circulation are amphoteric and help to stop bleeding. This is why Western herbalists have used Cayenne Pepper, taken internally and topically applied, for bleeding and hemorrhage. Hemorrhage is a localized pooling of blood which can be effectively treated by increasing blood circulation. Both Blood Stagnation and echymosis are commonly associated with hemorrhage since the blockage will cause the blood to seep out of its passageways. Tienchi ginseng (Radix Pseudoginseng) is the most representative herb that treats both internal and external injuries with associated bruising, clots and hemorrhage. It is also the most effective herb for dissolving blood clots. Another important herb that both removes clots and stops hemorrhages is cattail pollen (Pu Huang).

In cases of severe hemorrhage, hemostatic herbs and substances are indicated, followed by herbs that break up Blood Stagnation. In many cases the carbonized ash of astringent and hemostatic herbs and substances is most effective to stop bleeding. This includes the ashes of Mugwort (Ai Ye), Agrimony (Xian He Cao) and Human hair (Xue Yu Tan). Internally, 1 or 2 teaspoons of the ashes can be taken with a little water. The ashes are also effective when applied externally. Mugwort ashes, the residue of moxibustion, is saved by acupuncturists in the event that any abnormal bleeding occurs after treatment. Mugwort ashes are also very effective for diabetics with bleeding sores on their feet.

Herbs that invigorate Blood are classified as emmenagogues in Western Herbalism. In TCM they have many important uses, including to Warm and promote circulation of Blood in cardiovascular conditions or menstrual irregularities, treat sharp, acute pains caused by Blood Stagnation and break or crack Blood Stasis in the case of certain tumors, cysts and hardened clots and scar tissue.

HERBS THAT STOP BLEEDING

Typha Angustifolia (Pollen Typhae)   Pu Huang   (1)

Common Name: Cattail Pollen

Part Used: Pollen

Family: Typhaceae

Energy and Flavor: sweet and neutral

Organ Meridians Affected: Heart, Liver, Spleen and Pericardium

Actions: 1. Stops bleeding by Cooling pathogenic Heat; 2. Moves Blood and relieves Blood Stagnation.

Indications: 1. For bleeding, both by applying externally and taking as a tea internally; very good for traumatic injury and for nosebleeds, heavy or extended menstrual flow and vomiting blood; 2. For pain caused by Blood Stagnation with symptoms of chest pain, menstrual pain or delayed menstruation and pain after childbirth.

Contraindications: This herb should not be used during pregnancy.

Dosage: 5 - 10 grams

Notes: Cattails grow along stream banks and damp areas in many parts of the world. The carbonized herb is more effective to stop bleeding while the raw herb is used to relieve Stagnation and stop pain.

Agrimonia Pilosa   Xian He Cao (1)

Common Name: Agrimony

Part Used: Aerial portion (Herba)

Family: Rosaceae

Energy and Flavor: bitter and neutral

Organ Meridians Affected: Lung, Liver and Spleen

Actions: 1. Stops bleeding; 2. Stops diarrhea and helps dysentery; 3. Kills parasites.

Indications: 1. For bleeding of all kinds according to the other herbs used in the formula; 2. Helps alleviate diarrhea and other dysentery patterns; 3. For parasites such as trichomonas vaginitis, malaria and tapeworms.

Contraindications: This herb is generally very safe but should be used with caution in cases of extreme Heat or Fire symptoms.

Dosage: 6 - 15 grams; it can be used externally as a wash

Notes: To stop bleeding, the calcined ashes of the herb are most effective. For different kinds of bleeding conditions combine with Fresh

Rehmannia (Sheng Di Huang), Moutan Peony (Mu Dan Pi), Gardenia (Zhi Zi) and Mugwort (Ai Ye); for bleeding caused by Spleen Qi Deficiency combine with Ginseng (Ren Shen), Astragalus (Huang Qi) and Prepared Rehmannia (Shu Di Huang); for trichomonas (vaginal itching), make a strong decoction of 120 grams of the dried herb, soak a cotton ball and insert into the vagina overnight. In the morning douche with a combination of Agrimony and Yellow Dock decoction. In former times, Agrimony had a much wider therapeutic application than today, where it is mainly used as a hemostatic agent. It can be used to relieve pain and coalesce and strengthen the good cells of the body to resist all kinds of pathogenic influences. Agrimony flowers (He Cao Ye) taken in decoction (from 30 to 50 grams) is a specific treatment for worms, especially tapeworms. The tea should be taken in the morning, before breakfast. The tapeworm will be dislodged in 5 to 6 hours. Recent research has found it to be one of the valuable herbs for the treatment of cancer. It is used in the cancer formula called Ping Xiao Dan which contains Agrimony, Semen Strychni, Alumen, Radix Curcuma, Faeces Trogopterori, Fructus Aurantii Immaturus and Lacca Sinica Exsiccata (Shaanxi Traditional Chinese Medicine, Vol. 6, 1983).

Panax Notoginseng (Rx. Pseudoginseng) San Qi   (1)

Common Name: Tienchi ginseng, Notoginseng, Pseudoginseng

Part Used: Root (Radix)

Family: Araliaceae

Energy and Flavor: sweet, slightly bitter and Warm

Organ Meridians Affected: Liver and Stomach

Actions: 1. Stops bleeding and resolves Blood Stasis; 2. Reduces inflammation and associated pain.

Indications: 1. For bleeding, either externally caused by injury or internally for bleeding of any kind; it also breaks up Stasis that can cause symptoms such as chest pain and menstrual pain; 2. For inflammation and pain caused by injury such as sprained or broken bones as well as joint pain caused by Stagnant Blood.

Contraindications: This herb should not be used by pregnant women and should be used with caution by those with Blood Deficiency or Yin Deficiency or without Stagnation of Blood.

Dosage: 1 - 9 grams; 1 - 3 grams when taken as a powder; can be used topically

Notes: This is the quintessential herb for either internal or external hemorrhages. It stops bleeding by shortening the thrombin time. At the same time it is powerfully able to dissolve blood clots and normalize

circulation. It is a tonic that will lower blood pressure, increase coronary artery blood flow and lower cholesterol and other blood lipids.

I have used it singly in high daily dosage to dissolve dangerous life threatening blood clots with complete success, usually within a couple of weeks. Because it promotes blood circulation, it is able to relieve pain and is used with great effectiveness for Crohn's disease.

For hemorrhage or injuries it is usually used in a complex patented formulation called Yunnan Pai Yao.

Bletilla Striata   Bai Ji   (3)
Common Name: Bletilla Rhizome
Part Used: Rhizome (Rhizoma)
Family: Orchidaceae
Energy and Flavor: bitter, sweet and slightly Cold
Organ Meridians Affected: Liver, Lung and Stomach
Actions: 1. Stops bleeding in the Stomach and Lungs; 2. Reduces inflammation and aids in wound healing.
Indications: 1. For bleeding in the Stomach and Lungs such as ulcers and coughing up blood; 2. For external administration for traumatic injury with bleeding and inflammation, chronic sores that won't heal and wind/sun burned skin.
Contraindications: This herb should not be used by those who have bleeding from the Lungs or Stomach when there are true Heat signs of Excess, when there is coughing of blood with Externally contracted diseases or when there is Lung abscess. This herb should not be used with Aconite (Fu Zi or Wu Tou).
Dosage: 3 - 12 grams
Notes: for coughing or spitting of blood caused by Yin Deficiency combine with Donkey Skin Gelatin (E Jiao) and Stemonae (Bai Bu); for spitting of blood caused by Lung abscess and TB, combine with Fritillary (Chuan Bei Mu); for coughing of blood and phlegm, combine with Eriobotrya and Pinellia. Externally, powdered Bletilla can be applied as a powder or mixed with sesame oil for chapped and bleeding hands or feet.

Sanguisorba Officinalis   Di Yu   (3)
Common Name: Sanguisorba, Burnet-Bloodwort Root
Part Used: Root (Radix)
Family: Rosaceae
Energy and Flavor: bitter, sour, slightly Cold

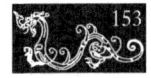

Organ Meridians Affected: Liver, Large Intestine, Stomach

Actions: 1. Reduces Heat in the Blood, drains Damp-Heat and stops bleeding; 2. Stops diarrhea; 3. Applied topically it reduces inflammation and aids in wound healing.

Indications: 1. For bleeding due to Heat in the Blood such as blood in the stool or urine, uterine bleeding, bleeding hemorrhoids and vomiting of blood; 2. For dysenteric disorders associated with diarrhea; 3. For injuries and burns as well as for sores that won't heal.

Contraindications: This herb should not be used when there is Cold or weakness, especially when there is Deficient Qi causing uterine bleeding.

Dosage: 6 - 12 grams

Notes: For uterine bleeding caused by Heat combine with Cattail Pollen (Pu Huang), Scutellaria (Huang Qin) and Unprepared Rehmannia (Sheng Di Huang); for bleeding hemorrhoids and dysentery combine with Sophora Flower (Huai Hua), Coptis (Huang Lian) and Pueraria (Ge Gen). It is broadly antimicrobial. Calcined and applied as a powder, it is most effective to stop bleeding. Dried and powdered, it can be applied topically for burns.

Biota Orientalis   Ce Bai Ye   (3)

Common Name: Biota Leaves

Part Used: Cacumen

Family: Cupressaceae

Energy and Flavor: bitter, slightly Cold, astringent

Organ Meridians Affected: Liver, Lung, Heart, Large Intestine

Actions: 1. Reduces Blood Heat and stops bleeding; 2. Cools Lung Heat, stops coughing and expels Phlegm; 3. Alleviates Wind-Damp Bi Pain; 4. Clears Heat on the skin and promotes the healing of burns.

Indications: 1. For bleeding due to Heat in the Blood with symptoms of coughing blood, bleeding gums, uterine bleeding and vomiting blood, it can also be used for bleeding with Cold symptoms when combined with the appropriate herbs; 2. For patterns of Lung Heat with blood streaked sputum and difficult to expectorate phlegm; 3. For Wind-Damp painful obstruction such as arthritis where there is Heat; 4. For burns where there is slight infection or the potential for infection, it speeds the healing of the burn.

Contraindications: This herb should not be used when there are no signs of Heat or Damp and should not be used over long periods of time.

Dosage: 6 - 12 grams

Notes: For coughing of blood, epistaxis, hematuria and uterine bleeding combine with Pollen Typhae (Pu Huang), Unprepared Rehmannia (Sheng

Di Huang), Mugwort (Ai Ye) and Lotus Node (Ou Jie); for bleeding caused by Coldness combine with Mugwort (Ai Ye), Ginger (Gan Jiang).

Artemisia Argyi   **Ai Ye** (1)
Common Name: Mugwort
Part Used: Foliage (Folium)
Family: Compositae
Energy and Flavor: bitter, acrid and Warm
Organ Meridians Affected: Liver, Spleen and Kidney
Actions: 1. Warms the channels and stops bleeding; 2. Warms the womb and calms the fetus; 3. Expels Cold and stops pain; 4. Calms cough, relieves asthma and breaks up Phlegm.
Indications: 1. For sterility, functional bleeding of the uterus and bleeding due to Cold from Deficiency causing heavy and extended menstrual bleeding; 2. For Cold in the womb causing the fetus to be restless, pain in the lower abdomen, threatened miscarriage and infertility; 3. For painful menstruation due to Cold from Deficiency; 4. For cough and asthma with Cold-Phlegm conditions.
Contraindications: This herb should not be used when there is Heat in the Blood due to Yin Deficiency and should be used with caution during pregnancy.
Dosage: 3 - 9 grams
Notes: This herb is used for moxabustion (a method of burning an herb on or near the skin to stimulate Qi and Blood circulation and relieve pain) by acupuncturists because of its blood circulating and Warm antispasmodic properties. The ashes should be saved because they are even more effective to stop bleeding than the Dry herb. The ashes can be applied to the toes and feet for non-healing sores associated with diabetes or other areas where bleeding occurs. For bleeding caused by Coldness and Blood Deficiency combine with Donkey Skin Gelatin (E Jiao) and Angelica sinensis (Dang Gui).

Crinis Carbonisatus Hominis   **Xue Yu Tan**   (2)
Common Name: Charred Human Hair
Family: Hominidae
Energy and Flavor: bitter and neutral
Organ Meridians Affected: Liver, Kidney and Heart
Actions: 1. Stops bleeding; 2. Encourages urination.
Indications: 1. For all kinds of bleeding, especially uterine bleeding and blood in the urine; 2. For painful urinary dysfunction with difficulty in urination and blood in the urine.

Contraindications: none noted

Dosage: 3 - 9 grams; the powder can be applied directly to a wound as needed.

Notes: For uterine hemorrhage combine with Angelica sinensis (Dang Gui) and Mugwort (Ai Ye).

Nelumbinis Nucifera   Ou Jie   (3)

Common Name: Lotus Rhizome Node

Part Used: Nodes (Nodus)

Family: Nymphaeaceae

Energy and Flavor: sweet, astringent and neutral

Organ Meridians Affected: Lung, Liver and Stomach

Actions: 1. Stops bleeding due to Heat in the Blood.

Indications: 1. For bleeding associated with Heat in the Blood such as extended menses, bleeding in the Lungs and Stomach and bleeding caused by both leakage and Stasis.

Contraindications: none noted

Dosage: 6 - 12 grams; the fresh juice is often used and is best in that form.

Notes: For uterine bleeding combine with Angelica sinensis (Dang Gui) and Motherwort (Yi Mu Cao).

Imperata Cylindrica   Bai Mao Gen   (2)

Common Name: Imperata, Woolly Grass, White Grass

Part Used: Rhizome (Rhizoma)

Family: Gramineae

Energy and Flavor: sweet and Cold

Organ Meridians Affected: Lung, Stomach and Urinary Bladder

Actions: 1. Stops bleeding due to Heat in the Blood; 2. Drains Heat and encourages urination; 3. Relieves Heat in the Stomach and Lungs.

Indications: 1. For bleeding associated with Heat in the Blood such as coughing, vomiting and urination of blood; 2. For patterns of Heat with symptoms such as Hot and painful urination with or without blood and edema; 3. For Heat in the Stomach and Lung with symptoms of thirst, nausea and wheezing.

Contraindications: This herb should not be used where there is Cold associated with Spleen Deficiency.

Dosage: 10 - 30 grams, more is often used when it is used by itself or if used fresh.

Notes: For hemorrhages caused by Blood Heat combine with Biota tops (Ce Bai Ye) and Unprepared Rehmannia (Sheng Di Huang); for blood

in the urine caused by Damp Heat, combine with Plantain seed (Che Qian Zi) and Lysimachia (Jin Qian Cao).

Rubia Cordifolia (Rubiae)   Qian Cao Gen (3)
Common Name: Madder root
Part Used: Root (Radix)
Family: Rubiaceae
Energy and Flavor: Cool, bitter and astringent
Organ Meridians Affected: Heart, Liver, Lung
Actions: 1. Cools Blood, stops bleeding; 2. Regulates Blood, disperses Blood Stagnation; 3. Stops coughs and expectorates phlegm.
Indications: 1. For conditions of bleeding with Blood Stagnation; 2. Bleeding from the Lungs, coughing blood.
Contraindications: Not for associated Cold conditions of the Stomach and Spleen.
Dosage: 6 to 12 grams

Notes: Different species of Madder root contain various pigments used for dyeing. A red dye is produced as a result of the presence of alizarin. Other colors from different species are purpurin for purple, rubiacin for orange and xanthin for yellow. For bleeding caused by Heat combine with Biota (Ce Bai Ye) and Imperata (Bai Mao Gen); for extravasation of blood caused by injuries and traumas, combine with Notoginseng (San Qi or Tian Qi), Angelica sinensis (Dang Gui), Ligusticum (Chuan Xiong), Safflower (Hong Hua) and Red Peony (Chi Shao).

Discrimination:
Pollen Typhae (Pu Huang) — removes Blood Stagnation.

Agrimonia Pilosa (Xian He Cao) — stops diarrhea and dysentery, kills parasites.

Notoginseng (Rx. Pseudoginseng) (San Qi or Tienchi) — resolves Stasis, reduces inflammation and pain.

Bletilla Striata (Bai Ji) — stops Stomach and Lung bleeding, anti-inflammatory, promotes wound healing.

Sanguisorba Officinalis (Di Yu) — removes Blood Heat, stops bleeding and diarrhea, promotes healing.

Cacumen Biota Orientalis (Ce Bai Ye) — Cools Lung Heat, expels Phlegm, relieves Wind-Damp Bi pain, clears Heat from the skin and promotes the healing of burns.

Artemisia Argyi (Ai Ye) — Warms the meridians, Warms the womb and calms the fetus, relieves menstrual cramps caused by Coldness.

Crinis Carbonisatus Hominis (Xue Yu Tan) – blood and pain in the urine, promotes urination.

Nodus Nelumbinis Nucifera (Ou Jie) – prolonged menstruation caused by Blood Heat, bleeding in the Lungs and Stomach.

Imperata Cylindrica (Bai Mao Gen) – drains Heat, diuretic, bleeding in the Stomach and Lungs.

Rubia (Qian Cao Gen) – Cools Blood, invigorates Blood, stops coughs and expectorates phlegm.

HERBS THAT INVIGORATE THE BLOOD

Ligusticum Chuanxiong   **Chuan Xiong** (1)

Common Name: Ligusticum, Szechwan Lovage Root, Cnidium

Part Used: Root (Radix)

Family: Umbelliferae

Energy and Flavor: acrid and Warm

Organ Meridians Affected: Liver, Gallbladder, Pericardium

Actions: 1. Regulates and moves the Blood; 2. Relieves Wind-Cold and pain; 3. Circulates the Qi in the Upper Burner, relieving headaches.

Indications: 1. Relieves dysmenorrhea, amenorrhea, difficult labor and retained placenta; 2. Relieves Blood Stagnation in the chest with symptoms of flank pain, chest pain and Blood Stagnation anywhere in the body; 3. Alleviates pain caused by external Wind-Cold with symptoms of body ache, dizziness and headaches; 4. Treats various skin problems associated with Wind.

Contraindications: Not to be used for headaches that occur because of Deficiency of Yin or from raising Liver Yang; it should not be used when there is abnormal bleeding or during pregnancy.

Dosage: 3 - 9 grams. In general, it is not good to prescribe a high dosage of this herb since its strong moving properties can injure Blood and Qi.

Notes: This herb is commonly used with Angelica sinensis to augment the Blood and Qi moving properties of a formula. However, it is also used for the treatment of irregular menstruation, especially combined with Red Peony (Chi Shao), Cyperus (Xiang Fu) and Motherwort (Yi Mu Cao).

For headache caused by Wind-Heat, it can be combined with Chrysanthemum Flower (Ju Hua) and Gypsum (Shi Gao); for headache caused by Wind-Cold-Damp it is combined with Notopterygium (Qiang Huo), Ligusticum root (Gao Ben) and Ledebouriella (Fang Feng); for Wind-Cold it is combined with Angelica dahurica (Bai Zhi) and Asarum (Xi Xin).

For Wind-Damp obstruction causing rheumatic and arthritic conditions, combine with Notopterygium (Qiang Huo), Angelica Du Huo (Du Huo), Ledebouriella (Fang Feng) and Cinnamon twigs (Gui Zhi).

Salvia Miltiorrhiza   Dan Shen   (1)

Common Name: Salvia Root, Red Sage Root
Part Used: Root (Radix)
Family: Labiatae
Energy and Flavor: bitter and slightly Cold
Organ Meridians Affected: Heart, Liver, Pericardium
Actions: 1. Invigorates the Blood and breaks up Stasis; 2. Clears Heat and calms restlessness.
Indications: 1. For delayed or slow menses, any pain due to Blood Stasis such as chest pain or menstrual cramps; 2. For inflammations including ulcers, boils and carbuncles; also for Heat and Stagnant Blood associated with insomnia, palpitations and irritability.
Contraindications: Do not use if there is no Blood Stasis. It should not be used in conjunction with Radix Veratri.
Dosage: 3 - 12 grams

Notes: One of the most valuable of all Chinese herbs, because its Cooling but circulating nature gives it a broader range of use for even Yin Deficient conditions. It stimulates blood circulation, breaks up congestion and clots, regulates cholesterol and blood triglycerides, removes angina and other pains caused by Blood Stagnation and calms the mind. This is the premiere herb for all heart problems, especially angina, for which it can be combined and taken with Motherwort (Yi Mu Cao) and Hawthorn (Shan Zha); for irregular menstruation with pain it can be combined with Motherwort (Yi Mu Cao) and Angelica sinensis (Dang Gui); for joint pains caused by Blood Stagnation combine with Angelica sinensis (Dang Gui), Ligusticum (Chuan Xiong) and Achyranthes (Niu Xi); for Blood Deficiency with Internal Heat with symptoms of palpitations, insomnia and irritability, combine with Jujube seeds (Suan Zao Ren) and the stems and leaves of Polygonum Multiflorum (Ye Jiao Teng).

Corydalis Yanhusuo   Yan Hu Suo   (1)

Common Name: Corydalis
Part Used: Rhizome (Rhizoma)
Family: Papaveraceae
Energy and Flavor: acrid, bitter and Warm

Organ Meridians Affected: Liver, Lung, Spleen and Heart

Actions: 1. Moves the Blood, breaks Stasis and reduces associated pain; 2. Regulates Stagnant Qi and reduces associated pain.

Indications: 1. For Stagnation of Blood with symptoms such as blocked menses, cramping due to Blood Stasis and traumatic injury; 2. For conditions of Stagnant Qi and pain such as epigastric pain, chest pain and menstrual pain.

Contraindications: This herb should not be used during pregnancy.

Dosage: 3 - 9 grams

Notes: This is an important reliever of pain caused by Blood Stagnation. Being in the poppy family, like many other plants in that group, besides its unique Blood moving properties, it has purely analgesic properties as well. For pains of all kinds combine with Angelica sinensis (Dang Gui), Myrrh (Mo Yao) and Frankincense (Ru Xiang). Grind all four herbs to a powder and mix with honey to form a pill about the size of a golf ball. Take one of these two or three times daily. For angina and chest pains combine with Red Sage root (Dan Shen); for stomach and abdominal pains combine with Licorice (Gan Cao) and White Peony (Bai Shao Yao); for menstrual pains combine with Angelica sinensis (Dang Gui) and Ligusticum (Chuan Xiong).

Curcuma Longa   Yu Jin   (2)

Common Name: Turmeric Tuber, Curcuma

Part Used: Tuber

Family: Zingiberaceae

Energy and Flavor: acrid, bitter and Cold

Organ Meridians Affected: Liver, Lung, Heart and Gallbladder

Actions: 1. Moves Blood, breaks Stasis and reduces associated pain; 2. Regulates the Liver and relieves patterns of Stagnant Qi with pain; 3. Clears the Heart and Cools the Blood; 4. Relieves Stagnation and clears Heat in the Liver and Gallbladder.

Indications: 1. Applied topically or taken internally for pain from Stagnant Blood due to traumatic injury; also for chronic sores; 2. For patterns of Stagnant Qi with menstrual, chest or abdominal pain; 3. For patterns of Phlegm-Heat blocking the orifices of the Heart and Heat in the Pericardium with symptoms of epilepsy, anxiety, seizures, delirium and mental derangement; 4. For gallstones and jaundice.

Contraindications: This herb should not be used during pregnancy or by those without signs of Stagnant Blood or Qi. It should also be used with caution by those with Yin Deficiency from blood loss. Turmeric should not be used with Flos and Fructus Caryophylli.

Dosage: 3 - 9 grams

Notes: For Qi and Blood Stagnation of the chest, combine with Red Sage (Dan Shen), Cyperus (Xiang Fu), Bupleurum (Chai Hu) and Bitter Orange (Zhi Shi); for dysmenorrhea caused by Qi and Blood Stagnation combine with Angelica sinensis (Dang Gui), Ligusticum (Chuan Xiong) and Cyperus (Xiang Fu). For mental derangement, the effects of intoxicating drugs such as marijuana and lack of focus, combine with Calamus (Shi Chang Pu).

Curcuma Longa **Jiang Huang** (2)
Common Name: Turmeric Rhizome
Part Used: Rhizome (Rhizoma)
Family: Zingiberaceae
Energy and Flavor: acrid, bitter and Warm
Organ Meridians Affected: Liver and Spleen

Actions: 1. Moves Blood and unblocks Stasis; 2. Facilitates the movement of Qi and eases pain; 3. Clears the meridians, expels Wind and moves Blood to relieve pain.

Indications: 1. For Stagnation of Blood associated with Cold with symptoms of late or slow menstruation, chest pain and abdominal pain; 2. For Stagnation of Liver Qi with symptoms of pain in the abdomen and epigastric region; 3. For Wind-Damp Bi Pain caused by Stagnation of Blood and Qi with symptoms of chronic pain such as arthritis, rheumatoid arthritis and other kinds of painful obstruction.

Contraindications: This herb should be avoided during pregnancy; it should not be used when there is Blood Deficiency with signs of Stagnation of Blood or Qi.

Dosage: 3 - 9 grams

Notes: Turmeric is one of the most useful and versatile of all herbs. This is because of its unique combination of properties, which are to normalize circulation, promote digestion and assimilation, and purify and detoxify the blood and liver. It is highly respected in Ayurvedic Medicine where it is known as "Haldi". Turmeric, together with Coriander and Cumin seeds,s comprise the three basic ingredients of Indian curry powder. It is one of the most effective herbs for the liver, increasing bile flow considerably, reducing SGOT and SGPT (liver enzymes), and preventing and dissolving liver and gall stones. It is one of the most effective and surest remedies, either singly or in combination with other herbs, for the treatment of gallstones and pain of the gallbladder and liver.

Curcumin, the compound responsible for its yellow color, is considered the primary anti-inflammatory component of turmeric. Even in high doses, curcumin has shown no toxicity. It is widely prescribed

for all inflammatory conditions such as sports injuries and other musculoskeletal traumas, inflammatory bowel disorders, arthritic and rheumatic conditions, for all of which it serves as an effective anti-inflammatory and analgesic.

Leonurus Heterophyllus   Yi Mu Cao   (1)
Common Name: Chinese Motherwort
Part Used: Aerial portion (Herba)
Family: Labiatae
Energy and Flavor: acrid, bitter and slightly Cold
Organ Meridians Affected: Heart, Liver and Urinary Bladder
Actions: 1. Moves and regulates Blood, breaks Stasis and regulates the menses; 2. Increases the flow of urine and reduces Stagnation of water.
Indications: 1. For Stagnation of Blood with symptoms of pain from Blood Stasis, late or slow menstruation, infertility, uterine bleeding, post partum pain and masses caused by Blood Stagnation; 2. For retention of water with symptoms of acute edema with or without Heat in the Kidney or Bladder, causing Blood in the urine.
Contraindications: Motherwort should not be used during pregnancy or by those with Blood Deficiency or Yin Deficiency.
Dosage: 9 - 30 grams

Notes: The Chinese name "Yi Mu Cao" literally translates as "Good for Mother" and attests to its long respect as a treatment for women's diseases. There are several different species of Motherworts; the European and the Chinese, however, are the primary ones used for treating menstrual and circulatory problems. As a member of the mint family, it is easily grown from seed in almost any soil condition. It is best harvested at the point when it is in full flower. Before blooming or after forming seeds, it is significantly lacking in its active constituents (benzoic acid). It has been shown to be effective for acute and chronic nephritis, irregular menstruation, postpartum uterine bleeding, incomplete involution of the uterus, excessive menstrual bleeding, hypertension and coronary disease.

It is a very effective herb for the heart, which gives rise to the Latin binomial, Leonurus cardiaca, for the European species. Chinese research substantiates its efficacy in the treatment of myocardial ischemia where it increases blood circulation in the coronary artery, lowers heart rate, improves microcirculation, and prevents platelet agglutination. A combination which I have used for heart conditions combines Hawthorn berries, Motherwort, Tienchi ginseng, Salvia milthiorhiza, all decocted

down to a syrup with honey or sugar. To this is added several drops of Peppermint oil to taste. A tablespoon is taken three times daily.

For edema caused by nephritis, a considerable amount is taken, from 90 to 120 grams of the herb slowly decocted in four cups of water down to two. One cup is taken twice daily. For difficult childbirth a strong dose consisting of the juice of the fresh herb or a handful of the dried herb is cooked down to one or two cups. Twenty seven grams of motherwort is also cooked with 9 grams of Angelica sinensis (Dang Gui) and is taken in three doses to help restore the womb after childbirth.

The seeds are also used as a sedative and/or in combination with Mulberry leaves and branches to reduce hypertension.

Lycopus Lucidum   Ze Lan   (3)
Common Name: Bugleweed
Part Used: Aerial portion (Herba)
Family: Labiatae
Energy and Flavor: acrid, bitter and Warm
Organ Meridians Affected: Liver, Spleen and Urinary Bladder
Actions: 1. Moves Blood, regulates the menstruation and breaks Stasis; 2. Increases the flow of urine.
Indications: 1. For Stasis of Blood with symptoms of blocked menstruation, post partum pain, irregular menstruation, abdominal pain and Stasis caused by traumatic injury; 2. For edema of any kind especially when Blood Stagnation is present; also for dripping of urine.
Contraindications: This herb should be used with caution during pregnancy and not be used when there is no Blood Stasis.
Dosage: 3 - 9 grams
Notes: North American Bugleweed (Lycopus virginicus) is similarly used for its sedative, astringent and mild narcotic properties. It can also be used for consumption and bleeding from the lungs. Chinese Bugleweed (Ze Lan) can be combined with Angelica (Dang Gui), Red Sage (Dan Shen) and Red Peony (Chi Shao).

Paeonia Rubra   Chi Shao   (1)
Common Name: Red Peony Root
Part Used: Root (Radix)
Family: Ranunculaceae
Energy and Flavor: sour, bitter and slightly Cold
Organ Meridians Affected: Liver and Spleen
Actions: 1. Moves Blood, relieves pain and reduces swelling; 2. Cools the Blood and the Liver.

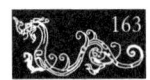

Indications: 1. For Stagnation of Blood with or without swelling, accompanied by symptoms of blocked menstruation, inflammation with pain, pain in the abdomen and pain caused by traumatic injury; 2. For Heat in the Blood or Liver with symptoms of fever, rashes, red and swollen eyes and bleeding due to Blood Heat.

Contraindications: This herb should not be used by those with Blood Deficiency.

Dosage: 6 - 12 grams

Notes: It is generally regarded that the difference between White Peony (Bai Shao Yao) and Red Peony (Chi Shao) is that the Red Peony is wild while the white is cultivated. It is used both internally and externally to relieve pain by promoting blood circulation.

Prunus Persica   Tao Ren   (1)

Common Name: Peach Kernel, Persica

Part Used: Seed (Semen)

Family: Rosaceae

Energy and Flavor: sweet, bitter and neutral

Organ Meridians Affected: Liver, Heart, Lung and Large Intestine

Actions: 1. Moves Blood and breaks up Stasis; 2. Moistens the Intestines.

Indications: 1. For Stagnation of Blood with symptoms of blocked menstruation, pain due to traumatic injury, pain in the abdomen and flanks and Lung and Intestinal abscesses; 2. For constipation due to Dryness, especially good for the elderly.

Contraindications: This herb should not be used by pregnant women.

Dosage: 5 - 10 grams

Notes: For dysmenorrhea or amenorrhea it can be combined with Angelica sinensis (Dang Gui), Safflower (Hong Hua), Motherwort (Yi Mu Cao) and Red Peony (Chi Shao). For constipation caused by Dryness and Blood Deficiency combine with Angelica sinensis (Dang Gui), Rhubarb (Da Huang) Cannabis seed (Huo Ma Ren) and Apricot seed (Xing Ren). The basic combination of Persica and Safflower (Hong Hua) is used to move and disperse Blood Stagnation.

Carthamus Tinctorius   Hong Hua   (1)

Common Name: Safflower, Carthamus

Part Used: Flower (Flos)

Family: Compositae

Energy and Flavor: acrid, bitter and Warm

Organ Meridians Affected: Heart and Liver

Actions: 1. Moves Stagnant Blood and regulates menses; 2. Relieves pain caused by Blood Stasis.

Indications: 1. For Blood Stagnation causing irregularity in the menses, or pain and masses in the abdominal region caused by Stagnation of Blood; 2. For pain due to traumatic injury with Stagnation of Blood or any other pain caused by Stagnation of Blood.

Contraindications: This herb should not be used by pregnant women.

Dosage: 3 - 9 grams

Notes: The best quality comes from higher plateaus of Tibet. The quality is determined by the concentration of its oils. I consider this herb to be similar to, but decidedly stronger than, Western Calendula (Calendula officinalis). For external or internal pains of all kinds it can be combined with Peach seed (Tao Ren), Angelica sinensis (Dang Gui), Ligusticum (Chuan Xiong), Corydalis (Yan Hu Suo) and Red Peony (Chi Shao).

Myrrha   Mo Yao   (2)

(Commiphora Myrrha)

Common Name: Myrrh

Part Used: Resin (Resina)

Family: Burseraceae

Energy and Flavor: bitter and neutral

Organ Meridians Affected: Heart, Liver and Spleen

Actions: 1. Moves Blood and relieves Stasis and pain caused by Blood Stasis; 2. Assists in wound healing.

Indications: 1. For any kind of Blood Stagnation including traumatic injury, blocked menses and painful obstruction; 2. Can by applied externally for chronic non healing wounds and sores.

Contraindications: This herb should not be used by pregnant women; it should not be taken internally for extended periods of time.

Dosage: 3 - 9 grams

Notes: This herb is commonly combined with Frankincense (Ru Xiang) to move Blood and stop pain. For general traumatic pain relief, combine Myrrh (Mo Yao), Frankincense (Ru Xiang), Angelica sinensis (Dang Gui) and Corydalis (Yan Hu Suo).

Olibanum   Ru Xiang   (2)

(Boswellia Carterii)

Common Name: Frankincense, Mastic

Part Used: Resin (Resina)

Family: Burseraceae

Energy and Flavor: acrid, bitter and Warm

Organ Meridians Affected: Heart, Liver, Spleen

Actions: 1. Moves Blood and Qi and relieves pain; 2. Disperses Wind-Damp from the meridians and relaxes the sinews; 3. Reduces swelling and aids in wound healing.

Indications: 1. For pain caused by either or both Stagnation of Blood and Qi with symptoms of menstrual pain, abdominal pain, traumatic injury, sores and swellings; 2. For Wind-Damp painful obstruction with symptoms of tightness and spasm; 3. Applied externally for pain and swelling such as traumatic injury, inflammation in the mouth or throat, carbuncles or chronic non healing sores.

Contraindications: This herb should not be used by pregnant women and should be used with caution by those with Spleen Deficiency.

Dosage: 3 - 9 grams

Notes: See Myrrh (Mo Yao)

Achyranthis Bidentata   Niu Xi   (1)

Common Name: Achyranthes Root

Part Used: Root (Radix)

Family: Amaranthaceae

Energy and Flavor: bitter, sour and neutral

Organ Meridians Affected: Liver and Kidney

Actions: 1. Moves Blood and relieves pain in the raw state; 2. Tonic to the Liver and Kidneys and strengthens the bones and sinews in the wine treated form; 3. Reduces Damp-Heat in the Lower Burner; 4. Regulates the flow of reckless Blood caused by either ascendant Liver Yang or Yin Deficient Fire.

Indications: 1. For pain caused by Blood Stagnation such as painful menstruation, blood trapped under the skin, difficulty with labor, Bi pain, traumatic injuries or post partum pain; 2. For weakness in the Liver and Kidney with symptoms such as atrophy of the limbs, bone pain and knee and lower back pain; 3. For Damp-Heat in the Lower Burner causing knee pain, painful urination, vaginal discharge or stones in the urine with bleeding; it is especially good for these ailments when they are accompanied by knee or lower back pain; 4. For reckless flow of Blood with symptoms of Liver Yang rising or Yin Deficient Fire accompanied by nosebleeds, vomiting of blood, dizziness, headache, toothache and bleeding gums.

Contraindications: This herb should not be used by pregnant women and should be used with caution by those with weak digestion and Spleen Deficiency.

Dosage: 6 - 9 grams

Notes: For dysmenorrhea or amenorrhea combine with Red Peony (Chi Shao), Angelica sinensis (Dang Gui), Ligusticum (Chuan Xiong); for lower back and knee pains combine with Loranthes (Sang Ji Sheng), Eucommia (Du Zhong) and Angelica Du Huo (Du Huo); for headache, vertigo, dizziness and blurred vision caused by Liver Yang (hypertension) combine with Ramulus cum Uncis Uncariae (Gou Teng), Chrysanthemum (Ju Hua) and Loranthes (Sang Ji Sheng).

Millettia Reticulata   Ji Xue Teng   (3)

Common Name: Ji Xue Teng

Part Used: Root and Stem (Radix et Caulis)

Family: Leguminosae

Energy and Flavor: bitter, sweet and Warm

Organ Meridians Affected: Heart, Spleen, Liver

Actions: 1. Regulates Blood; 2. Tonifies Blood; 3. Circulates Qi.

Indications: 1. For conditions requiring both circulation of Blood and Qi and tonification of Blood; 2. For paralytic conditions of the weak and elderly; 3. Sedative, lowers blood pressure; 4. Leukopenia caused by radiation therapy; 5. Aplastic anemia.

Contraindications: none.

Dosage: 9 - 30 grams.

Notes: This herb has both Blood moving and Blood tonifying properties. It can be combined with Angelica sinensis (Dang Gui) and Ligusticum (Chuan Xiong) to augment these functions. For soreness and pain of the joints caused by Wind-Cold-Damp with Blood Deficiency, combine with Angelica sinensis (Dang Gui) and Ligusticum (Chuan Xiong), Chaenomeles (Mu Gua), Loranthes (Sang Ji Sheng) and Achyranthes (Niu Xi).

Liquidambar Taiwaniana   Lu Lu Tong

Common Name: Liquidambar, Sweetgum fruit

Part Used: fruit

Family: Hamamelidaceae

Energy and Flavor: bitter and neutral

Organ Meridians Affected: Liver and Stomach

Actions: 1. Moves Qi and Blood, unblocks the channels; 2. opens the Middle Warmer; 3. relieves Wind-Dampness with painful obstruction and stiffness of the lower back and knees

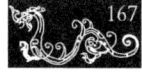

Indications: for congestion and blockage associated with abdominal blockage, irregular and scanty periods, injuries and traumas, lower back and joints, allergic rhinitis.

Dosage: 3-9 grams

Contraindications: Not for use during pregnancy. Be careful of the possibility that it may cause heart palpitations.

Notes: For abdominal pain, distention and irregular bowel movements combine with Lindera (Wu Yao), Saussurea (Mu Xiang), Citrus Aurantii (Zhi Ke); for irregular and scanty periods combine with Cyperus (Xiang Fu), Ligusticum (Chuan Xiong) and Angelica sinensis (Dang Gui); for trauma and injuries combine with Red Peony (Chi Shao), Corydalis (Yan Hu Suo), Artemisia anomalae (Liu Ji Nu) and Salvia milthiorrhiza (Dan Shen); for allergic rhinitis combine with Magnolia flower (Xin Yi Hua) and Xanthium (Cang Er Zi).

Manitis Penta-Dactyla   Chuan Shan Jia   (3)

Common Name: Pangolin (anteater) scales

Part Used: Scales (Squama)

Family: Manidae

Energy and Flavor: salty and Cold

Organ Meridians Affected: Liver, Stomach

Actions: 1. Disperses congealed Blood; 2. Promotes menses and lactation; 3. Reduces swelling and promotes the discharge of pus from boils, abscesses and carbuncles (can be topically applied); 4. Relieves rheumatic pains.

Indications: 1. Delayed or stopped menstruation; 2. Arthritic pains; 3. Pains from trauma and injuries; 4. Promotes the resolution and healing of boils, abscesses and ulcerated sores; 5. Stopped lactation.

Contraindications: Use with caution for the treatment of sores caused by Deficiency.

Preparation: Presoak in warm water for 2 hours, then simmer 1 to 3 hours.

Dosage: 3 - 9 grams

Notes: For amenorrhea combine with Angelica sinensis (Dang Gui), Ligusticum (Chuan Xiong) and Safflower (Hong Hua).

Artemisia Anomala   Liu Ji Nu

Common Name: Artemisia, Anomala

Part Used: the aerial portions

Family: compositae

Energy and Flavor: bitter, Warm

Organ Meridians Affected: Heart, Spleen

Actions: 1. Moves Blood, stimulates menstruation; 2. Relieves pain; 3. The ash can be topically applied to staunch bleeding of injuries, wounds and burns.

Indications: For pain caused by swelling, fracture, trauma combine with Drynaria (Gu Sui Bu), Corydalis (Yan Hu Suo), Dipsacus (Xu Duan); for amenorrhea or dysmenorrhea combine with Angelica sinensis (Dang Gui), Ligusticum (Chuan Xiong).

Dosage: 3-9 grams

Contraindications: Avoid during pregnancy, diarrhea, Spleen Deficiency, and in general for conditions of Qi and Blood Deficiency.

Notes: This herb has very similar properties to Artemisia Argyi, otherwise known as Artemisia Vulgaris or Mugwort (Ai Ye). The difference is that Artemisia Argyi may stop bleeding more. They can be used interchangeably, however.

Pyritum   Zi Ran Tong

Common Name: Pyritum, Pyrite

Energy and Flavors: pungent, bitter, neutral

Organ meridians Affected: Liver, Kidney

Actions and Indications: 1. Removes Blood Stagnation; 2. Promotes the healing of bones and ligaments; 3. Relieves the pain and swelling associated with traumatic injuries, especially fractures.

Dosage: 3-9 grams, cook for at least a half hour before ingesting. In pill or powder form use 0.3-0.6 grams.

Contraindications: Avoid for cases of Yin or Blood Deficiency with signs of Heat.

Notes: For pain, trauma and fractures combine with Drynaria (Gu Sui Bu), Dipsacus (Xu Duan), Corydalis (Yan Hu Suo), Olibanum (Ru Xiang) and Myrrh (Mo Yao); for pain caused by Blood Stagnation combine with Red Peony (Chi Shao).

Sanguis Draconis   Xue Jie

Botanical Name: Daemonorops Draco Bl. or Dracaena Cambodiana

Common Name: Dragon Blood, Calamus Gum

Part Used: gum resin

Family: Palmae (daemonorops); Liliaceae (dracaena)

Energy and Flavor: sweet, salty and neutral

Organ Meridians Affected: Heart and Liver

Actions: 1. Stop bleeding and promote the healing of wounds; 2. Invigorate and remove Blood Stagnation; 3. Alleviate pain

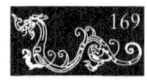

Indications: For hemorrhages caused from external injuries and to promote the healing of wounds, combine with Cattail Pollen (Pu Huang); for chronic ulcers, non-healing wounds combine with Olibanum (Ru Xiang) and Myrrh (Mo Yao) and apply externally.

Dose: 1 - 1.5 grams in pill form

Contraindications: Do not use if there are no signs of Blood Stagnation.

Notes: The red resinous secretion from the fruit and stem is harvested in the summer. It is then cooked down to a semi solid resin, spread out on a surface and dried. This is then pounded into a powder for use.

Lignum Sappan   Su Mu

Botanical Name: Lignum Sappan

Common Name: Sappan Wood

Part Used: the wood

Family: Leguminosae

Energy and Flavor: sweet, salty, mildly spicy, neutral

Organ Meridians Affected: Heart, Liver and Spleen

Actions: 1. Invigorate Blood and induce menstruation; 2. Alleviate pain and reduce swelling.

Indications: For Blood Stagnation with dysmenorrhea, amenorrhea or post partum pain, combine with Angelica sinensis (Dang Gui), Ligusticum (Chuan Xiong), Red Peony (Chi Shao) and Safflower (Hong Hua); for external injuries with swelling and pain, combine with Olibanum (Ru Xiang), Myrrh (Mo Yao) and Dragon's Blood (Xue Jie), mix with water or honey to form a paste and apply externally.

Dosage: 3 - 10 grams

Contraindications: Do not use during pregnancy

Vaccaria Segetalis   Wang Bu Liu Xing   (3)

Common Name: Vaccaria seed

Part Used: Seed (Semen)

Family: Caryophyllaceae

Energy and Flavor: bitter and neutral

Organ Meridians Affected: Liver, Stomach

Actions: 1. Invigorates Blood; 2. Promotes lactation and menstruation; 3. Reduces painful swelling of the breasts and testicles.

Indications: 1. Diseases caused by Blood Stagnation; 2. Amenorrhea and stopped lactation; 3. Painful and swollen glands, breasts or testicles; 4. Crush and mix with sesame oil and apply topically for shingles.

Contraindications: Do not use during pregnancy.

Dosage: 3 - 9 grams

Notes: For dysmenorrhea combine with Angelica sinensis (Dang Gui), Ligusticum (Chuan Xiong) and Safflower (Hong Hua); for insufficient lactation combine with Pangolin Scales (Chuan Shan Jia) or Astragalus (Huang Qi) and Angelica sinensis (Dang Gui) if the cause is Deficient Qi and Blood. For mastitis combine with Dandelion (Pu Gong Ying), Honeysuckle Flower (Jin Yin Hua) and Trichosanthes Fruit (Gua Lou).

Hirudo seu Whitmania   Shui Zhi (3)
(Hirudo Nipponia)
Common Name: Leech
Energy and Flavors: neutral, salty, bitter, toxic
Organ Meridians Affected: Liver and Bladder
Actions: 1. Breaks up Congealed Blood, immobile masses, tumors and Congealed Blood caused by injuries; 2. Promotes menstruation in conditions caused by Congealed Blood.
Indications: 1. Used for hardened swellings, cysts, tumors, fibroids, swollen blocked passages; 2. Used for amenorrhea caused by Blood Congealment.
Contraindications: Not for use in pregnancy nor for Blood Deficiency or conditions without Blood Stasis.
Toxicity: It is poisonous and should only be used for 2 or 3 days at a time.
Preparation: Hirudo has a strong anticoagulant called hirudin which interferes with the clotting effect of thrombin on fibrinogen. This principle is destroyed during prolonged cooking. Because of this, it should only be lightly toasted until yellow, ground to a fine powder and taken in pill or capsule form.
Dose: 1- 3 grams of the powder.

Notes: Live leeches are used in many cultures to extract bad blood. In Ayurvedic medicine leech therapy is extremely important, with entire Ayurvedic hospital wards dedicated to this single therapeutic approach. At an Ayurvedic hospital in Bangalore, India, I saw leeches used with immediate benefit for a variety of problems ranging from arthritic conditions to chronic skin conditions such as psoriasis. While bleeding, called vivisection, is generally effective for relieving pain associated with Excess and Stagnation, it is inappropriate for Deficiency conditions. Live leeches are therapeutically useful because they can suck out the dark colored, lactic acid saturated blood . They are stored in a dormant state in fluid containers. Before using, turmeric powder is rubbed on their abdomen to stimulate their appetite. They are then held next to the indicated area of the skin until they begin to take hold and suck.

  Chinese herbalism also uses dried and powdered leeches in capsules. These are then taken for amenorrhea, immobile abdominal masses caused

by Blood Stagnation and injury. For injuries they can be combined with Notoginseng (San Qi), Angelica sinensis (Dang Gui), Myrrh (Mo Yao) and Frankincense (Ru Xiang).

Trogopterori seu Pteromi   Wu Ling Zhi   (2)

Common Name: Flying Squirrel feces

Part Used: Excrement (Excrementum)

Family: Petauristidae

Energy and Flavors: Warm, bitter, sweet

Organ Meridians: Affected: Liver and Spleen

Actions: 1. Disperses congealed Blood in the lower abdomen and uterus and relieves pain; 2. Promotes childhood nutrition with Cold Stagnation and focal abdominal swelling.

Indications: Fibroids, ovarian and uterine cysts, tumors, swollen abdomen caused by mal-nutrition.

Contraindications: Avoid during pregnancy, and traditionally not to be used with Ginseng.

Dosage: 3 - 9 grams

Notes: For dysmenorrhea and amenorrhea caused by Blood Stagnation combine with Ligusticum (Chuan Xiong), Corydalis (Yan Hu Suo) and Motherwort (Yi Mu Cao); for epigastric pain caused by Blood and Qi Stagnation combine with Cyperus (Xiang Fu) and Saussurea (Mu Xiang); for excessive menstruation caused by Blood Stagnation combine with Donkey Skin Gelatin (E Jiao), Angelica sinensis (Dang Gui), Ligusticum (Chuan Xiong) and Red Peony (Chi Shao).

Discrimination:

Ligusticum Chuanxiong (Chuan Xiong) – Warm, regulates Qi.

Salvia Miltiorrhiza (Dan Shen) – Cooling and calming.

Corydalis Yanhusuo (Yan Hu Suo) – Warm, regulates Blood and Qi, reduces pain.

Curcuma Longa (Yu Jin) – Cool, regulates Qi of the Liver, relieves Heat Stagnation in the Liver and Gall Bladder, clears Heat and relieves Heart circulation.

Curcuma Longa (Jiang Huang) – removes blockage and Stasis, moves Qi, relieves pain, opens the meridians.

Leonurus Heterophyllus (Yi Mu Cao) – regulates menses, diuretic.

Lycopus Lucidum (Ze Lan) – regulates menses, diuretic, resolves edema.

Paeonia Rubra (Chi Shao) — Cool, regulates menses, treats inflammation, relieves pain.

Persicae (Tao Ren) — moistens the Intestines.

Carthamus Tinctorius (Hong Hua) — regulates menses, relieves pain.

Myrrha (Mo Yao) — relieves pain, treats traumatic injury, heals wounds and sores.

Olibanum (Ru Xiang) — relieves pain, disperses Wind-Damp from the meridians, reduces swelling from injuries.

Achyranthis Bidentata (Niu Xi) — relieves painful menses, tonic to Liver and Kidneys, treats lower back pain, strengthens bones and sinews, treats bone injuries and knee pains.

Millettia reticulata (Ji Xue Teng) — Tonifies Blood, circulates Qi, sedative, lowers Blood pressure.

Manitis (Chuan Shan Jia) — promotes menses and lactation, reduces swelling, discharges pus, relieves arthritic and rheumatic pain.

Vaccaria (Wang Bu Liu Xing) — promotes menses and lactation, reduces painful swelling of the breast, testicles and glands.

Hirudo seu Whitmaniae (Shui Zhi) — toxic, breaks Blood Stagnation, induces menstruation.

Trogopterori seu Pteromi (Wu Ling Zhi) — Dissolves Congealed masses, especially lower abdominal conditions, treats swollen abdomen caused by malnutrition.

HERBS THAT WARM THE INTERIOR AND EXPEL COLD

Herbs in this category are used for Internal Coldness with Qi and Yang Deficiency. Because Coldness is one indication of Yang Deficiency, they are often combined with Yang and Qi tonics. In cases of Yang collapse with convulsions or coma, these herbs are particularly indicated. In Western herbalism, Cayenne Pepper is often used to achieve this end; while in Ayurvedic herbalism a formula called Trikatu, consisting of equal parts black Pepper, Pippali long Pepper and Ginger is used.

Conditions of Deficient Yang or Qi commonly indicate a Deficiency of the Spleen and Kidney, so that many of the herbs in this category enter those Organ meridian channels.

Lateralis Aconiti   **Fu Zi** (1)
Common Name: Prepared Aconite
Part Used: Root (Radix)

Family: Ranunculaceae

Energy and Flavor: acrid, very Hot and toxic

Organ Meridians Affected: Heart, Kidney and Spleen

Actions: 1. Raises the collapse of Yang; 2. Warms the meridians and relieves pain caused by Cold; 3. Reduces Damp caused by Deficiency in Yang.

Indications: 1. For collapse of Yang with symptoms of Cold, extremely weak limbs with numbness, shock, diarrhea, faint pulse and a pale, swollen and moist tongue; this herb can also be used as a tonic for any kind of Deficiency of Yang, but should not be used for long periods as it will burn up the Yin. It is also a very important herb for critical situations where the Heart Yang has been impaired and it can not circulate through the meridians; 2. For pain anywhere caused by chronic conditions where Cold is the predominant factor; 3. For Dampness caused by Deficiency of Yang of the Spleen or Kidney with symptoms of diarrhea or edema.

Contraindications: This herb should not be used by those with Yin Deficiency, with true Heat, with false chills or during pregnancy.

Dosage: 3 - 9 grams, it should be decocted for 60 minutes before adding the rest of the herbs.

Notes: There are various methods of preparing this herb to neutralize its toxicity. In one method it is treated with salt and then boiled with Licorice and black soya beans.

This is the main herb for tonifying the Life Gate Fire (Ming Men) which is the origin for Yang Qi in the body. It is combined with Cinnamon Bark (Rou Gui) for conditions of metabolic Coldness caused by Yang Deficiency; this combination is also used to Warm the Kidneys and rescue the Yang.

There are different subspecies that are used. Sichuan Aconite, Chuan Wu, is used untreated and raw and is therefore very toxic. It enters the Heart, Spleen and Liver organ meridians and, while less tonifying, it has stronger Cold dispelling and pain relieving properties. It absolutely must be boiled for at least an hour or an hour and a half to neutralize its toxicity.

I was once asked to intermediate on behalf of a school, whose student practitioner failed to strongly inform a patient that Chuan Wu had to be pre-boiled for at least an hour before use. The patient had experienced long term debilitating side effects as a result and was threatening legal action. For this reason, I don't recommend my students to use Chuan Wu until they become very experienced with the use of Fu Zi. Even with this herb, it is the better side of precaution to tell the patient to pre-cook Fu Zi for an hour before use.

Aconite is the most Yang of all the materia medica; it is practically unimaginable to conceive of practicing Chinese medicine without it. Therefore, it is of great importance that it is put into the hands of practitioners who are trained in its proper use.

Having said this, I have heard of students who were admonished to use only the smallest amount of aconite for conditions such as intractable arthritis. After the admonition, a case such as the following, which is true, is told: A man went to several herbalists for his arthritis. The first gave the appropriate formula and dose of aconite and there was no change. Another gave a higher dose of aconite and still there was no change. Finally, the third herbalist recommended that the man cook 30 grams of Prepared Aconite with lamb (it was actually a higher dose than this) and finally the man's arthritis was completely cured.

There are various western species of aconite, commonly known as monkshood, that have been used by herbalists throughout the ages. It is usually given in very minute, prescribed doses and I have never heard of any western method for detoxifying it. One method for using Western aconite can be a model for the use of many therapeutically valuable but toxic plants. Five to thirty drops of 1:5 aconite liquid extract is mixed into an eight ounce glass of water. One teaspoon of this mixture is taken as needed.

For aconite toxicity, one of the most commonly recommended antidotes is mung bean congee. Clinically, the drug atropine is effective for treating aconite overdose. Regarding the case of the woman described above who experienced toxic side effects, the medical doctor she consulted was ill prepared for treating aconite poisoning. Even the national US poison control centers had little or no experience in being able to advise appropriate treatment. Atropine, a commonly prescribed drug of recent times, had nearly completely disappeared from the clinical experience of this general practitioner.

The addition of Licorice (Gan Cao) and Ginger (Gan Jiang) significantly lessens the toxicity of aconite in formulas. In my personal experience, I have used Prepared aconite (Fu Zi) very often, sometimes in high dosage, and have never encountered an adverse toxic reaction. I have seen where it is contraindicated for some individuals, especially those that are more Yin Deficient or whose lifestyle tends to be over stressed. In these, it can create a feeling of uncomfortable nervousness that precludes its appropriateness for that individual. While aconite is classified as Hot, Cinnamon bark (Rou Gui) is probably Hotter but has less of a Yang effect on the nervous system.

Zingiberis Officinalis   Gan Jiang   (1)
Common Name: Dried Ginger
Part Used: Rhizome (Rhizoma)
Family: Zingiberaceae
Energy and Flavor: acrid and Hot
Organ Meridians Affected: Heart, Lung, Spleen and Stomach

Actions: 1. Warms the Spleen and expels Cold; 2. Restores collapse of Yang and expels Interior Cold; 3. Warms the Lungs and assists expectoration of Cold Phlegm; 4. Stops chronic bleeding caused by Cold.

Indications: 1. For Cold in the Spleen and Stomach with symptoms of nausea, vomiting, diarrhea and pain in the abdominal region; also for improper function of the Spleen because of Deficiency of Spleen Yang; 2. For collapse of Yang with symptoms of Coldness and numbness in the limbs, shock and a very weak pulse; 3. For Cold Lung conditions where there is Phlegm obstruction with thin watery or white mucus, good for either chronic or acute ailments; 4. For chronic bleeding of the uterus and other bleeding caused by Cold where there is pale blood, cold limbs, dull facial color and a soggy thin pulse.

Contraindications: This herb should not be used by those with Yin Deficiency and Heat signs or bleeding associated with Hot Blood. This herb should be used with extreme caution during pregnancy.

Dosage: 3 - 9 grams

Notes: Fresh Ginger (Sheng Jiang) Warms the Exterior, while Dried Ginger Warms the Interior. It is added to any formula where there is Spleen and Stomach Coldness which can manifest as abdominal pains, vomiting, diarrhea, loose stool, poor appetite. For Cold phlegm in the Lungs with symptoms of clear or whitish mucus, chills, asthma, cough combine with Ephedra (Ma Huang), Asarum (Xi Xin) and Pinellia (Ban Xia) in Minor Blue Green Dragon Combination (Xiao Qing Long Tang).

Cinnamomum Cassia   Rou Gui   (1)
Common Name: Cinnamon Bark
Part Used: Bark (Cortex)
Family: Lauraceae
Energy and Flavor: acrid, sweet and very Hot
Organ Meridians Affected: Spleen, Liver, Kidney, Heart and Urinary Bladder

Actions: 1. Warms the Spleen and Kidneys and tonifies the Yang; 2. Expels Cold, Warms the meridians, promotes circulation of Qi and Blood and relieves pain; 3. Used with tonics to assist in the generation of Qi and Blood.

Indications: 1. For Cold and Deficiency of Yang with symptoms of cold limbs, chronic diarrhea, impotence, weakness and cold in the lower back, reduced appetite, frequent urination or wheezing due to the Kidneys not being able to grasp the Qi of the Lungs; 2. For pain and poor circulation of Blood and Qi caused by Cold, such as excessive or no menstruation, pain in the abdominal region, Damp-Cold Bi Pain or Yin sores that ooze a clear fluid and do not heal; 3. For assisting Qi and Blood tonics in the generation of Qi and Blood.

Contraindications: This herb should not be used by those with Yin Deficiency with Heat signs or when there is Interior Heat; it should be used with extreme caution during pregnancy.

Dosage: 1 - 6 grams

Notes: For Kidney Yang Deficiency combine with Prepared Aconite (Fu Zi), Prepared Rehmannia (Shu Di Huang) and Cornus (Shan Shu Yu) in Rehmannia Eight Combination (Ba Wei Di Huang Wan); for Cold Spleen, Stomach and Kidneys with abdominal pains, lack of appetite, loose stool, combine with Dried Ginger (Gan Jiang), Atractylodes (Bai Zhu), Ginseng (Ren Shen) and Prepared Aconite (Fu Zi) in Cinnamon, Aconite, Ginger and Ginseng Combination (Gui Zhi Fu Zi Li Zhong Wan); for Yin type boils combine with Astragalus (Huang Qi) and Angelica sinensis (Dang Gui).

Evodia Rutaecarpa   **Wu Zhu Yu**   (2)

Common Name: Evodia

Part Used: Fruit (Fructus)

Family: Rutaceae

Energy and Flavor: acrid, bitter, Hot and slightly toxic

Organ Meridians Affected: Liver, Spleen, Kidney and Stomach

Actions: 1. Warms the Spleen, expels Cold, relieves pain and helps the Liver; 2. Directs Rebellious Qi downward.

Indications: 1. For Cold and Phlegm obstructing the Spleen and Liver channels with symptoms of headaches, Cold and pain in the Stomach, daybreak diarrhea, loss of ability to taste, a pale moist tongue and a wiry or weak and slippery pulse; 2. For vomiting, nausea, flank pain, all caused by a disharmony between the Liver and Spleen.

Contraindications: This herb should not be used by those with Yin Deficiency, especially if Dryness is an issue, as this herb is very Drying and therefore should not be used for extended periods of time. It should not be used with Radix Salvia Miltiorrhiza (Dan Shen).

Dosage: 3 - 6 grams

Notes: For Coldness of the Spleen and Stomach with cold abdomen and epigastric pains combine with Dried Ginger (Gan Jiang), Saussurea (Mu Xiang) and Galangal (Gao Liang Jiang); for hernia caused by Cold Stagnation in the Liver meridian combine with Lindera (Wu Yao) and Fennel Fruit (Xiao Hui Xiang); for headache and vomiting caused by Deficiency of the Spleen and Stomach with Liver Qi rising combine with Ginseng (Ren Shen) and Fresh Ginger (Sheng Jiang) in Evodia Combination (Wu Zhu Yu Tang).

Foeniculum Vulgaris   Xiao Hui Xiang   (3)
Common Name: Fennel seed
Part Used: Fruit (Fructus)
Family: Umbelliferae
Energy and Flavor: acrid and Warm
Organ Meridians Affected: Liver, Kidney, Spleen and Stomach
Actions: 1. Expels Cold and relieves pain; 2. Regulates Qi of the Stomach.
Indications: 1. For any pain associated with Cold in the Lower Burner and abdominal region; also the stir-fried form of this herb is used for pain in the testicles; 2. For improper flow of Qi in the Stomach caused by Cold with symptoms of abdominal pain, nausea, vomiting and reduced appetite.
Contraindications: This herb should not be used by those with Yin Deficiency with Heat signs or by those with Excess Heat.
Dosage: 3 - 9 grams

Notes: For Cold Stagnation in the Liver meridian associated with hernia, it is combined with Cinnamon Bark (Rou Gui), Dried Ginger (Gan Jiang) and Saussurea (Mu Xiang). For Cold stomach combine with Pinellia (Ban Xia) and Fresh Ginger (Sheng Jiang).

Eugenia Caryophyllata   Ding Xiang
Common Names: Cloves, Caryophylli, Szygium aromaticum
Part Used: the flower
Family: Myrtaceae
Energy and Flavor: pungent, Warm
Organ Meridians Affected: Kidney, Spleen, Stomach
Actions: 1. Warms the Middle Warmer and directs the Qi downward; 2. Warms the Kidneys and boost Yang
Indications: For Cold Stomach and Spleen with abdominal pain, diarrhea and lack of appetite combine with Atractylodes (Bai Zhu), Amomum (Sha Ren) and Ginger (Gan Jiang); for hiccup caused by Cold Stomach combine with Diospyri (Shi Di) and Ginseng (Ren Shen); for male impotence, or clear vaginal discharge caused by Kidney Yang Deficiency, combine with Cinnamon Bark (Rou Gui) and Morinda (Ba Ji Tian).

Piper Longum   **Bi Ba** (3)

Common Name: Long Pepper Fruit, Pippali

Part Used: Fruit (Fructus)

Family: Piperaceae

Energy and Flavor: acrid and Hot

Organ Meridians Affected: Spleen, Lung, Kidney, Stomach and Large Intestine

Actions: 1. Expels Cold from the Middle and Lower burner and relieves pain; 2. Reverses the flow of Rebellious Qi; 3. Applied topically for pain.

Indications: 1. For pain caused by Cold in the Stomach and Intestines with symptoms of abdominal pain, nausea and vomiting; 2. For Rebellious Qi of the Stomach caused by Cold with symptoms of nausea, vomiting, belching, acid regurgitation and rumbling of the Stomach; 3. Can be applied topically for pain; is especially good for toothache.

Contraindications: This herb should not be used by those with Heat signs from either Excess or Deficiency.

Dosage: 1 - 3 grams

Notes: Pippali has similar properties to Black Pepper (Hu Jiao). In Ayurvedic medicine the two herbs are combined with dried Ginger in equal parts, powdered and mixed with honey and taken for Cold digestion, allergies with clear or whitish discharges, abdominal and other pains caused by Coldness. This mixture in Ayurveda is called Trikatu.

Alpinia Officinarum   **Gao Liang Jiang**   (3)

Common Name: Galangal, Lesser Galangal, Galanga

Part Used: Rhizome (Rhizoma)

Family: Zingiberaceae

Energy and Flavor: acrid and Hot

Organ Meridians Affected: Spleen and Stomach

Actions: 1. Warms the Middle Burner, expels Cold and relieves pain.

Indications: 1. For any conditions of Cold in the Middle Burner where there are symptoms such as pain in the abdominal region, vomiting, diarrhea and chronic inflammation in the digestive tract caused by Cold.

Contraindications: This herb should not be used by those with Deficiency with Heat signs or by those with true Heat signs.

Dosage: 3 - 6 grams

Notes: Similar to but more heating than Ginger. It is characteristically used in Thai cooking to aid and Warm digestion. For epigastric pain caused by Coldness, combine with Cyperus (Xiang Fu); for vomiting and nausea caused by a Cold Stomach combine with Pinellia (Ban Xia)

and Ginger (Gan Jiang). To promote appetite, combine with Chaenomeles (Mu Gua); to Warm the Stomach combine with Cyperus (Xiang Fu).

Discrimination:

Lateralis Aconiti (Fu Zi) – Yang collapse, extreme Cold and weakness.

Zingiberis Officinalis (Gan Jiang) – Coldness in the Spleen and Stomach, nausea, diarrhea.

Cinnamomum Cassia (Rou Gui) – very Hot, Warms the Spleen and Kidney, Cold extremities, circulates Qi and Blood.

Evodia Rutaecarpa (Wu Zhu Yu) – when Cold and Dampness cause headaches from obstruction of the Spleen and Liver channels, hernias, lowers Qi, relieves headaches, daybreak diarrhea, vomiting and nausea.

Foeniculum Vulgaris (Xiao Hui Xiang) – relieves pain in the Lower Warmer, regulates Stomach Qi.

Piper Longum (Bi Ba) – relieves abdominal pain in the Middle and Lower Warmer, lowers Qi for symptoms of nausea, vomiting, belching, topically for toothache.

Alpinia Officinarum (Gao Liang Jiang) – Warms the Stomach and Spleen, relieves pain.

TONIC HERBS

Herbs in this category are used for patterns of Deficiency. They are further subdivided into four subcategories: 1. Deficient Qi, 2. Deficient Blood, 3. Deficient Yin and 4. Deficient Yang. These four substances are called the Four Treasures and herbs assigned to them are not necessarily exclusive of each other and may be used for multiple Deficiencies, either singly as appropriate or in formulation. As one example, Ginseng, the most famous herb of this category, is considered to be useful for all Deficiencies even though it is classified according to its primary use as a Qi tonic.

Because, for some, tonics tend to be heavy and difficult to digest, one approach is to first give a Stagnation removing formula such as Stagnation Relieving Pills (Yu qu wan) for 1 to 3 days before administering a tonic. A standard approach found in most classical formulas is to add various Qi regulating herbs such as Citrus peel (Chen Pi) for Qi tonics and Ligusticum (Chuan Xiong) to accompany the use of Blood tonics. Similar approaches are used to counteract the heavy, cloying effect of Yin and Yang tonics.

Qi tonics are commonly sweet and slightly Warm. They enter the Spleen and Lungs because these organs are most involved with the production of Qi. Qi tonic herbs such as Astragalus, the most characteristic herb for the deep immune system (Wei Qi), can be used to tonify all four Deficiencies. Qi tonics may be used alone or in combination with Qi regulating herbs such as Saussurea (Mu Xiang) or Citrus peel (Chen Pi).

Blood tonics tend to be bitter-sweet with either a Warm or neutral nature. Because the Liver stores Blood, all Blood tonics enter that Organ meridian. They are often combined with Blood regulating herbs such as Ligusticum (Chuan Xiong) and Peony root (Bai Shao or Chi Shao). Blood is a part of Yin so that certain herbs, such as prepared Rehmannia (Shu di huang), are used to tonify both Blood and Yin. Both Blood and Yin tonics are indicated for Dryness, with the difference being that Yin Deficiency is associated with symptoms of Heat.

Yin tonics have a heavy, moist nature. They can be divided into two types, those that nourish the Kidneys and Liver and those that moisten the Lungs and Stomach. The Kidneys and Liver are the deepest aspects so that the deepest levels of Yin Deficiency always affect these Organs. Stomach and Lung Yin Deficiency are conditions that can evolve over time or result from the prolonged presence of a high fever or an acute viral disease.

Yang Tonics are generally used in combination with a small amount of Yin tonics. Yin is like the fluid in a container that receives and holds Qi or Yang. If Yin is depleted, neither Qi nor Yang herbs alone will be effective. Coffee is a substance that disperses Yang, ultimately in excess damaging both Yin and Yang. This, together with the Yang stress of contemporary life, is responsible for the Yin Deficient "burn out" syndrome that is so common among people today. Interestingly, many Yang tonics also have Yin lubricating properties and are used for constipation caused by Dryness and Deficiency of Yang motility. Other aspects of Yang Deficiency include their use for treating low libido and impotence. Two of the most common herbs added to formulas to tonify Yang are not listed in this category; they are Cinnamon bark (Rou Gui) and prepared Aconite (Fu Zi). Either or both of these powerfully Warm the Interior, stimulating overall Yang metabolism.

Tonics, therefore, should not be taken when there are patterns of Excess Stagnation. This is because instead of helping the body to overcome the Excess, they may aggravate the Excess symptoms. This is also true of the use of rich foods such as sugar, dairy, eggs and meat. One strategy to consider before administering tonics is to use a light vegetarian diet or

detoxifying herbs for one to three days before administering tonic herbs and formulas. Another, more common method, is to include smaller amounts of Qi or Blood moving herbs such as Ligusticum (Chuan Xiong) and Citrus peel (Chen Pi), as assistants with Qi or Blood tonics.

Individuals with weak digestion may find it difficult to digest tonics and even develop symptomatic Heat reactions such as dry mouth, irritability, insomnia, abdominal bloating, indigestion, nausea and loss of appetite. Food is considered the best tonic. Therefore, after a brief period of detoxification, the combination of tonic foods and herbs is superior and will often prevent adverse reactions when taking tonics. Even when taken with food, however, tonics may be better assimilated if they are combined with Qi and/or Blood regulating herbs such as Cardamon, Ginger and/or Ligusticum, for instance.

Most tonic herbs have a mild energy and can be cooked with rice or other cereals to make congee, as well as being used in various soups and stews. Following the Five Elements, salt goes to the Kidneys, so when tonifying the Kidneys it is always helpful to take the appropriate herbs with a pinch of salt. The sweet flavor goes to Earth-Spleen; thus for Spleen tonification a small amount of honey, barley or rice syrup or a raw unrefined sugar will serve as a carrier to the Spleen-Stomach.

The deepest levels of tonification will be more satisfactorily achieved if herbs are taken with animal protein. In Ayurvedic medicine, and for the general Hindu lacto-vegetarian diet, tonic herbs are usually combined with warm milk. In fact, Ayurveda predates Indian vegetarianism, so that its original texts describe the use of various flesh foods and animal parts to be used with herbs for Deficiency conditions. The Chinese Five Elements assign pork to the Kidneys and the cow, or beef, to the Spleen so that taking a minimum (say 2 to 4 ounces daily) of these corresponding flesh foods with the appropriate herbs will make them more powerfully assimilated and utilized. Many of the symptoms of Spleen Deficiency correspond in Western physiology to thyroid and pancreas weakness. This can be subclinical and may not be indicated in standard blood tests. It would be a good idea to combine the use of Spleen tonics with glandular extracts of thyroid and pancreas. For Kidney Deficiency, one should use adrenal extracts, the adrenal cortex extract for Yin Deficiency and the adrenal medulla extract for Yang Deficiency if they are available in this way. Similarly, combining organ extracts of Liver and Heart with corresponding tonic herbs will be more effective.

For Yang tonification, exercise is extremely important, while for Yin tonification, rest and sleep are best. Since Yin tonification cannot replace the value of sleep, prescribing calming and sedative herbs is

another method to indirectly tonify Yin. While tonics constitute the most renowned aspect of Chinese medicine, from a holistic perspective it is always a good idea to attempt to determine the underlying cause of a Deficiency. In most cases, Deficiencies are caused by stress, for which the best remedy is rest and good food.

QI TONICS

Panax Ginseng   **Ren Shen**   (1)

Common Name: Ginseng

Part Used: Root (Radix)

Family: Araliaceae

Energy and Flavor: sweet, slightly bitter and Warm

Organ Meridians Affected: Spleen, Lung and Heart

Actions: 1. Very strongly tonifies the Qi; 2. Tonifies the Lungs and Spleen; 3. Assists the body in the secretion of Fluids and stops thirst; 4. Strengthens the Heart and calms the Shen.

Indications: 1. For collapse of basal Qi with symptoms of very weak and thin pulse, abundant sweating, shallow breathing, extreme fatigue or shock; 2. For Deficiency of Lung and Spleen Qi with symptoms of shortness of breath, wheezing, difficulty in breathing, loss of appetite, diarrhea, fatigue and prolapse of the internal organs; 3. For wasting and thirsting disorder or dehydration in the aftermath of febrile diseases; 4. For weakness of the Heart caused by either Qi or Blood Deficiency with symptoms of palpitations, insomnia, restlessness and forgetfulness.

Contraindications: This herb should not be used by those with Yin Deficiency with Heat signs or by those with Heat because of Excess. It should also not be used when there are acute pathogenic conditions. It should be avoided by those with very high blood pressure.

Dosage: 3 - 9 grams, higher dosages are sometimes used for shock because of blood loss.

Notes: Ginseng is the premiere herb useful for all Deficiencies. It is, however, especially useful for Qi Deficiency. Add it to any formula for Qi tonification. Taken by itself, it is good for low energy caused by chronic weak digestion. There are different types of ginseng: Chinese white ginseng is somewhat Cooler than the precooked Chinese red ginseng; Korean red ginseng is considered even Warmer yet. American Ginseng (Panax Quinquefolium) is Cool and used to tonify Yin and Blood. The classics state that anyone past the age of 40 can take a little ginseng each day to maintain vitality and longevity. For optimum potency, ginseng needs to be at least 4 years old but the best is a minimum of 7 years. Wild ginseng is considered the most potent but at this point it is

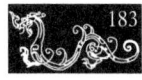

critically endangered, certainly in China, and now it is threatened in the United States. Ecologically minded consumers should insist on either woods grown or organically cultivated ginseng. Finally there is cultivated ginseng that comes in many grades and sizes. The most representative formula for Qi tonification is Four Major Herbs (Si Jun Zi Tang) which combines Chinese ginseng with Atractylodes (Bai Zhu), Poria (Fu Ling) and Licorice (Gan Cao).

Codonopsis Pilosula   **Dang Shen**   (1)
Common Name: Codonopsis
Part Used: Root (Radix)
Family: Campanulaceae
Energy and Flavor: sweet and neutral
Organ Meridians Affected: Spleen and Lung
Actions: 1. Tonifies the Spleen and Lung Qi; 2. Assists in the secretion of Bodily Fluids.
Indications: 1. For Deficiency of Spleen Qi with symptoms such as lack of appetite, fatigue, diarrhea, weakness of the limbs, and prolapse of internal organs; 2. For weakness of the Lungs with symptoms of shortness of breath, chronic cough or abundant sputum due to Spleen Qi Deficiency; 3. For Qi Deficiency that is not extreme or when there is Heat in the body that does not allow the use of radix Ginseng (Ren Shen);

4. For conditions such as wasting and thirsting disorder, dehydration resulting from febrile diseases and thirst due to injury to the Bodily Fluids; 5. This herb is sometimes given with herbs to release the Exterior or drain downward to protect the Righteous Qi when there are underlying indications of Qi Deficiency.

Contraindications: This herb should be used with caution when there is acute illness.

Dosage: 9 - 30 grams

Notes: Codonopsis is considered a milder substitute for ginseng (Ren Shen). To approximate the strength of ginseng, codonopsis is used in three times the amount. To restore the Qi, combine with Astragalus (Huang Qi); to stop urinary incontinence and excessive sweating combine with Astragalus (Huang Qi), Dragon Bone (Long Gu) and Oyster Shell (Mu Li); for Deficient Qi and Blood combine with Prepared Rehmannia (Shu Di Huang) and Angelica sinensis (Dang Gui); for lack of appetite and possibly loose stools and nausea, combine with Atractylodes (Bai Zhu).

Although it is often substituted for Ginseng (Ren Shen) in herbal patent medicine, this is primarily because it is cheaper. However, it is not nearly as strong in its tonifying properties.

Astragalus Membranaceus   Huang Qi   (1)
Common Name: Astragalus
Part Used: Root (Radix)
Family: Leguminosae
Energy and Flavor: sweet and slightly Warm
Organ Meridians Affected: Lung and Spleen

Actions: 1. Tonifies the Wei Qi and stops perspiration; 2. Tonifies the Spleen Qi and the Yang Qi of the Earth Element; 3. Tonifies the Qi and Blood; 4. Expels pus and assists in the healing of wounds; 5. Helps to regulate water metabolism in the body and reduce edema.

Indications: 1. For Deficiency of the Wei Qi and the Lungs (since the Wei resides in the Lungs) with symptoms of frequent colds and flus, shortness of breath, and spontaneous sweating; 2. For Deficiency of the Earth element with symptoms such as lack of appetite, prolapse of internal organs, diarrhea, fatigue and uterine bleeding; 3. For recovery from severe blood loss and postpartum bleeding; 4. For chronic abscesses and ulcers resulting from Deficiency; 5. For chronic Dampness and edema associated with Spleen Qi Deficiency.

Contraindications: This herb should not be used for case of Excess or Deficiency of Yin with Heat signs and should not be used when there is Stagnation of Qi with painful obstruction.

Dosage: 9 - 30 grams; much more can be used when indicated.

Notes: Astragalus tonifies the immune or "Wei Qi" and is a tonic herb for the prevention of colds, flus and other seasonal diseases. Wei Qi is that part of Yang that circulates just below the skin, imparting radiance and suppleness as well as being responsible for the reaction of goosebumps or shivers. By giving strength to the nervous system (the assumption is that a weakened immune system is concomitant with neurological weakness) and regulating the neurological reflex of the skin pores, it is able to contract the pores and regulate perspiration. Thus it prevents the penetration of the External Evils of Cold, Damp or Wind. For the prevention of colds and flus, combine it with Atractylodes (Bai Zhu) and Ledebouriella (Fang Feng) in the Jade Screen Combination (Yu Ping Feng San).

Wei is the functional, immunological or protective aspect of Qi and Yang, while Ying, associated with Blood and Yin, is the more substantive and nutritive aspect. These two qualities, Wei and Ying, are produced in the Lungs from the combination of Qi, extracted from air,

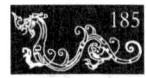

and food and fluid from the Spleen and Stomach. While Astragalus is a tonic, Cinnamon twigs (Gui Zhi) circulates Wei. Peony root (Bai Shao Yao), on the other hand, is used in many formulas to nourish the Ying, the physiological nutritive complement of Wei. These herbs are all combined together in Astragalus Combination (Huang Qi Jian Zhong Tang) that consists of Astragalus (Huang Qi), Maltose (Yi Tang), Cinnamon twig (Gui Zhi), White peony (Bai Shao Yao), Licorice (Gan Cao), Fresh Ginger (Sheng Jiang) and Jujube dates (Da Zao).

Astragalus, when combined with a smaller amount of Angelica sinensis (Dang Gui) is a blood tonic for treating anemia. Used either in formula or singly, it serves to regulate fluid metabolism, prevent bloating and counteract obesity. When combined with Licorice, it regulates blood sugar and is useful for both diabetes and hypoglycemia. It is commonly added to many tonic formulas, including those that contain Ginseng and/or Codonopsis (Dang Shen), to help the build immune system, stamina and endurance. A good combination for promoting health and longevity is Astragalus (Huang Qi) with Codonopsis (Dang Shen), Lycii berries (Gou Qi Zi), Polygonum multiflorum (He Shou Wu), and a small amount of both Angelica sinensis (Dang Gui) and Jujube dates (Da Zao). This can be made into a soup taken weekly or daily or cooked in rice congee (porridge).

Because of its popularity, there are many grades of Astragalus with a wide range of price. The best quality are large and long roots with a yellow pith and a sweet flavor when chewed. Chinese astragalus species are now under cultivation in North America.

Dioscorea Opposita   Shan Yao   (2)

Common Name: Dioscorea, Chinese Yam

Part Used: Root (Radix)

Family: Dioscoreaceae

Energy and Flavor: sweet and neutral

Organ Meridians Affected: Spleen, Lung, Kidney and Stomach

Actions: 1. Tonifies the Spleen and Stomach; 2. Tonifies the Lung Qi and nourishes the Lung Yin. 3. Nourishes the Kidneys and consolidates Jing; 4. Externally as a poultice.

Indications: 1. For Spleen and Stomach weakness with symptoms of chronic diarrhea, fatigue, loss of appetite, leukorrhea and spontaneous sweating; 2. For chronic cough due to Yin or Qi Deficiency, wheezing and asthma; 3. For weakness of the Kidney where the Kidney Qi is unable to hold the Jing with symptoms of spermatorrhea, frequent urination, vaginal discharge; also for wasting and thirsting disorders; 4. Can be applied externally as a poultice for carbuncles, boils and abscesses.

Contraindications: This herb should be used with caution when there is Excess Heat or Dampness, especially Dampness in the abdomen.

Dosage: 9-30 grams; a very large dosage can be used in special cases of wasting diseases.

Notes: The Chinese name translates as "mountain medicine" but it is also commonly known as "mountain potato", because it is widely used both in China and Japan as a food as well as a medicine. The tuber contains an abundance of starch, saponin, gum allantoin, choline, arginine, amino acids, amylase, protein, fat and other constituents. It is classified as sweet with a neutral energy, increasing its versatility as a nutritive tonic for the Lungs, Spleen and Kidneys.

This is a traditional food of Asian people and is currently being cultivated in Western herb gardens. In Asian cultures where both wild yam and soy products are regularly consumed, abnormal menopausal symptoms are practically unknown and the incidence of estrogen sensitive cancers such as breast cancer is much less. Because of both its delicious flavor and high nutrition, wild yam potato promises much wider acceptance throughout the West. This also offers the possibility of its eventually becoming a profitable cash crop. Each tuber is sizable and can be prepared in any manner that one might prepare the common potato: fried, baked or boiled in soups.

For lack of strength, general weakness, exhaustion and lack of appetite, powder 30 grams of Dioscorea (Shan Yao), add water and simmer until it is cooked. To this add rice wine or sweet wine to make a paste. This should be taken each evening on an empty stomach. Dioscorea can be made with sweet rice into a congee or simply added to soups. For urinary incontinence or lack of urine of the aged caused by debility and weakness, combine with Poria cocos (Fu Ling) and make into a similar paste described above. For diabetes combine 50 grams of Dioscorea tuber (Shan Yao), 15 grams each of Trichosanthes root (Gua Lou) and Adenophora (Nan Sha Shen), 10 grams of Anemarrhena (Zhi Mu) and 6 grams of Schisandra (Wu Wei Zi). This is decocted in 6 cups of water down to two or three cups which is taken daily in the same number of doses. For Kidney Deficiency combine Dioscorea with prepared Rehmannia (Shu Di Huang) and Cornus berries (Shan Zhu Yu). This can be taken for spermatorrhea and night sweats.

Atractylodes Macrocephala   Bai Zhu   (1)
Common Name: White Atractylodes
Part Used: Rhizome (Rhizoma)
Family: Compositae

Energy and Flavor: sweet, bitter and Warm

Organ Meridians Affected: Spleen and Stomach

Actions: 1. Tonifies the Spleen Qi; 2. Fortifies the Spleen Yang and dispels Damp; 3. Tonifies Qi and stops sweating; 4. Calms restless fetus when due to Deficiency of Spleen Qi.

Indications: 1. For Spleen Qi Deficiency with symptoms of lack of appetite, chronic diarrhea, fatigue, vomiting and abdominal distention; 2. For edema caused by retention of fluids and lack of urination; 3. For spontaneous sweating caused by Deficiency of Qi; 4. For restless fetus when caused by Deficiency of Spleen.

Contraindications: This herb should not be used by those with Yin Deficiency with Heat signs or with extreme thirst.

Dosage: 3 - 9 grams

Notes: Atractylodes (Bai Zhu) is one of the most revered tonic herbs of Chinese medicine. It is Warm and mildly stimulating to the Spleen and Stomach. As such it benefits digestion and regulates fluid metabolism. It can be used to regulate appetite and for weight control. It is commonly combined with Codonopsis (Dang Shen), Poria (Fu Ling) and Licorice (Gan Cao) for anorexia. This can be taken as a tea or a wine by soaking the powdered herbs in yellow rice wine for 10 days. This is then strained and bottled for use. A half cup can be taken 3 times daily on an empty stomach before meals.

Pseudostellaria Heterophylla   Tai Zi Shen   (3)

Common Name: Pseudostellaria

Part Used: Root (Radix)

Family: Caryophyllaceae

Energy and Flavor: sweet, slightly bitter and neutral

Organ Meridians Affected: Spleen and Lung

Actions: 1. Tonifies the Qi of the Lung and Spleen; 2. Assists the body in the production of Fluids.

Indications: 1. For Deficiency of Qi with symptoms of spontaneous sweating, fatigue and lack of appetite; 2. For injury to Bodily Fluids caused by febrile diseases, also for thirst.

Contraindications: This herb should not be used with Rhizoma et Radix Veratri (Li Lu).

Dosage: 9 - 30 grams

Notes: There is an herb called Starflower (Trientalis borealis) which I have used. It grows throughout the Pacific Northwest and has properties that are very similar to this herb.

Zizyphus Jujuba   **Da Zao**   (1)

Common Name: Jujube Date

Part Used: Fruit (Fructus)

Family: Rhamnaceae

Energy and Flavor: sweet and neutral

Organ Meridians Affected: Spleen and Stomach

Actions: 1. Tonifies the Spleen and Stomach Qi; 2. Tonifies the Blood; 3. Calms the Shen; 4. Moderates the actions of other herbs in formula.

Indications: 1. For Deficiency of Spleen and Stomach Qi with symptoms of fatigue, loose stools or diarrhea and lack of appetite; 2. For Deficiency of Blood where the Blood is unable to nourish the Organs; 3. For restless Shen with symptoms of irritability, palpitations and emotional distress; 4. Used to moderate the action of herbs in formula.

Contraindications: This herb should not be used when there are conditions of Dampness, Food Stagnation, intestinal parasites and dental diseases.

Dosage: 10 - 30 grams; this roughly calculates to 2 - 10 dates.

Notes: Jujube dates can be freely added to soups, rice congees (porridge) and to impart a pleasantly sweet flavor to herb teas. It is an inexpensive tonic that tonifies Qi and Blood, calms the spirit and generally strengthens the Stomach and Spleen. These trees are hardy in most temperate climates and produce an abundance of delicious fruits. They are available on special order from many commercial nursery outlets.

Polygonatum Sibiricum   **Huang Jing**   (3)

Common Name: Siberian Solomon Seal, Polygonatum

Part Used: Rhizome (Rhizoma)

Family: Liliaceae

Energy and Flavors: sweet, neutral

Organ Meridians Affected: Kidneys, Lungs and Spleen

Actions: 1. Tonifies the Spleen; 2. Moistens Dryness; 3. Tonifies the Kidneys and supplements Essence.

Indications: 1. For Spleen Deficiency with symptoms of fatigue and loss of appetite as well as the treatment of diabetes; 2. Dryness of the Lungs with Dry cough; 3. Kidney Qi Deficiency with Essence Deficiency, lower back pain, weakness of the legs and knees, exhaustion; 4. For wasting diseases such as TB and AIDS.

Contraindications: Not to be used for Spleen Deficiency with Dampness and poor digestion as this herb is very dampening.

Dosage: 6 to 20 grams. This herb has a mild energy and can be used as a tonic for several months if needed.

Notes: There are very similar species called Polygonatum biflorum that grow in the Northeastern to Midwest forests of North America. It was used by the natives in a similar manner as the Chinese species for general debility, indigestion, rheumatism, arthritis, lung disorders as well as for other conditions such as profuse menstruation, to promote sound sleep and externally to promote the healing of cuts and bruises. Northeastern American Polygonatum is probably as good or better than the imported Chinese variety.

Glycyrrhizae Uralensis   Gan Cao   (1)
Common Name: Chinese Licorice
Part Used: Root (Radix)
Family: Leguminosae
Energy and Flavor: sweet and neutral
Organ Meridians Affected: All 12 meridians

Actions: 1. Tonifies the Basal Qi and nourishes the Spleen Qi; 2. Clears Heat and dispels toxicity; 3. Moistens the Lungs; 4. Relieves spasms and alleviates pain; 5. Harmonizes and moderates herbs in formulas.

Indications: 1. For Deficiency of Spleen Qi with symptoms of shortness of breath, diarrhea, fatigue, palpitations and irregular pulse caused by either Qi or Blood Deficiency; 2. For Fire and toxicity with symptoms of sore throat, carbuncles or sores, it can be used both internally and externally for these symptoms; 3. For either Heat or Cold in the Lungs with symptoms of Dry cough and wheezing; 4. Mildly relieves spasms and thus pain in the abdomen or legs; 5. Used in many formulas to harmonize and moderate the action of the other herbs in the formula.

Contraindications: Licorice should not be used when there is Excess Dampness, nausea or vomiting and generally should be used with caution by those who tend to retain water.

Dosage: 2 - 9 grams

Notes: Licorice is one of the most commonly used of all Chinese herbs. However, it is generally used in small amounts because of its mineralocorticoid-like effects. These include the decrease of urinary output and sodium excretion and the increased secretion of potassium. For conditions such as Addison's disease, if Licorice is prescribed with cortisone, the dosage of cortisone can be reduced. Glycyrrhetinic acid, one of the constituents of Licorice, is anti-inflammatory but weaker than cortisone.

Because it can alleviate many allergic reactions and lessen the toxicity of many toxic substances (especially alkaloids which are found in many herbs), Licorice is commonly added to herbal formulas as an adjunctive

herb because it counteracts most possible adverse reactions either to herbs or their combinations in formulas. Licorice is contraindicated in individuals who are prone to edema or fluid retention. It also offers promise for helping to prevent a variety of allergic reactions to various substances such as foods and herbs. Because women are generally more prone to having an extra fat layer to prepare their body for childbirth, this being in the category of Dampness, this necessitates that Licorice be generally used in even smaller amounts and for shorter duration in women's formulas. When Licorice is intended for its Qi tonic properties, it is always taken in prepared form which is stir fried in honey. This is easily done by taking dry Licorice and mixing a little honey on it as it is gently heated in a wok or open skillet. The best quality honey fried Licorice is not too sticky, which makes it more difficult to handle. To prevent this, use less honey.

Saccharum Granorum   Yi Tang   (3)

Common Name: Maltose

Properties: Sweet, slightly Warm

Organ Meridians Affected: Lungs, Spleen and Stomach

Actions: 1. Fortifies Qi and tonifies the Spleen; 2. Soothes and tonifies the Middle Warmer; 3. Lubricates the Lungs.

Indications: 1. For exhaustion and fatigue of the Spleen with shortness of breath and low appetite; 2. For abdominal pains caused by Coldness and Deficiency of the Stomach; 3. For dry, unproductive coughs with labored, slow breathing caused by Lung Qi Deficiency.

Contraindications: Not to be used for symptoms of Dampness and Heat.

Dosage: 30 to 60 grams dissolved as an end process in a strained decoction.

Notes: Many are surprised to find that sugar is considered a Qi tonic. Maltose is a special form of sugar, however, made from malted barley. As such it has fuller nutritional value. Sugar can create heat in the body, and an excess of refined sugar especially is one of the most detrimental influences on our health. However, the use of whole, unrefined sugar from any natural source possesses all the minerals and accompanying nutrients of the whole plant and is a much more acceptable form to take it in.

Discrimination:

Ginseng (Ren Shen) — tonic for all Deficiencies, stops thirst, lubricates, calms Shen.

Codonopsis Pilosula (Dang Shen) — milder ginseng substitute.

Astragalus Membranaceus (Huang Qi) – tonifies Wei Qi (immune system) and Blood, stops perspiration, expels pus, regulates fluid metabolism.

Dioscorea Opposita (Shan Yao) – nourishes Lung Yin, nourishes Kidneys, consolidates Jing.

Atractylodes Macrocephala (Bai Zhu) – tonifies Spleen Yang, dispels Dampness, promotes digestion.

PseudoStellaria Heterophylla (Tai Zi Shen) – lubricates and supplements body fluids.

Zizyphus Jujuba (Da Zao) – nourishes Blood, calms Shen, harmonizes other herbs in formula.

Polygonatum Sibiricum (Huang Jing) – neutral energy, tonifies Kidneys and Essence.

Glycyrrhizae Uralensis (Gan Cao) – clears Heat, relieves pain, moistens the Lungs, harmonizes herbs in formulas.

Saccharum Granorum (Yi Tang) – supplements the Qi, moistens and lubricates.

HERBS THAT TONIFY THE BLOOD

Angelica sinensis   **Dang Gui**   (1)

Common Name: Dong Quai, Chinese Angelica

Part Used: Root (Radix)

Family: Umbelliferae

Energy and Flavor: sweet, acrid, bitter and Warm

Organ Meridians Affected: Heart, Liver and Spleen

Actions: 1. Tonifies the Blood; 2. Lubricates the Intestines; 3. Promotes circulation and dispels Bi Pain.

Indications: 1. For Deficiency of Blood with symptoms of pale complexion, blurred vision, menstrual disorders and palpitations; 2. For constipation due to Blood Deficiency; 3. Promotes circulation and nourishes the Blood for painful obstruction caused by Cold and Stagnation of Blood.

Contraindications: Not for those with diarrhea, abdominal distention caused by Dampness or those with Yin Deficiency with Heat signs.

Dosage: 3 - 9 grams

Notes: The Chinese name translates as "Ought-To-Return" which is connected with an ancient Chinese legend: Once there was a distant mountain upon which grew an abundance of precious herbs. Because it was so steep and dangerous, few attempted to scale its heights to bring back its herbal treasures. One young man, declaring himself the bravest

of all to his friends, boasted that he would climb the mountain to fetch some of the precious herbs. Since there was a good chance that the young man may never return from such a hazardous adventure, his mother insisted that he first marry the beautiful village maiden to whom he was betrothed. This was so that the young bride would be able to assist her in her old age.

As feared, the young man was gone a long time, for over three years, and everyone, including his mother, assumed that he must be dead. The mother, having grown fond of her devoted daughter in law, eventually told her that it would be good for her to remarry. The faithful wife at first hesitated in loyalty to her husband. Resigning herself to the fact that her husband indeed must be dead, she eventually married. The day after her marriage her first husband returned from the mountain. At first he was greeted by his friends and all the village folk for his courage and the wonderful herbs he brought back. The young woman, hearing of this, burst into tears of sadness and remorse which made her very sick. The young man knew that one of the herbs he had picked was the greatest of all women's tonics. Out of compassion, he decocted it into a tea and gave it to her to drink to alleviate her melancholy. The herb was, of course, the most famous herb of all for women, Dang Gui. As a result the woman soon recovered from her sickness and the people never forgot the power of Dang Gui for all women's complaints, including prolonged sadness and melancholy.

In commemoration of this event a Chinese poet wrote, "He ought to return sooner but failed, she ought to wait longer, but failed to wait." The herb has since been called "Dang Gui" meaning, "Ought-To-Return". — Paraphrased from *Legendary Chinese Healing Herbs* by Henry Lu, published by Sterling.

Dang Gui is one of the five most popularly used Chinese herbs. A closely related species, Angelica Acutiloba, is used as Dang Gui by the Japanese who regard it as superior to Angelica sinensis. This again denotes how there are often many subspecies that the Chinese use interchangeably. It is one of the unique herbs that contain vitamin B 12 and vitamin E. It also contains ferulic acid, succinic acid, nicotinic acid, uracil, adenine, butylidenephalide, ligustilide, folinic acid, and biotin, the combination of which encompasses a number of essential nutrients that are sold in health and natural food stores. Dang Gui has been extensively researched and studied. Two biochemical constituents have been found, one is a water-soluble and nonvolatile constituent that stimulates the uterus while the other is alcohol soluble and consists of an essential oil with a high boiling point. This second constituent has an opposite relaxing effect on the uterus as well as increasing DNA synthesis and the growth of uterine tissue.

The high content of vitamin B 12 (0.25 to 0.4 ug/100 g dried root) together with biotin and folic acid stimulates hematopoiesis in the bone marrow and has an antiplatelet action as well.

This herb figures in most prescriptions that require tonification and circulation of Blood. It is the most popular Chinese woman's herb but has many uses for certain conditions of men as well. It is used to stimulate blood production for anemia, regulate bleeding, relieve pain, and to relax the uterus. It is used for all types of anemia including pernicious anemia. One of the most common combinations used for Blood tonification is Dang Gui Four (Si Wu Tang) with Angelica sinensis (Dang Gui), Ligusticum (Chuan Xiong), Prepared Rehmannia (Shu Di Huang) and White Peony (Bai Shao).

Rehmannia Glutinosa — Shu Di Huang (1)

Common Name: Cooked Rehmannia

Part Used: Root (Radix)

Family: Scrophulariaceae

Energy and Flavor: sweet and slightly Warm

Organ Meridians Affected: Heart, Liver and Kidney

Actions: 1. Tonifies the Blood; 2. Tonifies the Yin of the Kidneys.

Indications: 1. One of the most commonly used herbs for Blood Deficiency. It can be used for any symptoms associated with Blood and Yin Deficiency provided it does not aggravate a tendency towards Spleen Dampness, as this herb is very heavy, sticky and damp and can be difficult to digest; 2. For Kidney Yin Deficiency with symptoms of night sweats, chronic low grade fever, dry mouth, tinnitus, premature graying of the hair and wasting and thirsting disorder.

Contraindications: This herb should be used with caution by those with weak digestion and Spleen Qi; it should be avoided by those with Stagnation of Qi or Phlegm.

Dosage: 9 - 30 grams

Notes: One of the most important and frequently prescribed herbs in Chinese herbalism. Rehmannia roots are prepared with rice wine and are often combined with Cardamon (Sha Ren) and tangerine peel (Chen Pi) to aid circulation and counteract its effect of causing digestive Stagnation. The roots are steamed and dried in the sun several times (nine times according to Chinese numerology, since the number nine signifies completion). It is a beautiful garden flower of which it and various related species (R. elata) are grown in the West as an ornamental.

Rehmannia is classified as a Blood tonic for symptoms of weakness and anemia, but it is used as much or more as a Kidney and Liver Yin

tonic for symptoms associated with aging, fatigue, Dryness, muscle, bone and joint problems, dizziness, vertigo, lower back and joint pains, hearing and eye problems. For gynecological problems and anemia it is combined with Angelica (Dang Gui), White Peony (Bai Shao) and Ligusticum (Chuan Xiong) for Blood tonification in the formula known as Dang Gui Four (Si Wu Tang). As a Kidney and Liver Yin Tonic, it is the major herb in Rehmannia Six (Liu wei di huang wan), with Cornus fruit (Shan Zhu Yu) and Dioscorea (Shan Yao). For Yin Deficiency it is combined with Tortoise plastron (Gui Ban), Anemarrhena (Zhi Mu) and Phellodendron (Huang Bai) in Anemarrhena and Phellodendron Combination (Zhi bai di huang wan).

Polygonum Multiflorum   He Shou Wu   (2)
Common Name: He Shou Wu, Fleeceflower, Ho Shou Wu, Fo Ti Tieng
Part Used: Root (Radix)
Family: Polygonaceae
Energy and Flavors: sweet, bitter, astringent and slightly Warm
Organ Meridians Affected: Liver and Kidney
Actions: 1. Nourishes the Liver, Kidneys and Essence; 2. Tonifies the Blood; 3. Moistens the Intestines; 4. The raw form of this herb is used for Fire and toxicity.
Indications: 1. For Deficiency of Yin or Blood with symptoms of dizziness, premature graying of the hair, soreness of the back or knees, blurred vision or insomnia; 2. For Deficiency of Blood; 3. For constipation due to either Blood or Yin Deficiency; 4. For symptoms of Fire and toxicity such as boils, abscesses, goiter and scrofula; the raw form of this herb is used for this application.
Contraindications: This herb should not be used by those with diarrhea or when there are Phlegm conditions associated with Spleen Deficiency.
Dosage: 9 - 30 grams. No form of He Shou Wu should ever be cooked in a metal container because the chemistry of the herbs is altered by metal.
Notes: This herb has mistakenly come to be known as Fo Ti Tieng, for which it is still popularly sold. The Chinese name He Shou Wu literally translates as He's Black Hair. It refers to an old legend of General He who was convicted of a serious crime and sentenced to confinement and death in a remote cell dug into the ground without food nor water. After a year, upon returning to remove his remains for burial, his executioners were surprised to find that not only had General He not died, but he had gone through a complete rejuvenation to the extent that even his hair regained its normal dark color. They had discovered that without food and water, General He was forced onto an exclusive diet of a vine-

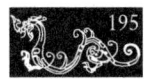

like herb which invaded the crevices of his cell. Since that time, the herb has been named He Shou Wu, in remembrance of General He's survival and physical rejuvenation.

Another somewhat different story reported by Li Ao in 813 A.D. describes how the properties of He Shou Wu restored the sexual potency of a man, allowing him to father a son, regain his normal hair color and live to the age of 160 years. While both stories are unsubstantiated, they both attest to the belief in the rejuvenative properties of He Shou Wu.

The chemistry of He Shou Wu resembles human adrenocortical hormones. These include chrysophenol, emodin, emodin methyl ester, rhein and the glycoside rhaphantin. In addition it contains a large quantity of lecithin and other glycosides. The herb is safe and non-toxic even for long term consumption. Because emodin has a slight laxative effect, to increase its tonic properties, He Shou Wu is steamed with black soya beans and Chinese yellow rice wine. This causes the dried pharmaceutical herb to have a characteristic reddish-brown color.

It is probably the lecithin contained in the herb that serves to impede the uptake of cholesterol from the plasma of the liver and prevent its deposit as plaque along the inner arterial walls. Because of this and other biochemical mechanisms, it seems to have the power to reduce the heart rate while at the same time slightly increasing the circulation of blood through the heart. It is also very good for lower back pain caused by Blood and Kidney Essence Deficiency.

He Shou Wu is a fast growing vine that has been recently grown in the West. It is very easy to cultivate from root cuttings. The stalk and leaves are also used both for insomnia and to clear inflammation, for the treatment of various skin diseases and itching.

Besides the legends surrounding the origin of its name, even further seeming miraculous properties are ascribed to the plant. In the Pent s'ao of Li Shi Shen, it is reported that "At fifty years of age, the root is as large as a fist and is called 'mountain slave'; if taken for one year, it will preserve the black color of the hair and mustache; at one hundred years, it is as large as a bowl and is called 'hill brother'. If taken for a year, a rubicund and cheerful countenance will be preserved. At one hundred and fifty years it is as large as a basin and is called 'hill uncle'. If this is taken for one year, the teeth will fall out and grow afresh. At two hundred years it is the size of a one peck osier basket and is called 'hill father'. If this is taken for a year the countenance will become like that of a youth and the gait will equal that of a running horse. Finally, at three hundred years it is the size of a three peck osier basket and it is called 'mountain spirit'. At this stage it is regarded as having a pure ethereal substance,

which if taken for an extended period of time, one becomes an earthly immortal."– Chinese Materia Medica by G.A. Stuart, reprinted by Southern Materials Center, Inc.

In 1930, papers throughout the Western world reported the death of master Li Ch'ing Yuen at the documented age of 252. Born in 1678, he became a practicing herbalist, renowned for his health and vitality. At the age of fifty, he met an older man who could outwalk him. Impressed, he came to appreciate the fact that a brisk daily walk was the best exercise for health and longevity. The older man also told him of the benefits of Lycii berries, which he daily consumed in a soup.

Throughout the years, Li Ch'ing Yuen attracted many followers. They were impressed with his ability to outwalk many who were but a fraction of his age. They also were amazed at the sharpness of his eyesight and of all his senses. During one of his walks Li Ch'ing Yuen met an old Taoist hermit who claimed himself to be 500 years of age. From this man, Li further learned secret Taoist Yoga practices called Chi Gong. This man recommended that Li Ch'ing Yuen consume little meat or root vegetables and limit his consumption of grains. Each day he was told by his mentor to take a small dose of Panax Ginseng and Polygonum Multiflorum. A simple but perfect combination, since one tonifies Qi while the other nourishes Blood. Whatever the reasons, Li Ch'ing Yuen was reported to have married 14 times and to have outlived eleven generations. For those of us who have had to survive the many feasts of birthdays and holidays, we can appreciate the fact that Li Ch'ing Yuen died after a banquet presented in his honor by a government official.

The caulis or vine of He Shou Wu, called Ye Jiao Teng, is sweet, slightly bitter and neutral. It enters the Heart and Liver Organ meridians and is used to nourish the Blood, calm the spirit, and alleviate itching when applied externally. The dose is 9-30 grams.

Paeonia Lactiflora   **Bai Shao** (1)

Common Name: White Peony

Part Used: Root (Radix)

Family: Ranunculaceae

Energy and Flavors: bitter, sour and slightly Cold

Organ Meridians Affected: Liver and Spleen

Actions: 1. Tonifies the Blood and preserves the Yin; 2. Nourishes the Liver and assists in the smooth flow of Qi.

Indications: 1. For menstrual disorders associated with Deficiency of Blood; 2. Stabilizes and supports the Yin for Exterior Wind-Cold conditions that do not resolve with sweating and for Yin Deficiency conditions where

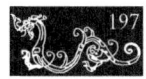

there is sweating; 2. For Deficiency of Liver Blood or Yin where the Liver Yang is aggressive, causing symptoms of pain in the flanks or abdomen, pain associated with menses, spasms throughout the body or "Liver attacking Spleen" conditions.

Contraindications: This herb should not be used by those with diarrhea and Spleen and Stomach Deficiency.

Dosage: 3 - 12 grams

Notes: Peony root combines antispasmodic, blood moving and blood nourishing properties. The North American Eclectic herbalists, as described in King's American Dispensatory, describe it as antispasmodic and tonic. He claims that it was successfully used by them "for chorea, epilepsy, spasms, and various nervous affections". This corroborates the use in traditional Chinese medicine, since by nourishing the Blood and the Fluids, the tension of the inner Organs is released, maintaining the integrity of their substance (Yin) and allowing for better functional coordination between them. Two forms of Peony are used, the red (Chi Shao) and the white (Bai Shao). In earlier times, there was no distinction between them. Only in more recent times has White Peony (Bai Shao) been distinguished as more of a Blood tonic and Red Peony (Chi Shao) as a Blood Moving herb.

For Deficient Blood, it is usually combined with Angelica (Dang Gui), Prepared Rehmannia (Shu Di Huang) and Ligusticum (Chuan Xiong); for muscle spasms of the extremities and abdominal cramps and pains it is combined with Licorice root; for Liver Qi Stagnation, it is combined with Bupleurum (Chai Hu) and Angelica (Dang Gui) in the formula Bupleurum and Peony Combination (Xiao Yao San). For weakness of the body caused by invasion of External evils of Wind and Cold, it is combined with Cinnamon twigs (Gui Zhi); for Deficient Blood and Yin causing the Yang to float upward to the surface giving rise to spontaneous perspiration, menopausal hot flashes and other superficial body symptoms, it is combined with Dragon Bone (Long Gu) and Sprouted Wheat (Fu Xiao Mai).

Lycii Barbarum   Gou Qi Zi (1)

Common Name: Lycii Berry, Chinese Wolfberry

Part Used: Fruit (Fructus)

Family: Solanaceae

Energy and Flavors: sweet and neutral

Organ Meridians Affected: Liver, Kidney and Lung

Actions: 1. Tonifies the Blood and Yin of the Liver and brightens the eyes.; 2. Tonifies the Yin of the Kidneys and Lungs.

Indications: 1. For Deficiency of the Liver with symptoms of blurred vision, poor night vision or any signs of Blood or Yin Deficiency of the Liver; 2. For Yin Deficiency of the Kidneys and Lungs with symptoms of dry consumptive cough, wasting and thirsting disorder, impotence, nocturnal emissions and sore lower back and knees.

Contraindications: This herb should not be used by those with patterns of Heat and Excess, nor should it be used when there is Spleen Deficiency with Dampness or loose stools.

Dosage: 6 - 18 grams

Notes: Lycii berries are most commonly classified as a Blood tonic but are more often used as a Yin tonic. The Chinese call them "red raisins" and add them freely to different types of soups and rice porridge. It is a nutritionally dense herb with beta carotene, thiamine, riboflavin, vitamin C, linoleic acid and the hormone precursor, beta sitosterol. It is a delicious food-grade herb that should be regularly used in every household along with other herbs that can be added to soups and cereals such as Astragalus root (Huang Qi), Codonopsis (Dang Shen), Dioscorea (Shan Yao), Jujube dates (Da Zao) and so on. Lycii berries were one of the herbs that the legendary Li Ch'ing Yuen, the Chinese Taoist who supposedly lived to 252 years of age, dying in 1930, took each day. Eventually he added Polygonum multiflorum (He Shou Wu) and Ginseng (Ren Shen), but this at least exemplifies the value and importance of Lycii berries.

They are combined with Chrysanthemum flowers (Ju Hua) for improving vision, relieving tinnitus, headache and as a Liver and Kidney Yin tonic. The best quality Lycii berries are large, soft and sweet. A species of this plant grows in the desert region of the Southwestern area of North America where they were harvested and eaten as a food by local Native Americans.

Gelatinum Corii Asini **E Jiao**

(Equus Asinus)

Common Name: Ass Hide Gelatin

Family: Equidae

Energy and Flavors: sweet, neutral

Organ Meridians Affected: Kidney, Liver, Lungs

Actions: 1. Tonifies and nourishes Blood; 2. Stops bleeding; 3. Moistens and lubricates Yin.

Indications: 1. Dizziness, pale complexion and palpitations; 2. Bleeding with coughing of blood, blood in the stool, excessive menstruation and uterine bleeding; 3. For Yin Deficiency with symptoms of irritability, insomnia and Yin Deficient Heat; 4. Coughs caused by Lung Yin Deficiency.

Preparation: It should be dissolved in the strained decoction, dissolved in red wine or taken in pills.

Contraindications: Not for External conditions or conditions associated with Dampness caused by Spleen Deficiency.

Dosage: 3 - 15 grams.

Notes: Originally only the black donkey skin was used, probably because the Chinese believe that black corresponds to the color of Kidney-Water which houses the source Qi. However, nowadays, probably any donkey skin is used. It is regularly taken by older women to counteract symptoms of Dryness associated with age. They dissolve a whole piece of gelatin in boiling water, keep it refrigerated in a jar and take daily spoonfulls as a Blood and Yin tonic. Interestingly, in the early part of this century, Gelatin taken with sweet port wine was considered a treatment for anemia. It is used for Blood Deficiency with anemia, heart palpitations, vertigo and pale complexion or insomnia with Blood vacuity accompanied with empty Heat. It is also used for spasms and trembling which are the result of Liver Blood or Yin Deficiency generating Liver Wind as well as constipation caused by Blood Deficiency and Dryness of the Large Intestine.

Arillus Euphoria Longanae   Long Yan Rou (3)

Common Name: Longan Berries, Dragon's Eye

Part Used: Fruit (Fructus)

Family: Sapindaceae

Energies and Flavors: sweet, Warm

Organ Meridians Affected: Heart, Spleen

Actions: 1. Nourishes the Blood; 2. Calms the spirit; 3. Relieves fatigue, especially mental fatigue.

Indications: 1. Can be used for anxiety, neurosis, insomnia, forgetfulness; 2. Heart palpitations caused by Heart Blood Deficiency; 3. Exhaustion and fatigue caused by Spleen Deficiency; 4. Exhaustion caused by worry, over-thinking or overwork.

Contraindications: Not for conditions of Dampness and Heat.

Dosage: 6 - 15 grams. They can also be eaten as a confection or food.

Notes: This herb is naturally high in glucose and sucrose which is responsible for its ability to nourish Heart Blood. Because the brain consumes a large amount of energy, individuals who study or excessively overuse their brain commonly have stronger-than-normal sugar cravings. As a result, the dried fruits are often consumed as a sweet confection.

For Deficient Qi and Blood with symptoms of palpitations, insomnia and forgetfulness, Longan berries are combined with Ginseng (Ren Shen), Astragalus root (Huang Qi), Angelica (Dang Gui) and Zizyphus seeds (Suan Zao Ren) in the formula called Ginseng and Longan Combination (Gui Pi Tang).

Morus Alba   Sang Shen   (3)

Common Name: Mulberry

Part Used: Fruit (Fructus)

Family: Moraceae

Energy and Flavors: sweet and Cold

Organ Meridians Affected: Liver, Heart and Kidney

Actions: 1. Tonifies the Blood and nourishes the Yin.

Indications: 1. For Deficiency of the Blood and Yin with symptoms of dizziness, tinnitus, constipation due to Blood Deficiency, wasting and thirsting disorder, insomnia and premature graying of the hair.

Contraindications: This herb should not be used by those with diarrhea due to Spleen Deficiency.

Dosage: 9 - 30 grams

Notes: Mulberries are a delicious way to supplement the Yin and nourish the Blood. For Liver and Kidney Yin Deficiency combine with Polygonum multiflorum (He Shou Wu), Eclipta (Han Lian Cao), and Ligustrum berries (Nu Zhen Zi); for thirst and dry mouth caused by Deficient Body Fluids or diabetes, combine with Ophiopogon (Mai Men Dong), Ligustrum fruit (Nu Zhen Zi) and Trichosanthes root (Tian Hua Fen); for constipation caused by Dryness of the Intestines combine with Black Sesame seeds (Hei Zhi Ma), Hemp seed (Huo Ma Ren), raw Polygonum multiflorum (He Shou Wu).

Discrimination:

Rehmannia Glutinosa (Shu Di Huang) – nourishes Kidney Yin.

Polygonum Multiflorum (He Shou Wu) – nourishes the Liver, Kidneys and Essence, lubricates the Intestines.

Angelica Sinensis (Dang Gui) – lubricates the Intestines, moves Blood, relieves pain, gynecological tonic.

Paeonia Lactiflora (Bai Shao) – preserves Yin, nourishes the Liver, helps smooth the flow of Qi.

Lycii (Gou Qi Zi) – tonifies Yin of Kidneys and Lungs, brightens vision.

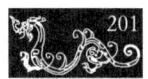

Gelatinum Corii Asini (E Jiao) – nourishes the Blood, stops bleeding, lubricates Yin.

Arillus Euphoria Longanae (Long Yan Rou) – nourishes the Blood, calms the Spirit, relieves mental fatigue.

Morus Alba (Sang Shen) – nourishes Yin, lubricates Dryness.

HERBS THAT TONIFY THE YANG

Cornu Cervi Parvum   Lu Rong   (1)
(Cervus Nippon)
Common Name: Deer Antler (Usually from the Sitka red deer)
Family: Cervidae
Energy and Flavors: sweet, salty, Warm
Organ Meridians: Affected: Kidneys and Liver

Actions: 1. Tonifies Kidney Yang; 2. Tonifies the Governor vessel (spine meridian); 3. Augments Essence and growth; 4. Strengthens the sinews and bones; 5. Treats infertility and impotence; 6. Tonifies Qi and Blood.

Indications: 1. For Kidney Yang Deficiency patterns including impotence, fatigue, Coldness, dizziness, tinnitus, weakness of the lower back and extremities, frequent, clear urination; 2. Maldevelopment of children, rickets, learning disabilities, mental retardation, failure to thrive; 3. Strengthens the bones (for healing fractures and osteoporosis) and ligaments; 4. Female infertility, uterine Coldness, Cold Deficient uterine bleeding and vaginal discharge; 5. Sores that do not heal.

Contraindications: This is a powerful Yang tonic and one should begin with a low dose and gradually increase. Too much can cause hyperactive Yang symptoms, including hypertension with dizziness, red eyes and conjunctivitis. It can also injure the Yin and cause hemorrhage. It is therefore strongly contraindicated in patients with Yin Deficiency with patterns of Heat.

Dosage: 3 - 9 grams as a powder divided into two or three daily doses. It can also be boiled into a tea or soaked in rice wine.

Notes: For Deficient Kidney Yang with Coldness, aversion to cold, impotence in men and frigidity in women, frequent urination, aching in the lower back and knees, dizziness, tinnitus, gradual hearing loss, lack of motivation and drive combine with Ginseng (Ren Shen), Eucommia (Du Zhong), Epimedium (Yin Yang Huo), Cuscuta seed (Tu Si Zi) and Prepared Rehmannia (Shu Di Huang). For Deficiency of Blood and Essence with weakness of the bones and maldevelopment in children, combine with Rehmannia Six Combination (Liu wei di huang wan).

Other antler byproducts: Antler from other deer species is a weaker substitute for Lu Rong, so the dosage used should be higher, 5 to 10 grams. Antler glue (Lu Jiao Jiao) is made from mature deer antlers. It is recommended for general bodily weakness, vomiting, epistaxis, uterine bleeding, blood in the urine and Yin boils. Dosage is again 5 to 10 grams. Deglutinated antler powder is the residue after a prolonged cooking of deer antler. It is similar to deer antler (Lu Jiao) but weaker.

Eucommiae Ulmoidis   Du Zhong   (1)

Common Name: Eucommia

Part Used: Bark (Cortex)

Family: Eucommiaceae

Energy and Flavors: sweet, slightly acrid and Warm

Organ Meridians Affected: Kidney and Liver

Actions: 1. Tonifies the Liver and Kidneys; 2. Calms ascendant Liver Yang (hypertension/high blood pressure); 3. Calms a restless fetus.

Indications: 1. For Deficiency of the Liver and Kidneys with symptoms of weak bones and muscles (especially the lower back and knees), fatigue, frequent urination and impotence. This herb is also sometimes used to assist the Liver with the smooth flow of Qi and Blood. 2. For ascendant Liver Yang with symptoms of dizziness and headache; 3. For Cold from Deficiency causing bleeding or threatened miscarriage, also good for pregnant women who have back pain due to Deficiency.

Contraindications: This herb should not be used by those with Heat signs associated with Yin Deficiency; it should not be used in conjunction with Radix Scrophularia ningpoensis (Xuan Shen).

Dosage: 6 - 12 grams

Notes: For impotence and frequent urination from Deficient Kidney Yang combine with Cornus (Shan Zhu Yu) and Cuscuta (Tu Si Zi); for lower back pain and weakness of the legs and knees combine with Psoraleae (Bu Gu Zhi) and Walnut (Hu Tao Ren); for threatened miscarriage combine with Dipsacus (Xu Duan) and Dioscorea (Shan Yao); for high blood pressure combine with Scutellaria (Huang Qin).

Dipsaci Asperi   Xu Duan   (1)

Common Name: Dipsacus, Teasel

Part Used: Root (Radix)

Family: Dipsacaceae

Energy and Flavors: bitter, acrid and Warm

Organ Meridians Affected: Kidney and Liver

Actions: 1. Tonifies the Liver and Kidneys; 2. Assists in the healing of bones; 3. Both stops bleeding and moves Blood; 4. Calms the fetus.

Indications: 1. For Deficiency of the Liver and Kidneys with symptoms such as weakness of the bones and sinews, stiffness of the joints and sore lower back and knees; 2. For fractures and tendon injuries; 3. For uterine bleeding caused by Deficiency, and both internally and externally for trauma as it moves Blood, reduces pain and assists in the healing process; 4. For restless fetus, threatened miscarriage and uterine bleeding during pregnancy.

Contraindications: This herb should not be used by those with Yin Deficiency with signs of Heat.

Dosage: 6 - 18 grams

Notes: The Chinese name "Xu Duan" means "Heal Fracture" and describes one of the most characteristic uses for this herb. It is one of the important herbs for back pain, weakness of tendons, bones, legs and knees. It is particularly useful because, having tonic and blood moving properties, it will not cause Stagnation.

Psoraleae Corylifoliae   Bu Gu Zhi   (2)

Common Name: Psoralea

Part Used: Fruit (Fructus)

Family: Leguminosae

Energy and Flavors: acrid, bitter and very Warm

Organ Meridians Affected: Kidney and Spleen

Actions: 1. Tonifies the Kidney Yang and augments Kidney Qi; 2. Tonifies the Spleen Yang; 3. Restrains leakage of Essence (Jing) and holds urine; 4. Applied topically for psoriasis and vitiligo.

Indications: 1. For Deficiency of Kidney Yang with symptoms of impotence, Cold and weak lower back and knees and weakness in the extremities; also for Kidney unable to grasp the Qi of the Lung; 2. For Deficiency of Spleen Yang where there is Cold diarrhea which is chronic and often "daybreak diarrhea," borborygmus and abdominal pain; 3. For leakage of Essence (Jing) and urine with symptoms of spermatorrhea, frequent urination, urinary incontinence and enuresis; 4. Has recently been used both topically and by injection for psoriasis, vitiligo and alopecia. It has anti-fungal properties.

Contraindications: This herb should not be used by those with Deficiency of Yin when there are Heat signs. It may be hard on the Stomach.

Dosage: 3 - 9 grams

Notes: For impotence, premature ejaculation and seminal emission make the following: Psoralea (Bu Gu Zhi) 12g, Euryale seed (Qian Shi) 12g, Lycii berries (Gou Qi Zi) 12g, Cuscuta seed (Tu Si Zi) 24g, Oyster shell

(Mu Li) 24g, Chinese Chives (Jiu Zi) 9g, taken once or twice daily or as needed. For enuresis and incontinence grind into a powder with equal parts Mantis Case (Sang Piao Xiao) and take 3 grams with salt water two or three times daily. For cock's crow diarrhea (before sunrise) caused by Deficient Kidney and Spleen Yang combine with Nutmeg (Rou Dou Kou), Schisandra (Wu Wei Zi) and Evodia (Wu Zhu Yu) in Four Miraculous Drugs Combination (Si Shen Wan). For impotence and seminal emission combine with Cuscuta (Tu Si Zi) and Walnut (Hu Tao Ren).

Juglandis Regiae   Hu Tao Ren   (3)
Common Name: Walnut
Part Used: Seed (Semen)
Family: Juglandaceae
Energy and Flavors: sweet and Warm
Organ Meridians Affected: Lung, Kidney and Large Intestine
Actions: 1. Tonifies the Kidney Yang; 2. Assists the Kidney Qi to grasp the Qi of the Lungs while Warming and astringent to the Lungs; 3. Lubricates the Intestines; 4. Helps with urinary stones; 5. Applied topically for superficial inflammation.
Indications: 1. For Deficiency of Kidney Yang with symptoms of sore and weak lower back and knees and frequent urination; 2. For Kidney failing to grasp the Qi of the Lungs and Cold and Deficiency in the Lung with symptoms of chronic cough, wheezing and asthma; 3. For constipation due to Dryness either from injured Fluids or Blood Deficiency, especially good for the elderly; 4. For stones in the urinary tract that originated in the Kidneys due to Cold; 5. Applied as a paste for inflammation of the skin and eczema.
Contraindications: This herb should not be used by those with Yin Deficiency when there are Heat signs present, nor should it be used when there is Phlegm Fire and cough.
Dosage: 9 - 30 grams

Notes: For frequent urination combine with Psoralea (Bu Gu Zhi); for cough and asthma caused by Lung Deficiency combine with Ginseng (Ren Shen); for constipation caused by Dryness of the Intestines combine with Cannabis Seed (Huo Ma Ren) and Cistanches (Rou Cong Rong).

Morinda Officinalis   Ba Ji Tian   (2)
Common Name: Morinda
Part Used: Root (Radix)
Family: Rubiaceae

Energy and Flavors: acrid, sweet and Warm

Organ Meridians Affected: Liver and Kidney

Actions: 1. Tonifies the Kidney Yang; 2. Expels Wind-Damp-Cold painful obstruction (Bi Pain).

Indications: 1. For Deficiency of Kidney Yang with symptoms of impotence, infertility, premature ejaculation, frequent urination, irregular menstruation, sore, cold and weak lower back and muscular atrophy; 2. For Wind-Damp-Cold painful obstruction (Bi Pain) of the back and legs.

Contraindications: This herb should not be used by those with either Heat signs caused by Yin Deficiency or Damp Heat patterns. It should not be used by those who are having difficulty urinating and should not be used in conjunction with Radix Salvia miltiorrhiza (Dan Shen).

Dosage: 3 - 12 grams

Notes: For lower back pain with weakness of the legs and knees, combine with Dipsacus (Xu Duan), Loranthes (Sang Ji Sheng) and Achyranthes (Niu Xi); for Deficient Kidney Yang with impotence, premature ejaculation and spermatorrhea combine with Psoralea (Bu Gu Zhi) and Cistanche (Rou Cong Rong); for female frigidity and infertility combine with Angelica sinensis (Dang Gui), Deglutinated Deer antler (Lu Jiao Shuang) and Psoralea (Bu Gu Zhi).

Epimedii Grandiflorum   **Yin Yang Huo** (2)

Common Name: Epimedium

Part Used: Aerial portion (Herba)

Family: Berberidaceae

Energy and Flavors: sweet, acrid and Warm

Organ Meridians Affected: Kidney and Liver

Actions: 1. Tonifies the Kidney Yang; 2. Expels Wind-Damp-Cold Bi Pain; 3. Strengthens Lung Qi and assists in expectoration.

Indications: 1. For Deficiency of the Kidney Yang with symptoms of impotence, frequent urination, seminal emission and pain and Cold in the lower back and knees; 2. For Wind-Damp-Cold painful obstruction with symptoms of joint pain, numbness and weakness of the extremities and cramping of the hands and feet; 3. This herb is useful in chronic Lung conditions such as chronic bronchitis.

Contraindications: This herb should not be used by those with Yin Deficiency with Heat signs. It should not be used for extended periods of time; using this herb inappropriately may result in dizziness, dry mouth, thirst, vomiting or nosebleed.

Dosage: 6 - 12 grams

Notes: For menopausal hot flashes combine with Morinda (Ba Ji Tian) in the formula Curculigo and Epimedium Combination (Er Xian Tang); for Wind-Cold-Damp arthritic conditions combine with Clematis (Wei Ling Xian), Eucommia bark (Du Zhong) and Cinnamon twigs (Gui Zhi); for cough caused by Deficient Yang combine with Psoralea (Bu Gu Zhi), Walnut (Hu Tao Ren) and Schisandra (Wu Wei Zi).

Gecko   Ge Jie   (2)
(Gecko Gecko)
Common Name: Gecko Lizard
Part Used: The whole male and female animal.
Family: Geckonidae
Energy and Flavors: salty and neutral
Organ Meridians Affected: Lungs and Kidneys
Actions: 1. Tonifies the Kidneys and Lungs; 2. Helps the Kidneys grasp Lung Qi; 3. Augments Essence.
Indications: 1. Asthma, emphysema, TB with cough, coughing blood; 2. Impotence and infertility; 3. Frequent urination with copious clear urine; 4. Daybreak diarrhea.
Contraindications: Not for coughs caused by External Wind Cold.
Preparation: Both the male and female Geckos are used simultaneously. The most active part is the tail, so the head and feet can be removed in decoctions. They can be taken as a powder or pill, soaked in wine or brewed in a water decoction.
Dosage: 9 - 30 grams

Notes: Gecko lizard is used to grasp the Yang in place because certain types of asthma, according to Chinese medical theory, arise as a result of weakness of Kidney Yang, causing the Qi to float upward and thus manifest as asthma. For asthma with cough caused by Deficient Kidney and Spleen Qi combine with Ginseng (Ren Shen), Schisandra (Wu Wei Zi), Walnut (Hu Tao Ren), Apricot Seed (Xing Ren) and Fritillary (Chuan Bei Mu). For impotence combine with Ginseng (Ren Shen), Epimedium (Yin Yang Huo) and Deer Antler (Lu Rong).

Cordyceps Sinensis   Dong Chong Xia Cao   (3)
Common Name: Cordyceps
Part Used: The entire fungus
Family: Clavicipitaceae
Energy and Flavors: sweet and Warm
Organ Meridians Affected: Lung and Kidney

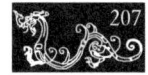

Actions: 1. Tonifies the Kidney Yang and assists the Lung Yin.

Indications: 1. For Deficiency of Kidney Yang with symptoms of impotence, weakness of the lower back and knees; 2. For chronic cough, wheezing and consumptive cough with blood streaked sputum due to Deficiency of Kidney Yang and Lung Yin.

Contraindications: This substance is very safe as it tonifies both Yin and Yang and can be used long term. This substance should be used with caution when there is an Exterior condition.

Dosage: 6 - 12 grams

Notes: To increase the effect of strengthening the immune system, this herb is cooked with duck. It tonifies both Kidney Yang and Lung Yin, clears Phlegm and stops bleeding. For blood streaked sputum from the Lungs combine with Glehnia (Sha Shen), Fritillary (Chuan Bei Mu) and Donkey Skin Gelatin (E Jiao). As with all the Kidney Yang formulas it can be combined with other Kidney Yang substances such as Deer Antler (Lu Rong) and Epimedium (Yin Yang Huo).

Trigonellae Foeni-Graeci   Hu Lu Ba   (3)

Common Name: Fenugreek Seeds, Trigonella

Part Used: Seed (Semen)

Family: Leguminosae

Energy and Flavors: bitter and Warm

Organ Meridian: Affected: Kidney and Liver

Actions: 1. Warms the Kidneys; 2. Disperses Dampness and Cold; 3. Relieves pain.

Indications: 1. Relieves hernial pains and pains of the abdomen and flanks; 2. Treats Kidney Yang Deficiency patterns including Coldness; 3. Regulates Qi.

Dosage: 3 - 9 grams

Contraindications: Not for symptoms of Heat or Damp-Heat caused by Yin Deficiency.

Notes: Fenugreek seeds are used as a condiment but have a special use for relieving the pain and condition associated with hernial disorders that involve the flanks, abdomen or testicles. For this, they can be combined with Fennel Seed (Xiao Hui Xiang) and Evodia (Wu Zhu Yu).

Alpiniae Oxyphyllae   Yi Zhi Ren   (3)

Common Name: Alpinia Oxyphylla, Black Cardamon, Bitter-Seeded Cardamon

Part Used: Fruit (Fructus)

Family: Zingiberaceae

Energy and Flavors: acrid, Warm

Organ Meridian: Affected: Kidney, Spleen

Actions: 1. Tonifies Kidney Yang and consolidates Kidney Qi; 2. Warms the Spleen and stops diarrhea and salivation.

Indications: 1. Enuresis; 2. Seminal emission; 3. Spermatorrhea; 4. Urinary incontinence; 5. Stomach pains caused by Coldness; 6. Chronic diarrhea and excessive salivation.

Dosage: 3 - 9 grams of the crushed seeds

Contraindications: Not for symptoms of vomiting, diarrhea and frequent urination caused by Internal Heat.

Notes: This herb has the properties of tonifying the Yang of the Spleen and Kidneys for symptoms of abdominal pain, nausea and vomiting. For this it is combined with Codonopsis (Dang Shen), Atractylodes (Bai Zhu) and Ginger (Gan Jiang). For diarrhea and excessive salivation or drooling caused by Spleen Deficiency combine with Codonopsis (Dang Shen), Poria (Fu Ling), Pinellia (Ban Xia) and Ginger (Gan Jiang).
For Kidney Deficiency with nocturnal urination and seminal emissions combine with Dioscorea (Shan Yao) and Lindera (Wu Yao).

Curculiginis Orchioidis **Xian Mao** (2)

Common Name: Curculigo orchioides, Circuliginis

Part Used: Rhizome (Rhizoma)

Family: Amaryllidaceae

Energy and Flavors: acrid, Hot, toxic

Organ Meridian: Affected: Kidney, Liver

Actions: 1. Tonifies Kidney Yang and treats Kidney Yang Deficiency patterns; 2. Strengthens the bones and sinews; 3. Clears Cold and Dampness.

Indications: 1. Impotence; 2. Urinary incontinence; 3. Cold intolerance; 4. Aching soreness of the lower back and knees; 5. Lower back pain; 6. Hypertension associated with menopause.

Dosage: 3 - 9 grams

Contraindications: Not for symptoms of Yin Deficiency.

Notes: This is an important Yang tonic and is particularly used for menopausal symptoms due to Deficiency of both Yin and Yang, frigidity and impotence. Its application clinically can be as an alternate Yang tonic when herbs such as Aconite and Cinnamon are too heating and stimulating to tolerate.

Cibotii Barometz **Gou Ji** (3)

Common Name: Cibotium Barometz

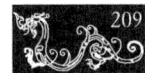

Part Used: Rhizome (Rhizoma)

Family: Dicksoniaceae

Energy and Flavors: bitter, sweet and Warm

Organ Meridians Affected: Kidneys and Liver

Actions: 1. Tonifies Kidney Yang and treats Kidney Yang Deficiency patterns; 2. Strengthens the Bones and Sinews; 3. Treats Cold, Wind-Dampness conditions with stiffness, soreness of the lower back and knees; 4. Treats urinary incontinence and chronic vaginal discharge.

Indications: 1. Promotes healing of the bones and ligaments from injuries; 2. Treats lower back and knee weakness; 3. Reduces edema of the legs; 4. Treats urinary incontinence and chronic vaginal discharge.

Dosage: 5 - 9 grams

Contraindications: Not for difficult urination caused by Yin Deficiency. It is also considered to be antagonistic with Herba cum radice Patrinia (Bai Jiang Cao).

Notes: For aching lower back, weakness of the legs and knees, combine with Eucommia (Du Zhong), Dipsacus (Xu Duan), Achyranthes (Niu Xi) and Loranthes (Sang Ji Sheng).

Drynariae Fortunei   Gu Sui Bu (3)

Common Name: Drynaria Fortunei

Part Used: Rhizome (Rhizoma)

Family: Polypodiaceae

Energy and Flavors: bitter, Warm

Organ Meridians Affected: Kidneys and Liver

Actions: 1. Tonifies Kidney Yang and treats Kidney Yang Deficiency patterns; 2. Promotes Blood circulation; 3. Heals bones and ligaments from injuries; 4. Stimulates hair growth.

Indications: 1. Lower back and knee weakness; 2. Diarrhea; 3. Tinnitus; 4. Failing hearing; 5. Bleeding gums from Kidney Deficiency; 6. Heals broken bones and torn ligaments from injuries; 7. Can be applied topically as a tincture for alopecia.

Dosage: 6 - 18 grams

Contraindications: Not for symptoms of Yin Deficiency or without Blood Stagnation.

Notes: For Kidney Deficiency with symptoms of lower back pain, tinnitus, hearing loss and toothache, combine with Prepared Rehmannia (Shu Di Huang), Cornus (Shan Zhu Yu), Walnut (Hu Tao Ren), Psoralea (Bu Gu Zhi) and Achyranthes (Niu Xi).

Cuscutae Chinensis   **Tu Si Zi**   (1)

Common Names: Cuscuta, Chinese Dodder Seeds

Part Used: Seed (Semen)

Family: Convolvulaceae

Energy and Flavors: acrid, sweet, neutral

Organ Meridians Affected: Kidneys, Liver

Actions: 1. Tonifies Kidney Yang and Essence; 2. Nourishes the Liver.

Indications: 1. Impotence, nocturnal emission, premature ejaculation, spermatorrhea, frequent urination; 2. Lower back pain; 3. Tendency to miscarriage; 4. Weak eyesight; 5. chronic diarrhea

Dosage: 9 - 15 grams

Contraindications: Not for use during pregnancy.

Notes: Specific for low sperm count and inactivity of the sperm. For this it can be combined with Psoralea (Bu Gu Zhi), Schisandra (Wu Wei Zi), Lycii Berries (Gou Qi Zi), Plantain Seeds (Che Qian Zi), Rubi (Fu Pen Zi), Alisma (Ze Xie), Cornus (Shan Zhu Yu), Dioscorea (Shan Yao), Prepared Rehmannia (Shu Di Huang), Poria (Fu Ling) in Five Seeds Formula (Wu Zi Wan).

Astragalus Complanati   **Sha Yuan Ji Li** (3)

Common Name: Astragalus Seed

Part Used: Seed (Semen)

Family: Leguminosae

Energy and Flavors: sweet, Warm

Organ Meridians Affected: Kidneys, Liver

Actions: 1. Tonifies Kidney Yang; 2. Consolidates Essence and semen; 3. Strengthens vision.

Indications: 1. Lower back pain; 2. Premature ejaculation, spermatorrhea, frequent urination; 3. Weak eyesight

Dosage: 9 - 15 grams of the crushed seeds

Contraindications: Not for symptoms of Heat in the Kidneys or Bladder

Notes: This herb is especially useful for seminal emissions, impotence, premature ejaculation, urinary incontinence and leukorrhea. For these conditions combine with Dragon Bone (Long Gu), Oyster shell (Mu Li) and Euryale seeds (Qian Shi).

Allium Tuberosi   **Jiu Zi** (3)

Common Names: Allium, Leek Seeds, Onion Seeds

Part Used: Seed (Semen)

Family: Liliaceae

Energy and Flavors: acrid, sweet, Warm

Organ Meridians Affected: Kidneys and Liver

Actions: 1. Tonifies Kidney Yang; 2. Treats Kidney Yang Deficiency patterns; 3. Warms the Stomach and Spleen.

Indications: 1. Treats impotence, premature ejaculation and spermatorrhea; 2. Treats urinary incontinence; 3. Treats chronic vaginal discharge; 4. Treats weakness and soreness of the lower back and extremities; 5. Relieves nausea and vomiting.

Dosage: 6 - 15 grams crushed seeds

Contraindications: Not for Yin Deficiency patterns with symptoms of Heat.

Notes: For Kidney Yang Deficiency with lower back pain, weakness of the legs and knees combine with Cistanche (Rou Cong Rong), Morinda (Ba Ji Tian), Psoralea (Bu Gu Zhi) and Cuscuta (Tu Si Zi). For frequent urination add Bitter Cardamon (Yi Zhi Ren) and Dioscorea (Shan Yao) to the above combination to supplement Spleen Yang.

Testis et Penis Otariae   **Hai Gou Shen** (3)

(Callorhinus Ursinus)

Part Used: The genitals (Testis et Penis)

Common Names: Seal and sea lion genitals

Family: Pinnipedae

Energy and Flavors: salty, Hot

Organ Meridians Affected: Kidneys, Liver

Actions: 1. Tonifies Kidney Yang; 2. Replenishes Essence and Marrow

Indications: 1. Impotence; 2. Fatigue, weakness of the lower back and extremities; 3. Abdominal pains caused by Coldness

Dosage: 3 - 9 grams

Contraindications: Not for an individual with symptoms of Heat or Yin Deficiency.

Notes: Following the principle of "like cures like," the reproductive organs of various animals are used as protomorphogens for impotence. These can be combined with Kidney Yang and Yin herbs such as Lycii (Gou Qi Zi), Cuscuta (Tu Si Zi) and Morinda (Ba Ji Tian).

Actinolitum   **Yang Qi Shi** (3)

Common Name: Actinolitum, Actinolite

Part Used: The powdered mineral

Energy and Flavors: salty, slightly Warm

Organ Meridians Affected: Kidneys

Actions: 1. Tonifies Kidney Yang (Ming Men); 2. Treats Deficient Yang patterns.

Indications: 1. Impotence; 2. Coldness; 3. Amenorrhea

Dosage: 3 - 9 grams

Contraindications: Not for Yin Deficiency symptoms.

Notes: Besides tonifying Kidney Yang conditions associated with male impotence, lower back pain, weak knees and legs, this mineral has a special function of warming the womb, increasing female libido and fertility and stopping uterine bleeding from a cold womb. For cold womb, it can be combined with Deer Antler (Lu Rong).

Stalactitum   E Guan Shi   (3)

Common Name: Stalactite

Part Used: The powdered mineral

Energy and Flavors: sweet, Warm

Organ Meridians Affected: Lungs

Actions: 1. Tonifies Yang; 2. Clears Phlegm and lowers Qi; 3. Promotes lactation.

Indications: 1. For asthma, chronic bronchitis, emphysema; 2. Insufficient lactation.

Preparation: Crush and powder before using, boil for at least 30 minutes before adding other herbs.

Dosage: 9 - 30 grams

Contraindications: Can cause Stomach Qi Stagnation; not for wheezing with blood.

Notes: Just as a stalactite is solidified minerals that drip down from the ceiling of a cavern, so also does its energy have a strong downward Qi useful for moving the Qi down from the Lungs and treating coughs and emphysema. For this it can be combined with Apricot seed(Xing Ren), Walnut (Hu Tao Ren), Pinellia (Ban Xia) and Ginger (Gan Jiang).

Hailong   Hai Long   (3)

(Solenognathus Hardwickii, Syngnathoides Biaculeatus, Syngnathus Cus)

Common Name: Pipe-Fish

Part Used: The whole animal

Family: Syngnathidae

Energy and Flavors: sweet, salty, slightly Warm

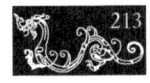

Organ Meridians Affected: Kidneys

Actions and Indications: 1. Tonifies Kidney Yang; 2. Treats impotence and general weakness in the elderly; 3. Reduces swelling and dissipates nodules.

Preparations: decoctions, powders or pills.

Dosage: 3- 9 grams

Contraindications: Not for use during pregnancy, not for Deficient Yin conditions, not for individuals with acute External diseases or weak digestion.

Notes: This can be added to most Kidney Yang formulas for the treatment of impotence.

Hippocampus   Hai Ma   (3)

(Hippocampus kellogii et al)

Common Name: Sea Horse

Part Used: The whole animal

Family: Syngnathidae

Energy and Flavors: sweet, salty, Warm

Organ Meridians Affected: Kidney, Liver

Actions: 1. Tonifies Kidney Yang; 2. Invigorates Blood and removes Stasis.

Indications: 1. Impotence; 2. Lower back pain and weakness of the lower extremities; 3. Urinary frequency; 4. Tumors, unripening boils; 5. Difficult childbirth

Dosage: 3 - 9 grams (It is best steeped in wine for impotence).

Contraindications: Not for pregnant women or individuals with hyperactive Yang-Fire symptoms.

Notes: Used with other Kidney Yang herbs for impotence. Combine with Jujube Dates (Da Zao) and Lycii Berries (Gou Qi Zi) for leaking conditions such as urinary incontinence and clear vaginal discharge.

Strichopus Japonicus   Hai Shen   (3)

Common Name: Sea Cucumber

Part Used: The whole animal

Family: Strichopae

Energy and Flavors: salty, Warm

Organ Meridians Affected: Heart, Kidneys

Actions: 1. Tonifies Kidney Yang; 2. Supplements Essence; 3. Stops Bleeding.

Indications: 1. Treats Kidney Yang patterns, impotence and Essence Deficiency; 2. Stops bleeding in consumption and hemophilia.

Dosage: 30 - 60 grams in decoction, much more can be eaten as a food

Contraindications: Not for Spleen Deficiency with diarrhea.

Notes: Used both as an herb and food for tonifying Kidney Yang and Essence for the treatment of impotence, seminal emission and frequent urination.

Cynomorium Songaricum   Suo Yang   (3)
Common Name: Cynomorium
Part Used: Aerial portion (Herba)
Family: Cynomoriaceae
Energy and Flavors: Sweet, Warm
Organ Meridians Affected: Large Intestine, Kidney, Liver
Actions: 1. Tonifies Kidney Yang; 2. Nourishes the Blood; 3. Lubricates the Intestines.
Indications: 1. Impotence, frequent urination, premature ejaculation and spermatorrhea; 2. Nourishes the Blood, strengthens the ligaments, treats paralysis caused by injured Essence and Blood; 3. Lubricates the Intestines, for constipation caused by Qi and Blood Deficiency.
Dosage: 6 - 15 grams
Contraindications: Not for symptoms of Kidney Yin Deficiency or diarrhea.

Notes: This herb is used with Rehmannia, Eucommia and Achyranthes for muscular atrophy caused by depletion of Kidneys and Liver. It can also be used with Astragalus complanati (Sha Yuan Ji Li) and Mantidis (Sang Piao Xiao) for urinary incontinence and premature ejaculation.

Cistanches Deserticolae   Rou Cong Rong   (2)
Common Name: Cistanche
Part Used: Aerial portion (Herba)
Family: Orobanchaceae
Energy and Flavors: sweet, salty and Warm
Organ Meridians Affected: Kidney and Large Intestine
Actions: 1. Tonifies Kidney Yang; 2. Lubricates the Intestines; 3. Warms the womb.
Indications: 1. For Deficiency of Kidney Yang with symptoms such as impotence, premature ejaculation, Cold and pain in the lower back and knees, urinary incontinence and post-urinary dripping; 2. For constipation due to lack of Fluids. This herb is useful for the aged, and those with Qi and Blood Deficiency; 3. For Cold and Deficiency of the womb with symptoms such as infertility, excessive white vaginal discharge and abnormal uterine bleeding.

Contraindications: This herb should not be used when there is Yin Deficiency with Heat signs or when there is diarrhea from either Deficient Spleen or Stomach or pathogenic Heat.

Dosage: 6 - 12 grams

Notes: For impotence and premature ejaculation combine with Prepared Rehmannia (Shu Di Huang), Cuscuta (Tu Si Zi), Morinda (Ba Ji Tian) and Schisandra (Wu Wei Zi); for frigidity and impotence combine with Epimedium (Yin Yang Huo), Antler Glue (Lu Jiao Jiao), and Human Placenta (Zi He Che); for constipation combine with Cannabis Seed (Huo Ma Ren), Walnut (Hu Tao Ren).

Placenta Hominis   Zi He Che   (3)

Common Name: Human Placenta

Family: Hominidae

Energy and Flavors: sweet, salty and Warm

Organ Meridians Affected: Lung, Kidney, Heart and Liver

Actions: 1. Tonifies the Liver and Kidneys and assists the Essence; 2. Tonifies the Qi and Blood.

Indications: 1. For Deficiency of the Liver and Kidneys with symptoms such as infertility, impotence, tinnitus, lower back pain, seminal emissions and vertigo; 2. For Deficiency of Qi and Blood with symptoms of fatigue, chronic cough and wheezing, insufficient lactation and Blood Deficiency.

Contraindications: The use of human placenta is very safe but should be used with caution when there is Heat from Yin Deficiency and for prolonged use.

Dosage: 1.5 - 4.5 grams

Notes: This is taken for Essence Deficiencies and can be combined with various tonic herbs according to what Organs are being treated. For Deficient Qi combine with Codonopsis and Astragalus, if there is chronic weakness caused by degeneration of Kidney and Liver Qi, combine with Prepared Rehmannia (Shu Di Huang) and Lycii Berries (Gou Qi Zi); for Blood Deficiency combine with Prepared Rehmannia (Shu Di Huang), Angelica sinensis (Dang Gui) and White Peony (Bai Shao); for Lung Deficiency with symptoms of shortness of breath, wheezing and cough, combine with Ophiopogon (Mai Men Dong), Schisandra (Wu Wei Zi).

Human placenta is one of the most nutrient rich substances possible. Many animals eat their placenta after childbirth to help the mother regain her strength. Some humans also wash it off and slice and stir fry it with some onions and/or garlic to replenish their strength. Placenta and colostrum (the liquid secreted by females before their milk sets in) has strong immune potentiating agents that make them useful for all

wasting and degenerative diseases including TB and AIDS. Human placenta can be frozen or sliced and dried for future use.

Discrimination:

Cornu Cervi Parvum (Lu Rong) – augments Essence, promotes normal development and growth, strengthens the sinews and bones, treats infertility and impotence, tonifies Qi and Blood.

Eucommiae Ulmoidis (Du Zhong) – relieves hypertension, treats lower back pain, calms a restless fetus.

Dipsaci Asperi (Xu Duan) – heals broken bones, treats back pain, stops bleeding and moves Blood.

Psoraleae Corylifoliae (Bu Gu Zhi) – treats back pain, impotence, tonifies Kidney Qi, restrains Essence, holds urine, topically for psoriasis and vitiligo.

Juglandis Regiae (Hu Tao Ren) – chronic cough, asthma, emphysema, wheezing, lubricates Intestines, relieves urinary stones.

Morinda Officinalis (Ba Ji Tian) – treats impotence, infertility, back, leg and knee pains, rheumatic complaints, menstrual irregularity.

Epimedii (Yin Yang Huo) – for impotence, premature ejaculation, treats lower back, legs and knee pains.

Gecko (Ge Jie) – tonifies the Lungs, treats asthma and wheezing.

Cordyceps Sinenis (Dong Chong Xia Cao) – nourishes Yin, impotence, chronic cough, raising bodily stamina.

Cistanches Deserticolae (Rou Cong Rong) – treats impotence, premature ejaculation, lower back, leg and knee pains, lubricates the Intestines.

Trigonellae Foeni-graeci (Hu Lu Ba) – disperses Cold Dampness, relieves hernia pains.

Alpinae Oxyphyllae (Yi Zhi Ren) – Warms the Spleen, stops diarrhea and salivation.

Curculiginis Orchioidis (Xian Mao) – Cold intolerance, strengthens bones and sinews, used for menopause.

Cibotii Barometz (Gou Ji) – heals bones and ligament injuries, reduces edema.

Drynariae Fortunei (Gu Sui Bu) – promotes blood circulation, heals bone and ligament injuries, externally to promote hair growth.

Cuscutae Chinensis (Tu Si Zi) – treats impotence, urinary incontinence, weak eyesight, tendency to miscarry.

Astragalus Complanati (Sha Yuan Ji Li) — urinary incontinence, premature ejaculation, weak eyesight.

Allium Tuberosi (Jiu Zi) — Urinary incontinence, chronic vaginal discharge, lower back pain, nausea and vomiting.

Testis et Penis Otariae (Hai Gou Shen) — impotence, weakness and fatigue, abdominal pains caused by Coldness.

Actinolitum (Yang Qi Shi) — treats impotence, amenorrhea.

Stalactitum (E Guan Shi) — clears Phlegm, lowers Qi, promotes lactation.

Hailong (Hai Long) — treats impotence, weakness in the elderly, reduces swelling and nodules.

Hippocampus (Hai Ma) — impotence, invigorates Blood circulation, frequent urination, unripening boils, difficult childbirth.

Strichopus Japonicus (Hai Shen) — treats impotence, stops bleeding, treats hemophilia.

Cynomorii Songarici (Suo Yang) — treats impotence, urinary incontinence, strengthens the ligaments, lubricates the Intestines.

Placenta Hominis (Zi He Che) — nourishes Essence, tonifies Qi and Blood, treats fatigue, chronic cough.

HERBS THAT TONIFY THE YIN

Panacis Quinquefolii   Xi Yang Shen   (1)

Common Name: American Ginseng

Part Used: Root (Radix)

Family: Araliaceae

Energy and Flavors: sweet, slightly bitter and Cool

Organ Meridians Affected: Lung, Heart, Kidney and Stomach

Actions: 1. Benefits the Qi, generates Fluids, nourishes the Yin; 2. Nourishes Lung Yin; 3. Calms restlessness

Indications: 1. For chronic coughs, tuberculosis, wasting disease; 2. For Yin Deficient symptoms including low grade afternoon fever and/or night sweats; 3. Tiredness and fatigue caused by consumptive wasting diseases such as tuberculosis or AIDS.

Contraindications: Use with caution for those with symptoms of a Cold Damp Stomach.

Dosage: 3 - 9 grams

Notes: North American Ginseng was once common and abundant in Northeastern forests. Its relative scarcity today makes it a point of ethics for environmentally responsible herbalists to use only organic

woodsgrown American Ginseng. It has a very different energy from Chinese Ginseng (Ren Shen) which tends to stimulate Qi and Yang and raise metabolism, while American Ginseng nourishes Blood and Yin and quiets metabolism. As such it is better for many to use on a daily basis to counteract the high paced stress of contemporary Western civilization.

>Asparagi Cochinchinensis   Tian Men Dong   (1)
>Common Name: Asparagus
>Part Used: Tuber
>Family: Liliaceae
>Energy and Flavors: sweet, bitter and Cold
>Organ Meridians Affected: Lung and Kidney
>Actions: 1. Nourishes Yin of the Lungs and Kidneys; 2. Expectorates phlegm
>Indications: 1. For afternoon tidal fever, night sweats, seminal emission and wasting of the muscles; 2. For dry throat, chronic cough with sticky phlegm, possibly streaked with blood; 3. For constipation caused by Dryness of the Intestines.
>Contraindications: Do not use for those with Deficiency of the Spleen and Stomach when there is presence of Cold accompanied by diarrhea; it should not be used for Wind-Cold cough.
>Dosage: 6 - 18 grams

Notes: A similar species of this herb is a common ornamental sold in nurseries as A. springerii. I once partially unearthed a specimen of this plant and found that it contained many watery tubers attached to the roots and that these had a sweet flavor similar to the Chinese species. Because this herb is believed to engender love and compassion, Chinese pharmacists prize it highly and routinely set aside some of the sweetest roots for their personal use. It is used for all types of Dry conditions, such as Dryness of the Lungs, Intestines and Kidneys for which it is often combined with Ophiopogon (Mai Men Dong). For diabetes, it is combined with Unprepared Rehmannia (Sheng Di Huang) and Ginseng (Ren Shen); for constipation caused by Dryness of the Intestines it is combined with Angelica (Dang Gui) and Cistanche (Rou Cong Rong). This herb is a well known Ayurvedic tonic called "Shatavari."

>Ophiopogonis Japonici   Mai Men Dong (1)
>Common Name: Ophiopogon
>Part Used: Tuber
>Family: Liliaceae

Energy and Flavors: sweet, slightly bitter and Cold

Organ Meridians Affected: Heart, Lung and Stomach

Actions: 1. Replenishes Yin Essence and promotes secretions; 2. Lubricates and nourishes the Stomach. 3. Soothes the Lung; 4. Nourishes the Heart.

Indications: 1. For chronic bronchitis, hemoptysis in pulmonary tuberculosis, restlessness, laryngitis, dry stool caused by Heat in the Stomach, palpitations, fearfulness and insomnia.

Contraindications: Not for those with weak Spleen and Stomach with Coldness and diarrhea.

Dosage: 6 - 12 grams

Notes: Ophiopogon (Mai Men Dong) is grown as a common ornamental, of which there are many species. One common name is Japanese Turf Lily, another is Mondo Grass. The part used is the small bulb-like tubers at the base of each plant. When freshly dug and eaten, they are remarkably sweet and one could imagine that they are used as a food in the part of the world where the plant naturally grows.

Ophiopogon is specific for Deficient Lung and Stomach Yin as well as Heart Yin, since it is able to relieve mental irritability (one of the symptoms of Heart Yin Deficiency). At the same time, it acts as a mild expectorant, clearing Hot Phlegm while lubricating the Lungs. For Dryness and Heat of the Lungs with dry cough and possible blood tinged sputum combine Ophiopogon (Mai Men Dong), Glehnia (Sha Shen), Asparagus (Tian Men Dong), Tendrilled Fritillary root (Chuan Bei Mu) and Unprepared Rehmannia root (Sheng Di Huang); for Deficient Stomach Yin the same combination is used without the Fritillary root (Chuan Bei Mu); for irritability and insomnia combine with Fresh Rehmannia root (Sheng Di Huang), Bamboo Leaf (Zhu Ye) and Coptis (Huang Lian); or for Heart Yin Deficiency combine with Fresh Rehmannia root (Sheng Di Huang) and Jujube seeds (Suan Zao Ren) as used in the formula Tian wang bu xin dan; for Dry constipation combine with Fresh Rehmannia (Sheng Di Huang) and Scrophularia (Xuan Shen).

Glehniae Littoralis   Bei Sha Shen (2)

Common Name: Glehnia (also called Adenophora).

Part Used: Root (Radix)

Family: Umbelliferae

Energy and Flavors: sweet, bland and Cool

Organ Meridians Affected: Lung and Stomach

Actions: 1. Nourishes Lung Yin and stops cough; 2. Nourishes Stomach Yin and generates Fluids.

Indications: 1. For Deficiency of Lung Yin with symptoms of dry throat, dry skin, chronic nonproductive cough and a red tongue with a thin coat; 2. For Heat caused by wasting of the Yin due to febrile diseases with symptoms such as dry mouth and throat and a red tongue with a bald or peeled Stomach/Spleen area.

Contraindications: This herb should not be used by those with conditions of Wind-Cold nor should it be used by those with a weak Cold Spleen.

Dosage: 6 - 12 grams

Notes: This herb has nearly identical properties and uses as North American Ginseng but is much cheaper. Adenophora (Nan Sha Shen) is another species and is considered less potent as a Qi tonic but stronger at stopping coughs. To lubricate the Lungs and generate Fluid, combine with Ophiopogon (Mai Men Dong).

Dendrobium Nobile (Dendrobii)   Shi Hu   (2)

Common Name: Dendrobium

Part Used: Aerial portion (Herba)

Family: Orchidaceae

Energy and Flavors: sweet, slightly salty, bland, Cold

Organ Meridians Affected: Lung, Kidney and Stomach

Actions: 1. Tonifies the Yin of the Lung and Stomach and assists in the generation of Fluids; 2. Clears Heat and nourishes the Yin; 3. Improves vision and strengthens the lower back.

Indications: 1. For Deficiency of the Lung and Stomach Yin with symptoms such as severe thirst, dry mouth, fever due to Yin Deficiency and a red tongue with little or no coat; 2. For Heat symptoms in the aftermath of febrile diseases due to wasting of the Yin, also for vomiting of blood and Wasting and Thirsting disorder.

Contraindications: This herb should not be used by those without signs of Heat and Dryness. It should not be used in the beginnings of febrile diseases.

Dosage: 6 - 18 grams

Notes: There are over 1000 species of these orchids. They are mostly epiphytic or lithophytic (rarely terrestrial) perennials that occur through eastern Asia to Australia. The term 'dendrobium' from the Greek means dendron 'tree,' and bios, 'life,' referring to its growth in the upper forest canopy.

This herb counteracts exhaustion and refreshes the Yin. It can be used for symptoms that occur after excessive activity such as hard ('back-breaking') labor, excessive sex and overwork. It is also effective to counteract the reactions to overly spicy or sweet foods and stimulants

such as sugar, coffee or alcohol. It is specifically indicated for conditions of Yin consumed by Stomach Heat with thirst, dry red tongue and scanty coating. One combination is to combine Dendrobium with Ophiopogon (Mai Men Dong), Glehnia (Sha Shen) and Raw Rehmannia root (Sheng Di Huang). For chronic Stomach Heat with inflammation of the face, mouth or gums, combine with Ophiopogon (Mai Men Dong). It is also effective for lower back ache from sudden bending and lifting combined with Loranthes (Sang Ji Sheng), Eucommia (Du Zhong), Dipsacus (Xu Duan), Achyranthes (Niu Xi) and Angelica Du Huo (Du Huo).

Polygonatum Odorati   Yu Zhu   (2)

Common Name: Solomon's Seal

Part Used: Rhizome (Rhizoma)

Family: Liliaceae

Energy and Flavors: sweet and slightly Cold

Organ Meridians Affected: Lung, Heart and Stomach

Actions: 1. Nourishes the Yin of the Lung and Stomach; 2. Generates Fluids and extinguishes Wind.

Indications: 1. For Deficiency of Lung and Stomach Yin with symptoms such as chronic dry cough, dry throat, Wasting and Thirsting disorder, insatiable appetite, and constipation; 2. For Yin Deficiency patterns with Internal Wind and pain and spasm in the sinews due to lack of Fluids; it can also be used for patients with Yin Deficiency with Exterior Wind-Heat patterns.

Contraindications: This herb should not be used by those with Cold Damp Phlegm in the Stomach.

Dosage: 6 - 18 grams

Notes: This herb is very similar to Polygonatum sibiricum (Huang Jing) except that Polygonatum (Yu Zhu) is Cooler and perhaps more lubricating. This exemplifies that there are many crossovers in terms of function and usage at least between some of the tonics. For Kidney Essence Deficiency manifested as aching sore back, dizziness and Heat on the soles of the feet, combine with Lycii Berries (Gou Qi Zi) and Ligustri Lucidum (Nu Zhen Zi).

Lilium Brownii (Lilii)   Bai He   (1)

Common Name: Lily Bulb

Part Used: Bulb (Bulbus)

Family: Liliaceae

Energy and Flavors: sweet, bland and slightly Cold

Organ Meridians Affected: Heart and Lung

Actions: 1. Clears Heat and stops cough due to either Lung Yin Deficiency or Lung-Heat; 2. Clears Heat from the Heart and calms the Spirit (Shen).

Indications: 1. For Heat in the Lung with symptoms such as cough, sore throat and blood streaked sputum; 2. For Heat in the Heart caused by either febrile disease or Yin Deficiency with symptoms such as insomnia, low-grade fever, irritability or palpitations.

Contraindications: This herb should not be used by those with Wind-Cold conditions when there is Phlegm, nor should it be used when there is Spleen Deficiency with diarrhea.

Dosage: 9 - 30 grams

Note: Just as the metaphor of a lily can conjure images of quiet serenity and beauty, the essence of Yin, Lily root has lubricating, demulcent properties that also calm and assuage the mind (Heart), fostering calm peacefulness beneficial for nervousness and insomnia. For the later stage of febrile diseases, with symptoms of exhaustion and irritability, combine with Anemarrhena (Zhi Mu) and Unprepared Rehmannia (Sheng Di Huang).

Sesami Indicum   **Hei Zhi Ma**   (2)

Common Name: Black Sesame Seed

Part Used: Seed (Semen)

Family: Pedaliaceae

Energy and Flavors: sweet and neutral

Organ Meridians Affected: Kidney and Liver

Actions: 1. Nourishes the Liver and Kidney Yin; 2. Nourishes the Blood; 3. Lubricates the Intestines.

Indications: 1. For Liver and Kidney Yin Deficiency with symptoms such as premature graying of the hair, tinnitus, blurred vision and dizziness; 2. For Deficiency of Blood with symptoms such as headache, dizziness and numbness of the limbs; 3. For constipation due to Blood Deficiency.

Contraindications: This herb should not be used by those with diarrhea.

Dosage: 9 - 30 grams

Notes: Sesame oil is high in essential fatty acids. Along with olive oil, it has a much longer shelf life than most other vegetable oils. For this reason, it is widely used for both cooking and medicine throughout Asian lands. The seeds are high in calcium which contributes to their tonic, nutritive properties. Black sesame seeds are a Kidney and Liver Yin tonic. They can be toasted, ground to a powder and mixed with

honey and eaten daily to restore hair color. To make it more potent, mix with powdered Polygonum Multiflorum (He Shou Wu). A similar healthful confection eaten in the Middle East is called Halvah.

Ecliptae Prostratae　　　　　　　**Han Lian Cao** (3)

Common Name: Eclipta

Part Used: Aerial portion (Herba)

Family: Compositae

Energy and Flavors: sweet, sour and Cold

Organ Meridians Affected: Liver and Kidney

Actions: 1. Tonifies Yin of the Liver and Kidneys; 2. Clears Blood Heat and stops bleeding.

Indications: 1. For Yin Deficiency of the Liver and Kidney with symptoms such as tinnitus, premature graying of the hair, loose teeth, dizziness and blurred vision; 2. For any bleeding disorder where there is Heat in the Blood such as vomiting blood, nosebleeds, blood in the urine and stool, uterine bleeding.

Contraindications: This herb should not be used by those with Cold Deficiency symptoms associated with the Spleen or Kidney.

Dosage: 6 - 18 grams

Notes: This is a common weed found growing in many parts of North America. It is used as a Liver and Kidney Yin tonic, restoring the color of premature graying hair, sharpening and improving all senses, treating dizziness, vertigo and blurred vision. For these conditions, combine it with Ligustri (Nu Zhen Zi) and Polygonum multiflorum (He Shou Wu). It can be topically applied to stop hemorrhage.

Ligustri Lucidum　　　　　　　**Nu Zhen Zi**　(1)

Common Name: Ligustrum, Privet

Part Used: Fruit (Fructus)

Family: Oleaceae

Energy and Flavors: sweet, bitter and neutral

Organ Meridians Affected: Liver and Kidney

Actions: 1. Nourishes Yin of the Liver and Kidneys; 2. Clears Yin Deficiency Heat (False Heat).

Indications: 1. For Liver and Kidney Yin Deficiency with symptoms such as premature graying of the hair, dizziness, spots in vision, loss of or diminished vision, and pain and weakness of the lower back; 2. For Heat symptoms caused by Deficiency of Yin.

Contraindications: This herb should not be used by those with Yang Deficiency of the Spleen with Cold and diarrhea.

Dosage: 6 - 12 grams

Notes: Japanese Privet is commonly grown both as a tree and a hedge throughout many countries of the world. The fruits are combined with Mulberry (Sang Shen), Eclipta (Han Lian Cao) and Lycii berries (Gou Qi Zi) for strengthening the eyes and senses. As an immune tonic they are used in "Fu Zheng" therapy (herbal immune tonic) to counteract the effects of radiation and/or chemotherapy. For this, they may be combined with Astragalus (Huang Qi), Ganoderma lucidum (Reishi or Ling Zhi) mushroom and other tonic herbs. For premature aging and gray hair combine with Polygonum multiflorum (He Shou Wu), Lycii Berries (Gou Qi Zi) and Ginseng (Ren Shen).

Fructificatio Tremellae Fuciformis   Bai Mu Er   (3)

Common Name: Wood Ear, Tremella

Part Used: The fruiting body (Fructificatio)

Family: Tremellaceae

Energy and Flavors: sweet, bland and neutral

Organ Meridians Affected: Lung, Kidney and Stomach

Actions: 1. Nourishes Yin of the Lung and Stomach.

Indications: 1. For Deficiency of Lung and Stomach Yin with ascendant Yang causing symptoms such as "Five Palm Heat" (heat sensation on the soles of the feet, palms of the hands and the chest signifying Yin Deficiency), Dry cough with or without blood streaked sputum and general wasting of the Yin.

Contraindications: This is a very safe herb and can be taken freely as food.

Dosage: 3 - 9 grams

Notes: Wood Ears or *white fungus* are purchased dry in Chinese markets and pharmacies. They are prepared by first soaking them in water until soft and then cooking in soups alone or with meat. They are also cooked with sugar into a sweet dessert-like recipe. They contain B vitamins and various trace minerals. They are very lubricating and used for Lung Dryness and consumptive diseases. They can be cooked with Lily bulb (Bai He) and Glehniae (Sha Shen) with rock candy for consumption and lung abscess.

Viscum Coloratum   Sang Ji Sheng   (1)

(Viscum album is also used for the source; also called Loranthus parasiticum)

Common Name: Mulberry Mistletoe

Part Used: Branches (Ramulus)

Family: Loranthaceae

Energy and Flavors: bitter, neutral

Organ Meridians Affected: Kidney, Liver

Actions: 1. Tonifies Liver and Kidneys; 2. Expels Wind and Dampness; 3. Nourishes the Blood; 4. Calms the womb; 5. Treats dry skin; 6. Relieves hypertension.

Indications: 1. Treats Bi syndrome with joint pains, numbness, weakness and atrophy; 2. Calms a restless fetus, stops bleeding during pregnancy; 3. Treats dry eczema; 4. Lowers hypertension.

Preparations: Fry in rice wine to enhance its ability to treat Wind-Dampness.

Dosage: 9 - 30 grams.

Contraindications: Overly large doses can be toxic.

Notes: Because it has a neutral energy, this is one of the most versatile herbs for relieving back and joint pains and/or stiffness with associated pain from various causes. For many the effects are almost immediate. Use it for those who experience gradual stiffness and aching pain of the lower back, with difficulty bending at the waist, and knee pains. For this purpose, it can be combined with Angelica Du Huo (Du Huo) and Achyranthes (Niu Xi) to promote flexibility and circulation of the joints and ligaments. It is similarly effective when combined with Turmeric root (Curcuma longa or Jiang Huang).

Plastrum Testudinis   Gui Ban   (2)

Common Name: Fresh Water Turtle

Family: Testudinidae

Part Used: Shell (primarily the ventral portion)

Energy and Flavors: salty, sweet, Cold

Organ Meridians Affected: Heart, Kidney, Liver

Actions: 1. Nourishes the Yin and holds down the Yang; 2. Strengthens the Kidneys and strengthens the bones; 3. Cools the Blood, stops uterine bleeding; 4. Nourishes the Heart; 5. Promotes Healing.

Indications: 1. Treats hypertension and other symptoms caused by Yin Deficiency such as night sweats, dizziness, tinnitus, steaming bone fever; 2. Treats facial spasms and tremors of the hands and feet caused by Internal Wind from Liver Yin Deficiency; 3. Treats aching soreness of the lower back and legs, retarded bone growth in small children, failure of the fontanel to close; 4. Cools the Blood and inhibits excessive menstrual or uterine bleeding; 5. Treats anxiety, insomnia and forgetfulness; 6. Non-healing sores and ulcers.

Preparation: Cook with vinegar to treat uterine bleeding.

Dosage: 9 - 30 grams

Contraindications: It is contraindicated during pregnancy; individuals with Cold and Dampness of the Spleen.

Notes: Only the ventral or lower part, facing the earth, is used in formula. It is used for treating high blood pressure caused by Yin Deficiency. For this condition it can be combined with Donkey Skin Gelatin (E Jiao), Fresh Rehmannia root (Sheng Di Huang) and Uncaria thorns (Gou Teng). For weakness of the lower back and knees, combine with Achyranthes (Niu Xi), Prepared Rehmannia (Shu Di Huang) and Loranthes (Sang Ji Sheng); for mental impairment caused by Yin Deficiency with symptoms of insomnia, forgetfulness, palpitations and paranoia, combine with Dragon Bone (Long Gu), Calamus root (Shi Chang Pu) and Polygala (Yuan Zhi).

Carapax Amydae Sinensis   **Bie Jia**   (2)

Common Name: Tortoise Shell

Part Used: Carapax (dorsal aspect)

Family: Trionychidae

Energy and Flavors: salty, neutral

Organ Meridians Affected: Liver, Spleen, Kidneys

Actions: 1. Nourishes Yin and subdues exuberant Yang; 2. Resolves hardness

Indications: 1. Yin Deficiency patterns including night sweats and chronic tidal fevers; 2. Reduces abdominal mass, enlarged Liver and Spleen.

Dosage: 9 - 30 grams

Contraindications: Not for use during pregnancy or diarrhea.

Notes: This Yin nourishing tonic offers a special form of calcium useful for severe Yin Deficiency with Dryness, Internal Wind with such varied symptoms as tremulous fingers, spasms and convulsions. For these conditions, it can be combined with Oyster shell (Mu Li), Fresh Rehmannia (Sheng Di Huang), Donkey skin gelatin (E Jiao) and White Peony (Bai Shao). For Yin Deficiency with Heat and fever, combine with Artemisia annua (Qing Hao) and Moutan Peony (Mu Dan Pi). If there are night sweats with afternoon fever, combine with Stellaria (Yin Chai Hu) and Lycii Bark (Di Gu Pi).

Momordicae Grosvenori   **Luo Han Guo**   (3)

Common Name: Momordica fruit

Part Used: Fruit (Fructus)

Family: Cucurbitaceae

Energy and Flavors: sweet, neutral

Organ Meridians Affected: Lungs and Spleen

Actions: 1. Lubricates and cools the Lungs; 2. Treats Lung Yin Deficiency; 3. Dissipates nodules and swollen glands.

Indications: 1. For Lung inflammation with Hot, Dry coughs, 2. Reduces lymphatic swelling.

Dosage: 9 - 15 grams

Notes: This is a common food herb eaten by the Chinese and often cooked with pork to tonify Lung Yin. It is frequently sold in Chinese markets as Winter melon.

Discrimination:

Panacis Quinquefolii (Xi Yang Shen) — nourishes Lungs, for chronic coughs, wasting diseases, fatigue.

Asparagi Cochinchinensis (Tian Men Dong) — nourishes Lungs and Kidneys, expectorant, lubricates Intestines.

Ophiopogonis Japonici (Mai Men Dong) — nourishes Lung Yin for chronic Dry Lung diseases, promotes secretions, lubricates the Stomach.

Glehniae (Bei Sha Shen) — Nourishes Lung Yin, Dry cough and skin, wasting diseases with Deficient Yin Heat.

Dendrobii (Shi Hu) — Nourishes Lung and Stomach Yin, generates Fluids, refreshes from overexertion, excess sex, clears Deficient Heat.

Polygonatum Odorati (Yu Zhu) — nourishes and lubricates Lung and Stomach Yin, treats Dry cough, treats Internal Wind caused by Yin Deficiency, also for Exterior symptoms with underlying Yin Deficiency.

Lilii (Bai He) — clears Heat, nourishes Lung Yin, calms the Heart and Shen.

Semen Sesami Indicum (Hei Zhi Ma) — nourishes Liver and Kidney Yin, tonifies Blood, lubricates the Intestines, restores hair color.

Ecliptae Prostratae (Han Lian Cao) — nourishes Liver and Kidney Yin, clears Blood Heat, stops bleeding, restores hair color, clears vision.

Ligustri Lucidum (Nu Zhen Zi) — nourishes Liver and Kidney Yin, clears Deficient Heat, restores hair color, clears vision, strengthens the lower back.

Fructificatio Tremellae Fuciformis (Bai Mu Er) — nourishes Lung and Stomach Yin, treats Deficient Heat, treats Dry cough with blood streaked sputum.

Sangjisheng (Sang ji Sheng) — Tonifies Liver and Kidneys, expels Wind-Dampness, nourishes Blood, relieves hypertension.

Plastrum Testudinis (Gui Ban) — Nourishes Yin, restrains Yang, stops bleeding, calms the Heart.

Carapax Amydae Sinensis (Bie Jia) — subdues hyperactive Yang, resolves hardness.

Momordicae (Luo Han Guo) — lubricates the Lungs, nourishes Lung Yin, resolves swollen glands, used as a Yin nourishing food.

HERBS THAT STABILIZE AND BIND

This category of herbs corresponds to astringents in Western herbalism and is used for treating abnormal discharges and displacement of organs. This includes conditions such as diarrhea, discharges from the vagina, penis or rectum. It also includes prolapse of the uterus or rectum, all of which are diseases associated with aging.

The herbs in this category are mostly sour and astringent and have various special functions: 1. Stopping abnormal sweating, 2. Stopping diarrhea, 3. Stopping frequent urination, and 4. Astringing abnormal menstrual bleeding and other bleeding from the Lower Warmer.

The herbs in this category only treat symptoms, so one should also use herbs to treat the underlying Deficiency.

Corni Officinalis   Shan Zhu Yu   (1)

Common Name: Cornus, Dogwood

Part Used: Fruit (Fructus)

Family: Cornaceae

Energy and Flavors: sour and Warm

Organ Meridians Affected: Liver and Kidney

Actions: 1. Preserves and tonifies the Kidney, Liver and Essence; 2. Stops sweating and benefits the Yang and Qi; 3. Assists menstruation and stops bleeding.

Indications: 1. For Deficiency of the Liver and Kidneys with symptoms such as frequent urination, inability to hold urine, impotence, sore and weak lower back and knees, dizziness, spontaneous sweating and nocturnal emissions; 2. For collapse of Yang or Qi with symptoms such as shock and excessive sweating; 3. For excessive uterine bleeding caused by Deficiency.

Contraindications: This herb should not be used by those with Fire symptoms or those with Damp-Heat and difficult or painful urination.

Dosage: 3 - 12 grams

Notes: Kidney Qi becomes exhausted when we over-extend ourselves either physically or emotionally. Kidney Yin or Yang tonics supplement precious hormonal Essence that becomes depleted from physical and mental stress. Cornus and Schisandra berries serve to help retain these secretions, creating a gathering and bracing effect through their sour and astringent flavors. This is why for shock, 30 to 60 grams of Cornus berries can be taken. While at best only mild tonics in themselves, when combined with Kidney Yin and Yang tonics their power is augmented.

For Deficient Liver and Kidneys with typical symptoms of lower back and joint pains, lack of libido, weakness of the knees and legs, dizziness, seminal emissions and impotence, combine with Prepared Rehmannia (Shu Di Huang) and Eucommia bark (Du Zhong); for impotence and lack of libido add Cuscuta (Tu Si Zi), Lycii berries (Gou Qi Zi, Deer Antler Gelatin (Lu Jiao Jiao) and Psoralea (Bu Gu Zhi). For abnormal sweating caused by general weakness, combine with Ginseng (Ren Shen), Astragalus (Huang Qi); for night sweats caused by Yin Deficiency combine with Angelica sinensis (Dang Gui) and Prepared Rehmannia (Shu Di Huang); for high blood pressure combine with Eucommia (Du Zhong) and Millettia (Ji Xue Teng). Cornus (Shan Zhu Yu) and Schisandra (Wu Wei Zi) can be combined for Kidney and Liver Deficiency by mutually augmenting each other's strengthening and astringent properties. This combination is useful for such symptoms as spontaneous sweating, palpitations, spermatorrhea and any other excretions or discharges caused by weakness.

Schisandrae Chinensis   Wu Wei Zi   (1)
Common Name: Schisandra, Five Flavored Fruit
Part Used: Fruit (Fructus)
Family: Magnoliaceae
Energy and Flavors: sour and Warm
Organ Meridians Affected: Lung, Heart and Kidney

Actions: 1. Tonifies the Kidneys and preserves the Essence; 2. Astringes the Lung Qi and stops coughing; 3. Retains Bodily Fluids and encourages their production; 4. Tonifies the Heart and calms the spirit (Shen).

Indications: 1. For Deficiency of Kidneys, leaking of Essence with symptoms such as excessive sweating and night sweats, nocturnal emissions, vaginal discharge, urinary incontinence and daybreak diarrhea; 2. For Lung Qi and Kidney Deficiency leading to chronic cough, especially dry cough, wheezing and asthma; 3. For spontaneous sweating, seminal emissions, night sweats, Wasting and Thirsting disorder and frequent urination; 4. For Deficiency of Heart Blood and Yin with symptoms such as palpitations, forgetfulness, insomnia and irritability.

Contraindications: This herb should not be used by those with Internal Heat nor by those with an Externally contracted disease.

Dosage: 2 - 9 grams

Notes: Schisandra has the ability to inhibit the loss of both physical and mental energy. Its spirit calming properties lie in its ability to heal and prevent the loss of psycho-physiological energy. It is useful for those individuals who tend to feel agitated and scattered. On a more purely physical level it can be used for all forms of leakages from spontaneous perspiration to premature ejaculation.

The complex five flavors of Schisandra are made more pleasant by the addition of a small amount of Citrus peel (Chen Pi) and Licorice (Gan Cao). This can be combined with Qi tonic herbs such as Codonopsis (Dang Shen) or Ginseng (Ren Shen) and/or Astragalus root (Huang Qi). Schisandra berry wine is taken to calm the Heart and quiet the spirit. It is made by soaking the powdered berries in good quality liquor such as rice wine or vodka in a wide mouthed jar, so that the fluid is approximately one or two inches above the settled herb mash. Shake daily for one month and strain through a fine cloth. Take one tablespoon twice daily.

Prunus Mume   Wu Mei   (2)

Common Name: Mume, Black Plum

Part Used: Fruit (Fructus)

Family: Rosaceae

Energy and Flavors: sour and Warm

Organ Meridians Affected: Liver, Lung, Spleen and Large Intestine

Actions: 1. Stabilizes Lung Qi and stops cough; 2. Stops diarrhea; 3. Retains Bodily Fluids and encourages their production; 4. Expels parasites and relieves vomiting.

Indications: 1. For chronic cough associated with Lung Deficiency; 2. For chronic diarrhea and blood in the stool, also for excessive uterine bleeding associated with Blood Deficiency; 3. For Heat from Deficiency of Yin or Wasting and Thirsting disorder; 4. For roundworms, tinea and ascariasis, also for vomiting; 5. Used topically for corns and warts.

Contraindications: This herb should not be used by those with Excess and Stagnation with Internal Heat nor when there is an External pathogenic influence present.

Dosage: 3 - 9 grams

Notes: These are the plums that are pickled in salt by the Japanese, and are used as an alkalinizing agent for digestion, popularly known as Umeboshi. They have many uses ranging from treating chronic Lung

Deficiency coughs when combined with Pinellia (Ban Xia), Citrus peel (Chen Pi), Fresh Ginger (Sheng Jiang) and Apricot Seed (Xing Ren); to the treatment of acute dysentery and intestinal parasites when combined with Coptis (Huang Lian) and Asarum (Xi Xin) in the formula Wu Mei Wan.

Ginkgo Biloba   **Bai Guo**   (3)

Common Name: Ginkgo Nut

Part Used: Seed (Semen)

Family: Ginkgoaceae

Energy and Flavors: sweet, bitter, astringent, neutral and slightly toxic

Organ Meridians Affected: Lung and Kidney

Actions: 1. Assists the Lung Qi, stops cough and expels Phlegm; 2. Stops leakage of Bodily Fluids.

Indications: 1. For coughing and wheezing with copious clear sputum due to Deficiency of Lung Qi; 2. For vaginal discharge, frequent urination due to either Deficiency or Damp-Heat.

Contraindications: This herb should not be used when there is Excess Cold-Damp; it should be used with caution when there is thick, difficult to expectorate sputum. This herb should not be used in large doses or for long periods of time.

Dosage: 6 - 9 grams

Notes: Ginkgo biloba is known as the oldest tree species on the earth today. Its hardiness is witnessed in its ability to survive the exhaust-filled streets of overcrowded cities, and also by the fact that a Ginkgo tree thrives today, surviving the Hiroshima atomic blast at the end of the 2nd World War. Ginkgo trees have been known to live well over an average of 1000 or more years, extending as far back as written history in China.

It has become one of the most popular herbs in the West because of the unique ability of the concentrated extract of the leaves (24 to 1) to improve blood circulation to the brain. As such it is useful for preventing and inhibiting the progression of senile dementia and possibly Alzheimer's disease. Its circulatory properties have many other practical applications such as the treatment of circulatory problems, dissolving blood clots, improving hearing, for the treatment of early stages of tinnitus (ringing in the ears), improving blood circulation to the eyes which helps in preventing macular degeneration, reducing asthma attacks and helping to prevent organ transplant rejection.

Much of its circulatory powers are due to its high flavonoid content which is highest in the yellow autumn harvested leaves. This aids in preventing the clumping of the blood that eventually can lead to congestive heart failure. Ginkgo is also able to increase acetylcholine levels, which improves the body's ability to transmit electrical impulses.

The ancient belief in the "Doctrine of Signatures" taught that what a thing resembles may be an indication of its use. In the Ginkgo tree, as one of the oldest surviving species on the earth, we have corroborated through extensive scientific research its value for treating conditions associated with aging.

Terminaliae Chebulae   He Zi   (3)

Common Name: Fructus Chebulae, Terminalia Fruit, Chebula Fruit, Sanskrit: Haritaki

Part Used: Fruit (Fructus)

Family: Combretaceae

Energy and Flavors: bitter, sour, astringent, neutral

Organ Meridians Affected: Lung, Stomach, Large Intestine

Actions: 1. Astringes the Intestines; 2. Astringes the Lungs.

Indications: 1. For chronic diarrhea, dysentery with either Hot or Cold patterns; 2. Stops coughing, fortifies the throat, treats wheezing and loss of voice.

Dosage: 3-9 grams

Contraindications: Not for cough caused by Exterior syndrome nor for Stagnation of Internal Damp Heat.

Notes: This herb has opposite, dual functions as used in Chinese herbalism and Ayurvedic Medicine. The way that it is used in Chinese herbalism is as an astringent for diarrhea and dysentery, especially when combined with Coptis (Huang Lian) and Saussurea (Mu Xiang) for Hot type dysentery, or with Poppy capsules (Ying Su Ke) and Dried Ginger (Gan Jiang) for Cold type dysentery. In Ayurveda its purgative properties are employed, especially when combined in the famous formula called Triphala.

Myristacae Fragrantis   Rou Dou Kou (3)

Common Name: Nutmeg Seeds

Part Used: Seed (Semen)

Family: Myristicaceae

Energy and Flavors: acrid, Warm

Organ Meridians Affected: Large Intestine, Spleen, Stomach

Actions: 1. Warms the Spleen and Stomach, circulates Qi; 2. Astringes the Intestines and stops diarrhea.

Indications: Intractable and chronic diarrhea caused by Cold Deficiency of the Spleen and Kidneys; 2. Promotes digestion, relieves epigastric and abdominal pains, stimulates appetite, stops nausea and vomiting caused by Coldness of the Stomach and Spleen.

Dosage: 3 - 9 grams of the crushed seeds

Contraindications: Not to be used for Damp Heat dysentery and diarrhea.

Notes: Nutmeg is used for Cold type dysentery and diarrhea caused by Deficient Spleen Qi. For this it can be combined with Codonopsis (Dang Shen) and Atractylodes (Bai Zhu). It is added to Cold-natured desserts and fruits to regulate Qi and aid digestion. For Qi Stagnation caused by Cold Stomach and Spleen, it can be combined with Pinellia (Ban Xia), Saussurea (Mu Xiang) and Fresh Ginger (Sheng Jiang); Cardamon seed (Sha Ren) and Massa Fermentata (Shen Qu) increase its Qi Regulating effect and this combination is especially effective for children.

Pericarpium Papaveris   **Ying Su Ke**   (3)

Common Name: Poppy Capsule

Family Name: Papaveraceae

Energy and Flavors: sour, astringent, neutral, toxic

Organ Meridians Affected: Lung, Large Intestine and Kidneys

Actions: 1. Astringes the Lungs; 2. Astringes the Intestines; 3. Stops pain.

Indications: 1. Chronic diarrhea and dysentery; 2. Chronic coughs; 3. Any kind of pain.

Contraindications: It is contraindicated for acute dysentery or coughs. Because it contains trace amounts of morphine, it should not be taken for a prolonged period and dosage should be strictly regulated.

Notes: Most poppies can be used either internally or externally for pain. Certain of them are, of course, the source for morphine. They are also effective for the treatment of diarrhea, especially when combined with Coptis (Huang Lian) and Saussurea (Mu Xiang). For coughs they can be combined with Mume Plum (Wu Mei).

Pericarpium Punicae Granati   **Shi Liu Pi**   (3)

Common Name: Pomegranate husk

Family: Punicaceae

Energy and Flavors: Sour, astringent, Warm, toxic

Organ Meridians Affected: Kidney, Large Intestine, Stomach

Actions: 1. Astringes the Intestines, stops diarrhea; 2. Retains Kidney Essence; 3. Kills parasites.

Indications: 1. Treats chronic diarrhea from Cold Deficiency, dysentery and prolapsed rectum; 2. Used for premature ejaculation, seminal emission, spermatorrhea, excessive uterine bleeding and vaginal discharge; 3. Kills and expels tapeworms and roundworms and amebic dysentery (an extract of this herb can be taken 3 times a day for 6 days to kill amebic dysentery; temporary side effects may be slight nausea and tinnitus); 4. Topically an alcoholic extract can be applied to treat ringworm.

Dosage: 3 - 9 grams

Contraindications: This herb should not be taken during the early stages of diarrhea and dysentery. When using it for parasites, it should not be taken with oils or fats to minimize absorption of the toxin into the system.

Notes: Pomegranate husk is a specific for the treatment for both tapeworms and roundworms. For this it can be combined with Areca Nut (Bing Lang). For dysentery and unrelenting diarrhea it can be combined with Myristacae (Rou Dou Kou), Coptis (Huang Lian) and Chebula (He Zi).

Ailanthi Altissimae   Chun Pi   (3)

Common Name: Ailanthus Bark

Part Used: Bark (Cortex)

Family: Simaroubaceae

Energy and Flavors: bitter, astringent, Cold

Organ Meridians Affected: Large Intestine, Stomach

Actions: 1. Clears Heat, dries Dampness and stops leukorrhea; 2. Astringes the Intestines; 3. Stops bleeding; 4. Kills worms.

Indications: 1. For Damp-Heat type diarrhea with Coptis (Huang Lian) and Scutellaria (Huang Qin); 2. For yellow leukorrhea with Phellodendron bark (Huang Bai); 3. For menorrhagia or uterine bleeding with Tortoise plastron (Gui Ban), Paeonia alba (Bai Shao) and Scutellaria (Huang Qin).

Dosage: 3 - 6 grams

Contraindications: Do not use if there are symptoms of Cold Deficiency of the Spleen and Stomach or noticeable Kidney Yin Deficiency.

Notes: For Damp Heat diarrhea or dysentery with symptoms of fever, rapid pulse and yellow tongue, Ailanthus can be combined with Coptis (Huang Lian), Scutellaria (Huang Qin) and Saussurea (Mu Xiang). For Damp Heat leukorrhea it can be combined with Phellodendron (Huang Bai). For menorrhagia and excessive uterine bleeding caused by Blood Heat, it is combined with Tortoise plastron (Gui Ban), White Peony (Bai Shao) and Scutellaria (Huang Qin).

Nelumbinis Nucifera   Lian Zi   (1)

Common Name: Lotus Seed

Part Used: Seed (Semen)

Family: Nymphaeceae

Energy and Flavors: sweet, astringent, neutral

Organ Meridians Affected: Heart, Kidney, Spleen

Actions: 1. Tonifies the Spleen, stops diarrhea; 2. Strengthens the Kidneys, reinforces Essence; 3. Nourishes the Blood and calms the mind.

Indications: 1. Used for Spleen Deficiency with chronic diarrhea and loss of appetite; 2. Prevents premature ejaculation, spermatorrhea, uterine bleeding and vaginal discharge; 3. Nourishes the Heart and calms the mind, for conditions caused by a lack of communication between Kidneys and Heart with symptoms of Deficiency irritability, anxiety and insomnia.

Dosage: 6 - 15 grams. This herb can be eaten as part of the diet cooked with other foods.

Contraindications: Not for individuals with constipation and abdominal distention.

Notes: Lotus seeds are used both in Chinese and Ayurvedic medicine as both a medicine and a food. As such, they are good for diarrhea and loose stool resulting from Spleen and Stomach Deficiency, for which they may be combined with Dioscorea (Shan Yao). Given the metaphor of the Lotus as a symbol of calm enlightenment, they are also used with Lily Bulb (Bai He), Glehnia (Sha Shen), Wild Jujube Seeds (Suan Zao Ren), Arborvitae Seeds (Bai Zi Ren) and Poria attached to the host-wood (Fu Shen) for irritability, restlessness, nervous anxiety and insomnia. They are also used to supplement Kidney Deficiency when combined with Cuscuta (Tu Si Zi) and Euryale seed (Qian Shi) for symptoms of leukorrhea and seminal emissions. Lotus seeds are highly nourishing and are often added to various therapeutic food recipes with Euryales (Qian Shi). In India, they are roasted and made into a popped cereal and used for recovery from childbirth or sickness.

Euryales Ferocis   Qian Shi   (1)

Common Name: Foxnut

Part Used: Seed (Semen)

Family: Nymphaceae

Energy and Flavors: sweet, astringent, neutral

Organ Meridians Affected: Kidney, Spleen

Actions: 1. Tonifies the Spleen and stops diarrhea; 2. Strengthens the Kidneys and restrains Essence; 3. Dispels Dampness and relieves leukorrhea.

Indications: 1. Stops diarrhea, especially good for children; 2. For nocturnal emission, premature ejaculation, spermatorrhea and urinary incontinence; 3. For clear or whitish vaginal discharge.

Dosage: 9 - 15 grams. This herb is very similar to Lotus seed and they are frequently used together.

Contraindications: None

Notes: Euryale, or Foxnuts, have the same use as Lotus seed (Lian Zi) except they are not used so much for calming the mind.

Rosa Laevigatae   **Jin Ying Zi**   (2)
Common Name: Rosehip
Part Used: Fruit (Fructus)
Family: Rosaceae
Energy and Flavors: sour, astringent and neutral
Organ Meridians Affected: Bladder, Kidneys, Large Intestines
Actions: 1. Controls Essence; 2. Astringes the Intestines and stops diarrhea; 3. Decreases urination.

Indications: 1. For seminal emissions and clear leukorrhea, combine with Euryales seed (Qian Shi) and Dodder seed (Tu Si Zi); 2. For chronic diarrhea caused by Deficient Spleen combine with Codonopsis (Dang Shen), Atractylodes (Bai Zhu) and Dioscorea (Shan Yao).

Dosage: 6 - 9 grams

Contraindications: Not for acute conditions caused by Excess Heat.

Notes: Rosehips are commonly used in the popular Western herb market as a healthful beverage with high vitamin C content. Taken with some of the stems and leaves, they are also very effective for acute postpartum uterine hemorrhage. For nocturnal emission and urinary incontinence, combine with Euryale ferox (Qian Shi).

Rubi Chingii   **Fu Pen Zi**   (2)
Common Name: Chinese Raspberry
Part Used: Fruit (Fructus)
Family: Rosaceae
Energy and Flavors: sweet, astringent, slightly Warm
Organ Meridians Affected: Kidney, Liver
Actions: 1. Augments the Kidneys, restrains Essence; 2. Supports Yang.

Indications: 1. For seminal emissions, premature ejaculation, spermatorrhea, enuresis, urinary frequency caused by Deficient Kidneys; 2. Improves eyesight, treats aching lower back and impotence caused by Kidney and Liver Deficiency.

Combinations: 1. Combine with Ootheca mantidis (Sang Piao Xiao) for urinary frequency; 2. Take with Schisandra berries (Wu Wei Zi), Lycii berries (Gou Qi Zi), Cuscuta seed (Tu Si Zi) and Plantaginis seed(Che Qian Zi) for impotence, spermatorrhea, premature ejaculation, weak and low sperm count; 3. Take with Eucommiae ulmoides (Du Zhong) and Dipsacus (Xu Duan) for lower back pain and weakness of the lower extremities caused by Kidney Deficiency.

Contraindications: Use with caution for Yin Deficiency patterns.

Ephedrae Sinensis   Ma Huang Gen   (3)

Common Name: Ephedra root

Part Used: Root (Radix)

Family: Ephedraceae

Energy and Flavors: sweet, neutral

Organ Meridians Affected: Lungs

Actions: 1. Stops sweating caused by Yin Deficiency.

Indications: It is useful for spontaneous sweating, night sweats and postpartum sweating caused by Yin Deficiency.

Dosage: 3 - 9 grams

Contraindications: Not for Exterior conditions.

Notes: While the upper part of Ephedra (Ma Huang) has a stimulating, dispersing and upward energy, the root is contracting and astringent. To inhibit excessive sweating caused by Deficient Qi and Blood, combine with Astragalus (Huang Qi) and Angelica sinensis (Dang Gui); if there is Deficient Kidney Yin, combine with Raw Rehmannia (Sheng Di Huang) and Oyster shell (Mu Li).

Oryza Glutinosa   Nuo Dao Gen Xu   (3)

Common Name: Glutinous Rice Root

Part Used: Root and Rhizome (Radix et Rhizoma)

Family: Graminaceae

Energy and Flavors: sweet, neutral

Organ Meridians Affected: Kidneys, Liver, Lungs

Actions and Indications: 1. Stops sweating caused by Yin Deficiency; 2. Treats Yin Deficient fevers.

Dosage: 15 - 60 grams.

Contraindications: None

Notes: Glutinous Rice roots can be combined with Light Wheat (Fu Xiao Mai) and Oyster shell (Mu Li) for abnormal sweating caused by weakness and Deficiency. For fever and Heat caused by Yin Deficiency, it can be combined with Glehnia (Sha Shen) and Lycii bark (Di Gu Pi).

Tritici Levis   **Fu Xiao Mai**

Common Name: Light Wheat

Family: Graminae

Energy and Flavors: sweet and Cool

Organ Meridians Affected: Heart

Actions: 1. Tonifies Qi and clears Heat; 2. Stops excessive sweating.

Indications: 1. For fatigue and tiredness caused by both Qi and Yin Deficiency; 2. Calms the spirit and nourishes the Heart; 3. Children's bedwetting.

Notes: For abnormal sweating and night sweats caused by weakness and Deficiency, combine with Oyster shell (Mu Li), Astragalus (Huang Qi) and Ephedra root (Ma Huang Gen) in the formula called Mu li san. For emotional instability, nervousness and insomnia combine with Licorice (Gan Cao) and Jujube Dates (Da Zao).

Os Sepiae seu Sepiellae   **Hai Piao Xiao** (3)

Common Name: Cuttlefish Bone

Family: Sepiidae

Energy and Flavors: salty, astringent, slightly Warm

Organ Meridians Affected: Kidney, Liver and Stomach

Actions: 1. Astringes and stops bleeding; 2. Controls Essence and relieves leukorrhea; 3. Counteracts stomach acidity and stops pain; 4. Heals ulcers.

Indications: 1. It stops uterine bleeding and vaginal discharge; the powder can also be applied topically to stop bleeding from wounds and injuries; 2. Controls gastrointestinal acidity and relieves abdominal pains; 3. It resolves Dampness and the powder can be topically applied to promote the healing of wounds, sores and weeping eczema; 4. It is effective for the treatment of diarrhea and dysentery caused by Deficiency with pressure sensitivity around the navel.

Dosage: 6 - 12 grams

Contraindications: It should not be used for conditions of Deficient Yin and Excessive Heat.

Notes: Powder of Cuttlefish bone is taken alone or in combination with Fritillary (Chuan Bei Mu) for stomach acidity and pain. For excessive

uterine bleeding it can be combined with Rubiae cordifoliae (Qian Cao Gen) and Donkey Skin Gelatin (E Jiao). For Kidney Deficiency with symptoms of seminal emissions or leukorrhea it is combined with Cornus (Shan Zhu Yu), Dioscorea (Shan Yao), Cuscuta (Tu Si Zi) and Oyster shell (Mu Li). Externally it can be applied as a healing antimicrobial powder with Phellodendron (Huang Bai) and Indigo (Qing Dai).

Ootheca Mantidis   **Sang Piao Xiao** (2)

Common Name: Mantis Egg-Case, Mantis

Family: Mantidae

Energy and Flavors: sweet, salty, neutral

Organ Meridians Affected: Kidney, Liver

Actions: 1. Tonifies Kidneys and strengthens Yang; 2. Restrains Essence and decreases urination.

Indications: 1. For seminal emission, nocturnal enuresis, urinary incontinence, premature ejaculation and clear or whitish leukorrhea, combine with Dragon's bone (Long Gu), Oyster shell (Mu Li), Dodder seed (Tu Si Zi) and Psoralea fruit (Bu Gu Zhi).

Dosage: 3 - 9 grams

Contraindications: Not to be used for Excessive Fire or Deficient Yin patterns or cystitis.

Notes: The egg case is collected in the Fall or Spring. It is then either boiled or steamed and dried for use. Its main use is for leakages of all kinds. For seminal emissions, urinary incontinence and leukorrhea caused by Kidney Yang Deficiency, combine with Dragon Bone (Long Gu), Oyster shell (Mu Li), Cuscuta (Tu Si Zi) and Psoralea (Bu Gu Zhi).

Discrimination:

Fructus Corni Officinalis (Shan Zhu Yu) – preserves Kidney and Liver Yin and Essence, treats impotence, stops sweating, aids menstruation and stops bleeding.

Fructus Schisandrae Chinensis (Wu Wei Zi) – Preserves Essence, protects and holds the Qi, prevents leakage, stops cough, calms the mind.

Fructus Prunus Mume (Wu Mei) – stops coughs, stops diarrhea, retains Bodily Fluids, relieves vomiting, expels parasites

Semen Ginkgo Biloba (Bai Guo) – stops chronic cough, expels phlegm, restrains leakage for urinary incontinence or clear leukorrhea.

Fructus Terminaliae Chebulae (He Zi) – for chronic diarrhea caused by either Heat or Coldness, stops coughing, improves the voice.

Semen Myristacae Fragrantis (Rou Dou Kou) – for chronic diarrhea, warms the Spleen and Stomach, promotes digestion, stops nausea and vomiting.

Pericarpium Papaveris (Ying Su Ke) – for chronic diarrhea and dysentery, chronic coughs, pain.

Pericarpium Punicae Granati (Shi Liu Pi) – astringes the Intestines, treats premature ejaculation, vaginal discharge and abnormal vaginal bleeding, kills and expels worms and amebas.

Cortex Ailanthi Altissimae (Chun Pi) – clears Damp Heat, stops leukorrhea, astringes the Intestines, stops bleeding, kills worms.

Semen Nelumbinis Nucifera (Lian Zi) – tonifies Spleen, stops diarrhea, strengthens the Kidneys, reinforces Essence, nourishes the Blood and calms the mind.

Semen Euryales Ferocis (Qian Shi) – similar to Semen Nelumbinis (Lian Zi) except it clears Dampness more.

Fructus Rosa Laevigatae (Jin Ying Zi) – restrains Essence, for seminal and vaginal discharge, stops diarrhea, decreases urination.

Fructus Rubi Chingii (Fu Pen Zi) – augments Kidneys, impotence, restrains Essence, seminal emission and vaginal discharge, improves eyesight.

Radix Ephedrae (Ma Huang Gen) – sweating caused by Yin Deficiency.

Radix et Rhizoma Oryza (Nuo Dao Gen Xu) – stops sweating, treats Yin Deficiency fevers.

Fructus Tritici Levis (Fu Xiao Mai) — stops sweating, tonifies Qi.

Os Sepiae seu Sepiellae (Hai Piao Xiao) – stops bleeding, treats stomach acidity, relieves leukorrhea, promotes healing of ulcers.

Ootheca Mantidis (Sang Piao Xiao) – tonifies Kidneys, strengthens Yang, decreases urination.

SUBSTANCES THAT CALM THE SPIRIT

These herbs are substances that calm the spirit, tranquilize the mind and treat symptoms of Deficient Heart Blood and Qi and upflaring of Heart Fire with symptoms such as restlessness, palpitations, anxiety, insomnia, dream-disturbed sleep, convulsions, epilepsy and manic-psychotic disorders.

This category is subdivided into substances that settle the spirit and those that nourish the Heart and calm the spirit. Herbs that settle the spirit are the more potent sedatives and are primarily heavy minerals and shells which have the power to sedate by weighing the Qi downwards. Included in this category are several toxic heavy metals such as Cinnabaris (which contains mercury). These should be used with great reservation and for a limited time only.

Herbs that nourish the Heart and calm the spirit are more tonifying than the preceding. These herbs calm and sedate by tonifying Heart Yin and Blood as well as Liver Yin. By so doing they can be used for Deficiency conditions with symptoms of anxiety, insomnia, neurosis, manic depression and schizophrenia.

The herbs should be selected according to their indications. If, for example, any of these symptoms are accompanied by Yin or Blood Deficiency, they should be combined with herbs and substances that nourish Yin and Blood. In treating symptoms of Internal Wind such as epilepsy and convulsions, one should primarily use herbs that resolve Phlegm and open the Orifices as well as subduing Internal Liver Wind as the primary herbs, with tranquilizing herbs added as assistants. If there is a hyperactivity of Liver Yang, use herbs that subdue uprising of Liver Yang in combination with herbs that calm the spirit.

SUBSTANCES THAT ANCHOR, SETTLE AND CALM THE SPIRIT

Os Draconis   Long Gu   (1)

Common Name: Dragon Bone

Energy and Flavors: sweet, astringent and neutral

Organ Meridians Affected: Liver, Heart and Kidney

Actions: 1. Calms the spirit; 2. Anchors ascendant Liver Yang; 3. Stops leakage of Bodily Fluids.

Indications: 1. For disturbance of the spirit (Shen) with symptoms such as palpitations, emotional issues, restlessness, insomnia and dream disturbed sleep; 2. For ascendant Liver Yang with symptoms such as emotional outbursts, irritability, headache, dizziness and blurred vision; 3. For spontaneous and night sweats, nocturnal emissions, urinary dribbling, vaginal discharge and uterine bleeding.

Contraindications: This herb should not be used by those with symptoms of Damp-Heat.

Dosage: 15 - 30 grams; it should be cooked for 30 - 45 minutes before the other herbs are added.

Notes: Dragon Bone represents the fossilized bones and vertebrae of prehistoric mammals and reptiles. There are several large deposits of these in different parts of China, including one place outside of Beijing known as Dragon Bone Mountain. I have heard reports of such a deposit somewhere in Florida with one company marketing a powder of the substance as a source of calcium. Dragon Teeth (Long Chi) are the fossilized teeth of prehistoric animals. They are more expensive and are regarded as having stronger sedative properties, especially for sleep that is disturbed by dreams. Dragon Bone is described as "anchoring the Yang"which means that it brings the ascendant Yang down to its source, just as its counterpart, Oyster shell (Mu Li), "anchors the Yin" and is used for treating Yin Deficiency. These are often combined together in many formulas because of their close synergistic effects, with Dragon Bone (Long Gu) being somewhat "drier" and Oyster shell (Mu Li) considered more "slippery".

These two are combined with Haematitum (Dai Zhe Shi), Prepared Rehmannia (Shu Di Huang) and Dioscorea (Shan Yao) for hypertension caused by Yin Deficiency with Liver Yang rising, with symptoms of blurred vision, insomnia, irritability and dizziness. For abnormal sweating and night sweats combine with Oyster shell (Mu Li) and Schisandra (Wu Wei Zi); for palpitations with insomnia combine with Oyster shell (Mu Li), Polygala (Yuan Zhi) and Zizyphus seeds (Suan Zao Ren); for night sweats caused by Yin Deficiency combine with Cornus (Shan Zhu Yu) and Prepared Rehmannia (Shu Di Huang); for leukorrhea caused by Deficient Kidneys combine with Oyster shell (Mu Li), Dioscorea (Shan Yao) and Cuttlefish bone (Wu Zei Gu).

Concha Ostreae   Mu Li   (1)
Common Name: Oyster Shell
Family: Ostreidae
Energy and Flavors: salty, astringent and slightly Cold
Organ Meridians Affected: Liver and Kidney
Actions: 1. Calms and anchors the spirit; 2. Moistens Dryness; 3. Softens and moves lumps.
Indications: 1. For disturbance of Shen with symptoms such as headache, insomnia, palpitations and restlessness; 2. For loss of vital Fluids through night sweats, unabating sweating, nocturnal emissions, vaginal discharge and uterine bleeding; 3. For lumps of the neck such as scrofula and goiter.
Contraindications: Oyster shell should not be used by those who are Cold and weak nor by those with high fever without sweating.

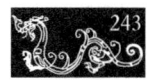

Dosage: 15 - 30 grams; it should be cooked for 30 - 45 minutes before the other herbs are added.

Notes: For Liver and Kidney Yin Deficiency with flaring of Yang manifesting with dizziness, vertigo, blurred vision, tinnitus, palpitations, irritability and insomnia combine with Dragon Bone (Long Gu), Tortoise Plastron (Gui Ban) and White Peony (Bai Shao); for inflamed swollen glands and lymph nodes combine with Fritillary (Chuan Bei Mu) and Scrophularia (Xuan Shen).

Cinnabaris   Zhu Sha   (3)

Common Name: Cinnabar

Part Used: mineral of red mercuric oxide

Energy and Flavors: sweet, Cool and toxic

Organ Meridians Affected: Heart

Actions: 1. Calms the spirit and Heart; 2. Stops convulsions; 3. Clears Heat and toxins.

Indications: 1. For disturbance of Shen associated with Excess Heat, Hot Phlegm or Blood Deficiency with symptoms such as palpitations, insomnia, restlessness and dream disturbed sleep; 2. For convulsions associated with high fever in infants, or epilepsy; 3. Applied externally for boils, carbuncles, mouth sores and snakebite.

Contraindications: Cinnabar should not be used by those without Heat signs. Because of its toxicity, it should not be used in large doses or for extended periods of time. It should only be taken in powdered form. DO NOT COOK as this will increase its toxicity.

Dosage: 0.3 - 2 grams

Notes: For Spirit disturbance associated with Heart Fire, combine with Coptis (Huang Lian) and Licorice (Gan Cao); if there is also Blood Deficiency add Angelica Sinensis (Dang Gui) and Unprepared Rehmannia (Sheng Di Huang); for insomnia and palpitations caused by Blood Deficiency combine with Angelica Sinensis (Dang Gui), Zizyphus Seeds (Suan Zao Ren) and Biota (Bai Zi Ren).

Magnetitum   Ci Shi   (3)

Part Used: Powdered or crushed mineral

Energy and Flavors: spicy, salty

Organ Meridians Affected: Kidneys, Liver, Lung and Heart

Actions: 1. Calms and sedates the spirit; 2. Calms the Liver and lowers rising Liver Yang; 3. Helps the Kidneys grasp Lung Qi.

Indications: 1. For insomnia, restlessness, tremors and convulsions; 2. For irritability, dizziness, vertigo, tinnitus and blurred eyesight; 3. Treats asthma caused by Kidney Deficiency.

Preparation: Crush into a fine powder and simmer several hours before adding other herbs to the formula.

Dosage: 9 - 30 grams

Contraindications and Toxicity: It should only be used for short periods because of the presence of heavy metals.

Notes: For tinnitus caused by Kidney Deficiency combine with Schisandra (Wu Wei Zi), Prepared Rehmannia (Shu Di Huang), Cornus (Shan Zhu Yu) and Dioscorea (Shan Yao); for dizziness and vertigo caused by Yin Deficiency with upflaring Yang, combine with Dragon Bone (Long Gu) and Oyster shell (Mu Li).

Haematitum   Dai Zhe Shi   (3)

Common Name: Red Ochre, Hematite

Part Used: Crushed or finely ground mineral

Energy and Flavors: bitter, Cold

Organ Meridians Affected: Liver, Stomach, Pericardium, Heart

Actions: 1. Calms the Liver, anchors uprising Yang and clears Liver Fire; 2. Moves Qi downward; 3. Cools the Blood, stops bleeding.

Indications: 1. Hyperactive Liver Yang caused by Yin Deficiency with symptoms of irritability, dizziness, vertigo, tinnitus and blurred vision; 2. Treats acute asthma, vomiting, nausea and hiccup by descending Rebellious Qi; 3. Treats nosebleeds, coughing up of blood and uterine bleeding.

Preparation: Crush to a fine powder and cook for 2 hours before adding other herbs to the formula.

Dosage: 9 - 30 grams

Contraindications and Toxicity: Do not use during pregnancy. Because it most likely contains traces of arsenic, it should only be used for short periods.

Notes: For Kidney and Liver Yin Deficiency with Yang rising (high blood pressure), combine with Dragon Bone (Long Gu), Oyster shell (Mu Li), White Peony (Bai Shao), Tortoise Plastron (Gui Ban) and Achyranthes (Niu Xi); for cough caused by rebellious Qi, possibly with vomiting, belching or hiccup, combine with Inula flowers (Xuan Fu Hua), Pinellia (Ban Xia) and Fresh Ginger (Sheng Jiang); for asthma caused by Lung and Kidney Deficiency combine with Ginseng (Ren Shen) and Cornus (Shan Zhu Yu).

Pteria Margaritifera (Margarita)   Zhen Zhu Mu (3)
Common Name: Mother of Pearl
Family: Pteriidae
Energy and Flavors: sweet, salty, Cold
Organ Meridians Affected: Heart, Liver
Actions: 1. Subdues Liver Yang; 2. Clears Liver Heat and brightens the eyes.
Indications: 1. Sedates the Heart, settles tremors and palpitations, 2. Used for Deficient Liver and Kidney Yin with hyperactive Yang and symptoms of headache, dizziness, vertigo, tinnitus, restlessness, anxiety and insomnia; 3. Promotes healing and generates flesh; 4. Topically it can be made into a paste to clear blemishes on the skin caused by Heat; 5. It can also be used to treat Heat toxins.
Contraindications: Not for Cold conditions.
Dosage: 0.3 - 0.9 grams in pill or powder form.
Notes: For Deficient Liver and Kidney Yin with Yang rising (high blood pressure), with symptoms of headache, dizziness, vertigo, tinnitus, irritability and insomnia combine with Unprepared Rehmannia (Sheng Di Huang), White Peony (Bai Shao), Haliotis (Shi Jue Ming) and Dragon Bone (Long Gu); for Deficient Liver Blood with blurred and impaired night vision, combine with Black Atractylodes (Cang Zhu), calf, pig, chicken and/or deer liver; to Calm Heart spirit, take the powder with honey; for childhood convulsions, palpitations, seizures and anxiety, combine with Succinum (Hu Po), Dragon Bone (Long Gu) and Cinnabaris (Zhu Sha). Mother of Pearl powder can be topically applied anywhere on the body to relieve inflammation. It can also be made into a salve for burns and clearing the complexion. Drops of the strained and cooled decoction can be placed in the eyes to clear Heat and treat conjunctivitis.

HERBS THAT NOURISH THE HEART AND CALM THE SPIRIT
Zizyphus Spinosae   Suan Zao Ren (1)
Common Name: Zizyphus, Wild Jujube Seed
Part Used: Seed (Semen)
Family: Rhamnaceae
Energy and Flavors: sweet, sour and neutral
Organ Meridians Affected: Liver, Heart, Spleen and Gallbladder
Actions: 1. Nourishes the Heart Yin and calms the spirit; 2. Contains Fluid leakage.

Indications: 1. For Deficiency of either Blood or Yin with symptoms such as insomnia, palpitations, irritability and restlessness; 2. For night sweats and spontaneous sweating.

Contraindications: This herb should not be used when there is extreme Fire in the body nor in cases of severe diarrhea.

Dosage: 6 - 18 grams

Notes: This is one of the most commonly used substances for symptoms of nervousness, anxiety and insomnia. The seeds can be used raw for a stronger sedative effect, or toasted for Stomach and Spleen Deficiency with night sweats. For insomnia, take 1.5 to 3 grams of the crushed seeds in capsules or in a cup of hot water before bed. For Deficiency of Liver and Heart Blood combine with Angelica sinensis (Dang Gui), Polygala (Yuan Zhi), White Peony (Bai Shao Yao), Longan berries (Long Yan Rou) and Polygonum stems (Ye Jiao Teng); for insomnia caused by Spleen Qi and Heart Blood Deficiency combine with Codonopsis (Dang Shen) and Poria with Host-wood (Fu Shen).

Polygalae Tenuifoliae   Yuan Zhi   (1)
Common Name: Polygala, Chinese Senega
Part Used: Root (Radix)
Family: Polygalaceae
Energy and Flavors: bitter, sweet and Warm
Organ Meridians Affected: Heart, Lung and Kidney
Actions: 1. Calms the spirit; 2. Expels Phlegm from the Heart orifices; 3. Expels Phlegm from the Lungs; 4. Diminishes abscesses.

Indications: 1. For disturbance of the Shen with symptoms such as palpitations, insomnia, excessive brooding, restlessness and forgetfulness; 2. For Phlegm masking the Heart with symptoms of emotional instability and seizures; 3. For cough with copious sputum that is difficult to expectorate; 4. For abscesses, boils, ulcers and swollen painful breasts, this herb is either applied externally as a powder or taken as a tincture.

Contraindications: This herb should not be used by those with Yin Deficient Heat signs.

Dosage: 3 - 9 grams

Notes: This herb has related species that grow in North America that have similar properties. One that is found in the Northeast is commonly known as Senega Snake root (Polygala senega) and was used by the Native Americans as an expectorant. The Chinese species is also an expectorant but is highly regarded for its antispasmodic properties that seems to exert a positive relaxing influence on the Lungs and Heart. It is also capable of counteracting negative emotions and enhancing more

positive feelings. Combined with the part of the Poria mushroom that is attached to the root (Fu Shen) and Zizyphus seeds (Suan Zao Ren) it is effective for nervous irritability, anxiety and insomnia; for cough caused by Cold Phlegm with tight wheezing and congestion, combine with Pinellia (Ban Xia) and Fritillary (Chuan Bei Mu).

Biota Orientalis   Bai Zi Ren   (2)

Common Name: Biota Seed

Part Used: Seed (Semen)

Family: Cupressaceae

Energy and Flavors: sweet and neutral

Organ Meridians Affected: Heart, Liver, Kidney and Large Intestine

Actions: 1. Nourishes the Heart and calms the spirit; 2. Moistens the Intestines and relieves constipation.

Indications: 1. For Deficiency of Heart Blood with symptoms such as palpitations, insomnia, anxiety and forgetfulness; 2. For constipation due to Blood or Yin Deficiency.

Contraindications: This herb should not be used by those with diarrhea nor should it be used for conditions of Phlegm.

Dosage: 3 - 15 grams

Notes: The fruit is gathered in the autumn. These are then shelled and dried in the shade. The seeds are further crushed and broken for use. For irritability, insomnia, palpitations and anxiety, combine with Zizyphus seeds (Suan Zao Ren), Schisandra (Wu Wei Zi) and Polygala (Yuan Zhi); for night sweats caused by Yin Deficiency combine with Oyster shell (Mu Li), Ginseng (Ren Shen), Schisandra (Wu Wei Zi); for constipation of post partum women or the elderly, combine with Cannabis (Huo Ma Ren) and Walnut (Hu Tao Ren).

Albizziae Julibrissan   He Huan Pi

Common Name: Mimosa tree, Albizzia

Part Used: The bark of the tree

Family: Leguminosae

Energy and Flavors: sweet, neutral

Organ Meridians Affected: Heart, Liver

Actions: 1. Tranquilizes the mind and relieves depression, 2. Invigorates Blood, relieves pain and reduces swelling.

Indications: 1. For anger, depression with forgetfulness combine with Biota (Bai Zi Ren), Polygonum (He Shou Wu) and Zizyphus seeds (Suan Zao Ren); 2. For pain and swelling caused by external injury as well as pain associated with chronic degenerative diseases combine with Angelica sinensis (Dang Gui), Olibanum (Ru Xiang), Myrrh (Mo Yao) and Corydalis (Yan Hu Suo).

Notes: The translation of the Chinese, "happiness bark," refers to its use to help counteract feelings of anger and depression.

Polygonum Multiflorum   Ye Jiao Teng   (3)

Common Name: He Shou Wu Stem

Part Used: Stem (Caulis)

Family: Polygonaceae

Energy and Flavors: sweet, slightly bitter and neutral

Organ Meridians Affected: Heart and Liver

Actions: 1. Nourishes the Heart Blood and calms the spirit; 2. Tonifies Blood, improves circulation and dispels Wind; 3. Applied externally, it relieves itches and rashes.

Indications: 1. For dream disturbed sleep, palpitations, insomnia and restlessness associated with Yin or Blood Deficiency; 2. For sore, aching and tired limbs associated with Blood Deficiency where Internal Wind has arisen due to the Deficiency; 3. Applied externally as a wash for rash with itch.

Contraindications: This herb should not be used by those with diarrhea.

Dosage: 9 - 30 grams

Notes: This herb has been recently introduced in many Western gardens and is increasingly available from nurseries and herb growers. It is one of the fastest growing vine-like plants and can be somewhat invasive. A strong decoction of the leaves and stems can be taken as a tea for insomnia or topically applied as a wash to relieve itching and skin rashes. For insomnia cased by Deficient Heart Blood combine with Zizyphus seeds (Suan Zao Ren), Biota (Bai Zi Ren) and Angelica sinensis (Dang Gui); for sore and tired limbs caused by Blood Deficiency combine with Angelica sinensis (Dang Gui), Millettia (Ji Xue Teng), White Peony (Bai Shao) and Salvia (Dan Shen).

Discrimination:

Os Draconis (Long Gu) – anchors the ascendant Yang, stops leakage of Bodily Fluids.

Concha Ostreae (Mu Li) – anchors the ascendant Yang, lubricates, softens hard lumps.

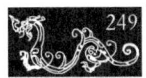

Cinnabaris (Zhu Sha) — clears Heart Heat, stops convulsions.

Magnetitum (Ci Shi) — calms Liver Yang, helps Kidneys grasp Lung Qi downwards, treats tinnitus.

Haematitum (Dai Zhe Shi) — calms Liver Yang, directs Qi downwards, cools the Blood and stops bleeding.

Margarita (Zhen Zu Mu) — calms Liver Yang, sedates the Heart and relieves palpitations, for patients who are easily frightened, relieves Heat.

Zizyphus Spinosae (Suan Zao Ren) — nourishes Blood, Liver and Heart Yin, astringes Fluids, inhibits night sweats.

Polygalae Tenuifoliae (Yuan Zhi) — expectorates Phlegm from the Lungs, treats disturbed Shen (spirit) of the Heart.

Biota Orientalis (Bai Zi Ren) — nourishes Heart Yin, lubricates the Intestines.

Albizziae Julibrissin (He Huan Pi) — calms the spirit, relieves anger and depression, invigorates Blood and relieves pain.

Polygonum Multiflorum, Stem (Ye Jiao Teng) — nourishes Heart Blood, improves circulation, treats arthritic and skin conditions caused by Blood Deficiency.

AROMATIC SUBSTANCES THAT OPEN THE ORIFICES

Herbs in this category are used to help revive conditions associated with central nervous system collapse, including strokes and coma. There are two important differentiations: closed Orifices caused by Heat and closed Orifices caused by Cold. Many herbs in this category can be used for both but must be combined with appropriate Cooling or Heating herbs.

Herbs that open the Orifices are strongly dispersing and should not be used if the underlying cause is Collapse of Yang from severe Yang Deficiency. It this is the cause, then Yang and Qi tonics should be taken instead.

Secretio Moschus   She Xiang   (1)
Common Name: Musk
Family: Cervidae
Energy and Flavors: acrid and Warm
Organ Meridians Affected: Heart, Spleen and Liver

Actions: 1. Opens the Orifices and awakens the spirit; 2. Moves Blood and reduces inflammation and pain. 3. Moves downward, assisting the delivery of late or stillborn babies.

Indications: 1. For Heat or Phlegm Fire and high fever which cause loss of consciousness, convulsion or seizures; 2. For either internal or external application for Heat and toxicity associated boils, carbuncles, traumatic injury and painful obstruction; 3. For delayed birth or to assist the passage of stillborn or placenta.

Contraindications: This herb should not be used by pregnant women nor should it be used in cases of Yin Deficiency with Heat signs. It should be used with caution by those with high blood pressure.

Dosage: 0.075 - 0.15 grams

Notes: For unconsciousness caused by high fever, combine with Ox Gallstone (Niu Huang) and Rhinoceros Horn (Xi Jiao) (Water Buffalo Horn can be substituted); for unconsciousness caused by a stroke combine with Styrax (Su He Xiang) and Cloves (Ding Xiang); for sudden and severe chest and abdominal pain combine with Saussurea (Mu Xiang) and Corydalis (Yan Hu Suo); to expel a dead fetus or placenta after childbirth, combine with Cinnamon bark (Rou Gui).

Benzoinum   **An Xi Xiang**   (2)

Common Name: Benzoin

Family: Styracaceae

Energy and Flavors: acrid, bitter and neutral

Organ Meridians Affected: Heart, Liver and Spleen

Actions: 1. Opens the Orifices and moves Blood and Qi.

Indications: 1. For obstruction of the Orifices where there is Stagnation of Blood or Qi with symptoms such as coma, focal distention or pain in the chest or abdomen or loss of consciousness.

Contraindications: This herb should not be used by those with Yin Deficiency with Fire.

Dosage: 0.3 - 1.5 grams

Notes: For severe abdominal pains caused by Cold, combine with Ginger (Gan Jiang), Saussurea (Mu Xiang), Agastache (Huo Xiang) and Fennel seed (Xiao Hui Xiang).

Borneol   **Bing Pian**   (1)

Common Name: Borneol

Family: Dyptercarpaceae or Compositae

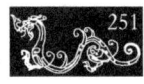

Energy and Flavors: acrid, bitter and slightly Cold

Organ Meridians Affected: Heart, Lung and Spleen

Actions: 1. Opens the Orifices and awakens the spirit; 2. Clears Heat and relieves pain.

Indications: 1. For loss of consciousness and convulsions caused by very high fever; 2. Used topically for swollen sore throat, vaginal inflammation, skin sores and photophobia.

Contraindications: This herb should not be used by those with Qi or Blood Deficiency, it should not be used during pregnancy and should not be exposed to extreme Heat or flame. Like many of the substances in this category, it should not be taken over a prolonged period.

Dosage: 0.03 - 0.9 grams

Notes: For unconsciousness caused by high fever combine with Musk (She Xiang) and Ox Gallstone (Niu Huang) in the patented formula Angong Niuhuang Wan.

Liquidambar Orientalis — Su He Xiang

Common Name: Styrax

Part Used: The resin or sap is collected from the bark in autumn

Family: Hamamelidaceae

Energy and Flavors: pungent, sweet and Warm

Organ Meridians Affected: Heart and Stomach

Actions: 1. Opens the Orifices and clears the mind; 2. Stops pain.

Indications: For sudden coma caused by Qi Stagnation or stroke, combine with Musk (She Xiang), Cloves (Ding Xiang) and Borneol (Bing Pian); for stifling and tight feeling in the chest combine with Borneol (Bing Pian), Sandalwood (Tan Xiang) and Cloves (Ding Xiang).

Notes: For fainting, coma, infantile convulsions and seizures, combine with Musk (She Xiang), Benzoinum (An Xi Xiang) and Flos Caryophylli (Ding Xiang).

Acori Graminei — Shi Chang Pu

Common Name: Sweetflag

Part Used: Rhizome (Rhizoma)

Family: Araceae

Energy and Flavors: acrid and Warm

Organ Meridians Affected: Heart, Liver and Stomach

Actions: 1. Opens the Orfices, awakens the spirit and expels Wind-Damp Phlegm; 2. Harmonizes the Earth element and dispels Damp; 3. Applied internally or externally for Wind-Cold-Damp painful obstruction.

Indications: 1. For Phlegm masking the Heart with symptoms such as loss of consciousness, deafness, seizures, insanity and forgetfulness; 2. For Damp obstructing the Earth Element with symptoms such as loss of appetite and distention and/or fullness of the chest and abdomen; 3. For internal or external application for Wind-Damp-Cold painful obstruction or trauma pain.

Contraindications: This herb should not be used by those with Yin Deficiency with Heat signs and should be used with caution by those with excessive sweating or spermatorrhea.

Dosage: 3 - 9 grams

Notes: For unconsciousness caused by Damp Heat Phlegm blockage of the Pericardium, combine with Bamboo juice (Zhu Li) and Curcuma (Yu Jin); for Damp Heat blocking the Middle Warmer with dysentery and vomiting combine with Coptis (Huang Lian); for Cold Dampness blocking the Middle Warmer combine with Citrus (Chen Pi) and Magnolia bark (Hou Po); for insomnia, forgetfulness, tinnitus and deafness combine with Polygala (Yuan Zhi), Poria (Fu Ling) in the Chinese patented formula Anshen Dingzhi Wan.

SUBSTANCES THAT PACIFY INTERNAL LIVER WIND AND STOP TREMORS

Herbs that pacify Internal Liver Wind and stop tremors are used for tremors, spasms, convulsions, dizziness and vertigo caused by hyperactive Liver Yang. Internal Liver Wind can arise from Heat, Deficient Yin or Blood, and herbs in these categories should be used in the prescriptions. As an example, if Internal Liver Wind is caused by Heat, herbs that Clear Heat should be added. Herbs that tonify Yin or Blood should be used if Deficiency of either of these is the cause. Many substances in this category are insects and generally are considered to be in the category of "strange proteins". Primarily they seem to have a powerful antispasmodic effect on the nervous system. They can also be used for their anti-toxic and anti-carcinogenic properties.

Uncariae Rhynchophylla   Gou Teng   (1)

Common Name: Gambir, Hook Vine

Family: Rubiaceae

Part Used: Branch with Thorn (Ramulus cum Uncis)

Energy and Flavors: sweet and slightly Cold

Organ Meridians Affected: Heart, Liver and Pericardium

Actions: 1. Calms Liver Wind and relieves spasms; 2. Clears Liver Heat and sedates Liver Yang.

Indications: 1. For Liver Heat causing Internal Wind with symptoms such as convulsion, tremors and seizures; 2. For Liver Heat and Yang rising with symptoms such as headache, hypertension, irritability and dizziness.

Contraindications: None noted.

Dosage: 6 - 15 grams. Do not cook this herb for more than 10 minutes.

Notes: Chinese Uncaria clears Excess Liver Heat and hyperactive Liver Yang (high blood pressure). Its antispasmodic properties, however, makes it useful for assisting the treatment of Deficient Kidney and Liver Yin patterns with symptoms such as dizziness, vertigo, blurred vision, headache and hypertension. For these conditions, it can be combined with Prunella (Xia Ku Cao), Scutellaria (Huang Qin), Haliotis (Shi Jue Ming) and Chrysanthemum flower (Ju Hua). If there are pronounced symptoms of Liver Heat with high fever, spasms and convulsions, add Antelope's horn and Gypsum (Shi Gao). South American Cat's Claw is one of a number of Uncaria species, found mostly in tropical and subtropical parts of the world, that share similar anti-inflammatory properties with the Chinese variety.

Gastrodiae Elatae   Tian Ma   (1)

Common Name: Gastrodia

Part Used: Rhizome (Rhizoma)

Family: Orchidaceae

Energy and Flavors: sweet and neutral

Organ Meridians Affected: Liver

Actions: 1. Calms Liver Wind, sedates Liver Yang and relieves convulsion; 2. Relieves Wind and stops pain.

Indications: 1. For patterns of Wind caused by Excess Heat or Cold or by Deficiency of Blood with symptoms such as headache, convulsions in children, dizziness, facial paralysis, epilepsy or Wind-stroke; 2. For Wind with symptoms such as headache, dizziness and arthritic conditions; also for Wind-Phlegm migraine headaches.

Contraindications: This herb should not be taken in large doses or for extended periods of time.

Dosage: 3 - 9 grams

Notes: Gastrodia is similar to Uncaria (Gou Teng) except that its sweet flavor causes it to possess more Yin tonic properties. For Internal Liver Wind with spasms and convulsions it can be combined with Uncaria (Gou Teng) and Scorpion (Quan Xie); for migraine headache it can be combined with Ligusticum (Chuan Xiong) and Achyranthes (Niu Xi); for headache caused by hyperactive Liver Yang with hypertension, combine with Uncaria (Gou Teng), Scutellaria (Huang Qin) and Achyranthes

(Niu Xi); for dizziness and vertigo caused by Spleen Dampness with Stagnant Liver Qi, combine with Pinellia (Ban Xia), White Atractylodes (Bai Zhu), Poria (Fu Ling); for joint pains caused by Wind-Damp obstruction combine with Frankincense (Ru Xiang) and Ligusticum (Chuan Xiong); for numbness of the limbs and extremities combine with Angelica sinensis (Dang Gui), Ligusticum (Chuan Xiong) and Achyranthes (Niu Xi).

Tribuli Terrestris   Bai Ji Li   (2)

Common Name: Puncture Vine Fruit, Tribulus

Part Used: Fruit (Fructus)

Family: Zygophyllaceae

Energy and Flavors: acrid, bitter and Warm

Organ Meridians Affected: Liver and Lung

Actions: 1. Calms the Liver Yang; 2. Clears Wind-Heat and clears the eyes; 3. Assists the Liver in the smooth flow of Qi.

Indications: 1. For Liver Yang rising patterns with symptoms such as headache, dizziness and vertigo; 2. For Wind-Heat with symptoms such as red, painful and swollen eyes with excessive tearing; 3. For Stagnation of Liver Qi with symptoms such as pain and fullness in the chest and flanks and poor lactation.

Contraindications: This herb should not be used by women during pregnancy nor should it be used by those with either Yin or Blood Deficiency.

Dosage: 3 - 9 grams

Notes: This herb is a common weed sometimes called "puncture weed" because the hard thorny seed is commonly responsible for injuries to bare feet and bicycle tires that happen to ride over them. For hyperactive Liver Yang with dizziness, vertigo, distention, pain in the head from hypertension, combine with Uncaria (Gou Teng), Chrysanthemum flower (Ju Hua) and White Peony (Bai Shao); if there is pronounced redness of the eyes with tearing add Chaste Tree (Man Jing Zi) and Cassia seed (Jue Ming Zi); for Liver Qi Stagnation with stifling sensation in the chest combine with Bupleurum (Chai Hu), Tangerine leaf (Ju Ye), Green Tangerine peel (Qing Pi) and Cyperus (Xiang Fu); for Wind and Heat in the Blood combine with Cicada (Chan Tui), Ledebouriella (Fang Feng) and Schizonepeta (Jing Jie).

Concha Haliotidis   Shi Jue Ming   (1)

Common Name: Abalone Shell

Family: Haliotidae

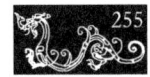

Energy and Flavors: salty and Cold

Organ Meridians Affected: Liver, Kidney and Lung

Actions: 1. Clears Heat and calms ascending Liver Yang; 2. Clears Liver Heat that is obstructing the vision.

Indications: 1. For Liver Yang rising with symptoms such as headache, dizziness and vertigo; 2. For Liver Heat rising with symptoms such as blurred vision, red eyes and photophobia.

Contraindications: This herb should not be used by those without true Heat signs.

Dosage: 9 - 30 grams

Notes: Abalone shell is specifically used for bringing down hyperactive Liver Yang with symptoms of hypertension. If the cause is Liver and Kidney Yin Deficiency with dizziness, vertigo and blurred vision, combine with Oyster shell (Mu Li), White Peony (Bai Shao) and Tortoise Plastron (Gui Ban); if there are feelings of pain and distention of the head, reddening of eyes and face, add Uncaria (Gou Teng), Chrysanthemum (Ju Hua), Scutellaria (Huang Qin) and Cassia seed (Jue Ming Zi); for blurred vision with dryness of the eyes caused by Deficiency of Liver Blood, combine with Prepared Rehmannia (Shu Di Huang) and Lycii berries (Gou Qi Zi).

Cornus Saigae Tataricae **Ling Yang Jiao** (3)

Common Name: Antelope's horn

Family: Bovidae

Energy and Flavors: salty, Cold

Organ Meridians Affected: Heart, Liver

Actions: 1. Clears Internal Liver Wind, subdues Yang; 2. Clears Liver Fire and brightens the eyes; 3. Eliminates toxins and reduces fever.

Indications: 1. For high fever with spasms, convulsions, delirium, mania and loss of consciousness; 2. For high blood pressure with dizziness and blurred vision; 3. For headache, eye inflammation and pains.

Dosage: 0.9 - 3 grams when taken in powders or pills; 1.5 to 3 grams when taken in decoctions. It should be cooked for one hour before other ingredients are added.

Notes: Because of ecological considerations, Goat horn (Cornus Naemorhedis - Shan Yang Jiao) is more commonly used as a substitute for Antelope. While having similar properties, Goat horn is significantly weaker, necessitating the use of a significantly higher dosage of 9-15 grams. For high fever, spasms and convulsions combine with Uncaria (Gou Teng), Chrysanthemum (Ju Hua) and Unprepared Rehmannia (Shu Di Huang) in Antelope and Uncaria Combination (Ling Jiao Gou

Teng Tang); for hyperactivity of Liver Yang with dizziness, distended feeling in the head and blurred vision, combine with Haliotis (Shi Jue Ming), Prunella spike (Xia Ku Cao) and Chrysanthemum (Ju Hua); for Liver Fire rising with hypertension, red, painful and swollen eyes, with headache combine with Gardenia (Zhi Zi), Gentian (Long Dan Cao) and Cassia seed (Jue Ming Zi); for high fever with loss of consciousness associated with conditions such as meningitis and encephalitis, combine with Rhinoceros horn (Xi Jiao), for which Water Buffalo horn can be substituted, and Gypsum (Shi Gao).

Lumbricus — Di Long (2)

Common Names: Earthworm, Lumbricus

Family: Megascolecidae

Energy and Flavors: salty and Cold

Organ Meridians Affected: Liver, Spleen and Bladder

Actions: 1. Clears Heat and calms Internal Liver Wind; 2. Soothes asthma; 3. Opens the channels.

Indications: 1. For convulsions and spasms caused by high fever, use with Uncaria (Gou Teng), Silkworm (Jiang Can) and Scorpion (Quan Xie); 2. For asthma, use with Ephedra (Ma Huang) and Apricot seed (Xing Ren); 3. For hemiplegia caused by blockage of the meridians, Lumbricus (Di Long) is used in Tonify Yang to Restore Five Decoction (Bu yang huan wu tang); 4. For cystitis and urinary stones combine with Plantain seed (Che Qian Zi), Achyranthes (Niu Xi), Lysimachiae (Jin Qian Cao) and Semen Abutili seu malvae (Dong Kui Zi).

Notes: Earthworms are used as an inexpensive protein source in certain cultures. The use of worms and insects in Traditional Chinese Medicine has its counterpart in the traditional medicine of Western Europe as recent as 500 years ago, if not even in more recent times. Insects represent the essence of pure neurological instinct reaction that is akin to the manifestation of involuntary reflexes such as spasms, seizures, shaking, and stroke, all associated with Internal Wind patterns. Described as "strange proteins", these seem to have a corrective effect on the nervous system. Today, it is customary to administer insects as a powder taken in capsules.

Buthus Martensi — Quan Xie (2)

Common Names: Scorpion, Buthus

Family: Buthidae

Energy and Flavors: pungent, neutral and toxic

Organ Meridians Affected: Liver

Actions: 1. Antispasmodic, subdues Internal Wind; 2. Clears toxins; 3. Stops pain.

Indications: 1. Stops tremors and convulsions in conditions such as opisthotonos, tics, and epilepsy; 2. It detoxifies sores, swellings and swollen glands; 3. It opens the channels and stops pain for the treatment of stubborn headaches such as migraines and other Wind Damp pains.

Dosage: 2 to 5 grams or 0.6 - 1 gram of the powder.

Contraindications: It is toxic and overdose should be avoided. It should not be used in patients with Blood Deficiency. It is contraindicated during pregnancy.

Notes: For spasms, rigidity, muscle twitches throughout the body and convulsions, combine with Centipede (Wu Gong) and Uncaria (Gou Teng); for stubborn or migraine headache as well as rheumatic pains combine with Silkworm (Jiang Can), Centipede (Wu Gong) Gastrodia (Tian Ma) and Ligusticum (Chuan Xiong); for cancer and tumors make into a powder together with Silkworm (Jiang Can) and Centipede (Wu Gong), suspend in the water in a small cloth bag while cooking an egg. Eat the egg and drink the broth. In certain areas of China, people believe that consuming 10 roasted Scorpions a month is protective from all disease.

Scolopendra Subspinipes   Wu Gong (2)

Common Name: Centipede, Scolopendra

Family: Scolopendridae

Energy and Flavors: pungent, Warm and toxic

Organ Meridians Affected: Liver

Actions: 1. Antispasmodic, subdues Internal Wind; 2. Clears toxins; 3. Opens the channels and stops pain.

Indications: 1. For spasms, tetany, convulsions and epilepsy; 2. Treats venomous bites and stings, clears toxins and reduces swollen glands; 3. Treats stubborn migraine headaches and rheumatic pains.

Dosage: 1 - 3 grams or 0.6 to 0.9 grams as a powder.

Contraindications: This is a toxic substance and the dosage should be conservative. It is contraindicated during pregnancy.

Bombyx Batryticatus   Jiang Can (2)

Common Name: Silkworm

Family: Bombycidae

Energy and Flavors: acrid, salty, neutral

Organ Meridians Affected: Liver and Lung

Actions: 1. Antispasmodic, subdues Internal Wind; 2. Expels Wind and stops pain; 3. Clears toxins and dissipates nodules.

Indications: 1. It is used for childhood convulsions, Bell's palsy, epilepsy and tetanus; 2. It is effective for migraine headaches, sore throat, conjunctivitis and eye pains as well as rheumatic pains; 3. It can be used for toxic swellings and swollen glands.

Dosage: 3 - 10 grams; as a powder only 0.9 to 1.5 grams is taken.

Contraindications: Traditionally is contraindicated with Platycodon (Jie Geng), Poria (Fu Ling), Dioscorea hypoglauca (Bei Xie), and Ootheca mantidis (Sang Piao Xiao).

Notes: For convulsions with high fever and epileptic spasms, combine with Gastrodia (Tian Ma), Arisaema with bile (Dan Nan Xing) and Ox Gallstone (Niu Huang); for chronic childhood convulsions with diarrhea caused by Spleen Deficiency, combine with Codonopsis (Dang Shen), Atractylodes (Bai Zhu) and Gastrodia (Tian Ma); for stroke with facial spasms, mouth and eye deviation, combine with Scorpion (Quan Xie) and Typhonium tuber (Bai Fu Zi); for sore throat caused by Wind Heat combine with Platycodon (Jie Geng), Ledebouriella (Fang Feng) and Licorice (Gan Cao); for swollen glands combine with Fritillary (Chuan Bei Mu) and Prunella (Xia Ku Cao); for rubella and itching, combine with Cicada slough (Chan Tui), Arctium (Niu Bang Zi) and Mentha (Bo He).

Discrimination:

Uncariae Rhynchophylla (Gou Teng) – antispasmodic, clears Liver Heat, sedates Yang.

Gastrodiae Elatae (Tian Ma) – calming, antispasmodic, stops pain, for either Heat or Cold.

Tribuli Terrestris (Bai Ji Li) – calming, Clears Wind-Heat from the eyes, smoothes Liver Qi.

Haliotidis (Shi Jue Ming) – clears Heat, calming, anti-hypertensive, clears the vision.

Lumbricus (Di Long) – clears Heat, soothes asthma, opens the meridians.

Buthus Martensi (Quan Xie) – clears toxins, stops pain.

Scolopendra Subspinipes (Wu Gong) – clears toxins, opens the channels, stops pain.

Bombyx Batryticatus (Jiang Can) – clears Phlegm Heat toxins, dissipates nodules, stops pain.

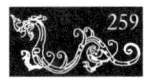

HERBS THAT EXPEL PARASITES

Herbs in this category are used to treat roundworms, tapeworm, pinworm, hookworm and other intestinal parasites. The herbs are selected according to the constitution and the type of parasite. In most cases, these herbs should be combined with other herbs to assist their action, such as purgatives, Qi tonics to protect the righteous energy and possibly carminatives. Some of these herbs are toxic and should only be prescribed for a short period.

Quisqualis Indicae   Shi Jun Zi   (1)

Common Name: Quisqualis, Rangoon Creeper

Part Used: Fruit (Fructus)

Family: Combretaceae

Energy and Flavors: sweet and Warm

Organ Meridians Affected: Spleen and Stomach

Actions: 1. Kills parasites; 2. Improves children's digestion.

Indications: 1. For all kinds of parasites, especially roundworms; 2. For malnutrition and digestive disorders in children with symptoms such as poor appetite, abdominal distention and pain and general weakness of the digestive organs.

Contraindications: This herb should not be used by those with weak Spleen from Cold nor should it be used by those with diarrhea.

Dosage: 6 - 12 grams

Notes: For roundworm combine with Melia (Ku Lian Gen Pi) and Areca seed (Bing Lang).

Melia Toosendon   Ku Lian Gen Pi   (2)

Common Name: Melia, Chinatree, Chinaberry

Part Used: Bark (Cortex)

Family: Meliaceae

Energy and Flavors: bitter, Cold and toxic

Organ Meridians Affected: Liver, Spleen and Stomach

Actions: 1. Kills parasites; 2. Applied topically for skin ailments.

Indications: 1. For infestation of parasites in the intestinal tract or vagina; 2. Applied topically for tinea infections and other skin ailments.

Contraindications: This herb should not be taken for long periods of time and should be used with extreme caution by those with weak constitutions or by those with Liver problems.

Dosage: 6 - 12 grams

Notes: For roundworm use Melia alone; for hookworm combine with Areca seed (Bing Lang); for pinworms combine with Stemona (Bai Bu) and Black Plum (Wu Mei). Make into a strong decoction and inject as an enema each of two to four consecutive nights.

Areca Catechu   Bing Lang

Common Name: Areca nut, areca seed, betel nut

Part Used: Seed (Semen)

Family: Palmae

Energy and Flavors: pungent, bitter and Warm

Organ Meridians Affected: Stomach and Large Intestine

Actions: 1. Destroys parasites; 2. Regulates Qi circulation; 3. Promotes urination.

Indications: For tapeworm combine with Pumpkin seeds (Nan Gua Zi); for Food Stagnation with bloating and constipation combine with Saussurea (Mu Xiang), Bitter Orange (Zhi Shi) and Rhubarb (Da Huang); for edema combine with Poria (Fu Ling) and Alisma (Ze Xie); for swollen and painful legs combine with Citrus (Chen Pi) and Chaenomelis (Mu Gua).

Torreyae Grandis   Fei Zi   (2)

Common Name: Torreya

Part Used: Seed (Semen)

Family: Taxaceae

Energy and Flavors: sweet, astringent and neutral

Organ Meridians Affected: Lung, Large Intestine and Stomach

Actions: 1. Kills parasites; 2. Lubricates the Lungs.

Indications: 1. For all kinds of intestinal parasites; 2. For mild cases of Dry Lungs with cough.

Contraindications: None noted.

Dosage: 6 - 12 grams

Notes: For hookworm, combine with Areca seed (Bing Lang); for tapeworm combine with Pumpkin seeds (Nan Gua Zi) and Areca seed (Bing Lang); for roundworm, combine with Quisqualis fruit (Shi Jun Zi), Melia (Ku Lian Pi) and Black Plum (Wu Mei).

Daucus Carota   He Shi

Common Name: Wild Carrot

Part Used: Seeds (Semen)

Family: Umbelliferae

Energy and Flavors: bitter, pungent, neutral, slightly toxic

Actions: Kills parasites and relieves pain

Indications: For all intestinal worms combine with Quisqualis fruit (Shi Jun Zi), Areca seed (Bing Lang) and Pumpkin seeds (Nan Gua Zi).

Cucurbitae Moschatae   Nan Gua Zi (1)

Common Name: Pumpkin Seed

Part Used: Seed (Semen)

Family: Cucurbitaceae

Energy and Flavors: sweet and neutral

Organ Meridians Affected: Large Intestine and Stomach

Actions: 1. Expels parasites; 2. Assists post partum fluid metabolism and poor lactation.

Indications: 1. For roundworm and tapeworm in the Intestines; 2. For postpartum swelling of the hands and feet as well as poor lactation.

Contraindications: None noted.

Dosage: 30 - 60 grams

Notes: Pumpkin seeds can be taken alone or with Areca catechu (Bing Lang) to dislodge tapeworm. This is followed a few hours later with a purgative of Rhubarb root (Da Huang), Mirabilitum (Mang Xiao), Citrus Peel (Chen Pi) and Garlic (Da Suan). Pumpkin seeds are also effective for the treatment of benign prostatic hypertrophy (B.P.H.).

Allium Sativus   Da Suan   (1)

Common Name: Garlic

Family: Liliaceae

Part Used: Bulb (Bulbus)

Energy and Flavors: acrid and Warm

Organ Meridians Affected: Lung, Spleen, Large Intestine and Stomach

Actions: 1. Kills parasites; 2. Relieves food poisoning.

Indications: 1. For all kinds of intestinal parasites as well as parasites in other areas of the body including the vagina and skin; 2. For food poisoning from shellfish.

Contraindications: This herb should not be used by those with Yin Deficiency and Heat signs. It should not be applied topically for long periods of time, as it destroys tissue.

Dosage: 6 - 15 grams

Notes: The prevention and elimination of parasites is one of many medicinal and culinary uses for garlic. For pinworms and yeast overgrowth

(candida albicans), a decoction can be made and injected into the Large Intestine once or twice daily. At the same time, one clove should be taken and chewed three or four times daily. Garlic cloves can also be crushed and mixed with sesame oil to be applied directly to toxic swellings.

Discrimination:

Fructus Quisqualis Indicae (Shi Jun Zi) — kills roundworms, treats malnutrition, especially of children.

Cortex Melia Radicis (Ku Lian Gen Pi) — kills roundworms, hookworms and pinworms.

Semen Torreyae Grandis (Fei Zi) — kills worms.

Semen Cucurbitae Moschatae (Nan Gua Zi) — for worms, especially tapeworm.

Bulbus Allium Sativus (Da Suan) — intestinal parasites as well as parasites throughout the body.

SUBSTANCES FOR EXTERNAL APPLICATION

Herbs in this category are primarily used externally in the form of powders, pastes, ointments, liniments and fomentations. As such they are used to treat trauma, inflammation, swelling, bruises, bleeding, pain and so forth. Because most of them are toxic, they should be used internally with great caution and only sparingly for a brief period of a few days. They can be used singly or in combinations as a carrier for other medicines. In general all herbs in this category are contraindicated during pregnancy.

Alumen   **Ming Fan**   (1)

Common Name: Alum

Energy and Flavors: sour, astringent and Cold

Organ Meridians Affected: Lung, Liver, Spleen and Large Intestine

Actions: 1. Stops itching, relieves Damp-Heat inflammation and kills parasites; 2. Stops bleeding; 3. Relieves diarrhea; 4. Clears Heat and relieves Wind-Phlegm.

Indications: 1. Applied topically for Damp-Heat itching and rashes and infestation of parasites; 2. For blood in the stool, uterine bleeding as well as applied topically for all kinds of bleeding; 3. For chronic diarrhea. 4. For Wind-Phlegm conditions with symptoms such as convulsions, irritability and difficult to expectorate sputum.

Contraindications: This herb should not be used when there is no Dampness or Heat. This herb should be used with caution when used internally.

Dosage: 1 - 3 grams internally

Notes: For chronic vaginal discharge with itching combine with Cnidium (She Chuang Zi) and Alumen (Ming Fan); for eczema, swelling and irritation of the nose and middle ear combine with Borneol (Bing Pian).

Borax   **Peng Sha**   (3)

Common Name: Borax

Energy and Flavors: sweet, salty and Cool

Organ Meridians Affected: Lung and Stomach

Actions: 1. Applied externally for Heat and toxins; 2. Clears Hot-Phlegm in the Lungs.

Indications: 1. For pain and swelling with symptoms of open sores, athlete's foot with associated sores, white draining vaginal lesions and sores in the mouth and throat; 2. For Hot-Phlegm in the Lungs that is difficult to expectorate.

Contraindications: This herb should not be used by pregnant women and should be used with caution internally and should not be used internally for more than five days and preferably only three. Long term use of more than a week or so at a time can cause damage to the kidneys.

Dosage: 2 - 5 grams internally

Notes: For general sores, or nasal, pharyngeal and vaginal sores apply a powder alone or combined with Borneol (Bing Pian) and Alumen (Ming Fan); for Phlegm Heat with cough and difficult expectoration combine with Fritillary (Chuan Bei Mu) and Trichosanthes fruit (Gua Lou).

Cnidii Monnieri   **She Chuang Zi**   (1)

Common Name: Cnidium Seed

Part Used: Fruit (Fructus)

Family: Umbelliferae

Energy and Flavors: acrid, bitter and Warm

Organ Meridians Affected: Kidney and Spleen

Actions: 1. Applied topically it clears Damp-Heat on the skin and kills parasites; 2. Tonifies Kidney Yang; 3. Warms and dries Wind-Damp-Cold.

Indications: 1. For external application as a powder, wash or ointment for any kind of Damp-Heat skin affliction, especially in the genital area (yeast or fungal infections); 2. For impotence and infertility due to Cold in the Kidney or womb; 3. For Damp-Cold or Wind-Damp-Cold with symptoms of vaginal discharge or sore lower back.

Contraindications: This herb should not be used by those with conditions of Internal Damp-Heat nor by those with Yin Deficiency with Heat signs.

Dosage: 6 - 12 grams

Notes: This herb is also used internally as a Kidney Yang tonic. For trichomonas and vaginal itch combine with Alumen (Ming Fan), Phellodendron (Huang Bai), Borneol (Bing Pian) and use as a douche; for weeping eczema, genital and anal itch and scabies apply topically as a wash or powder with Sophora root (Ku Shen), Stemona (Bai Bu), Alumen (Ming Fan), Borneol (Bing Pian) and Calomelas (Qing Fen); for impotence and/or infertility caused by Kidney Deficiency take internally with Cuscuta (Tu Si Zi), Psoralea (Bu Gu Zhi) and Schisandra (Wu Wei Zi); for lower back pain caused by Kidney Deficiency use internally with Loranthes (Sang Ji Sheng), Eucommia (Du Zhong), Gentiana (Long Dan Cao) and Achyranthes (Niu Xi).

Momordicae Cochinchinensis   Mu Bie Zi (3)

Common Name: Momordica Seed

Part Used: Seed (Semen)

Family: Cucurbitaceae

Energy and Flavors: bitter, sweet, Warm and toxic

Organ Meridians Affected: Liver, Large Intestine and Stomach

Actions: 1. Clears Heat and reduces inflammation; 2. Moves Blood and reduces inflammation.

Indications: 1. For inflammation due to toxicity with symptoms such as breast abscesses, non-healing sores and scrofula; 2. For Stagnation of Blood due to traumatic injury with pain and inflammation.

Contraindications: This herb should not be used by pregnant women nor by those who are in weak condition. This herb should not be taken with pork.

Dosage: .5 - 1.5 grams internally

Notes: For chronic abscesses apply topically as a wash or powder with Scutellaria (Huang Qin), Phellodendron (Huang Bai), Sophora (Ku Shen) and Trichosanthes root (Tian Hua Fen); for sore throat combine with Borneol (Ping Pian), Alumen (Ming Fan) and Borax (Peng Sha); for acne rosacea apply topically with Calomelas (Qing Fen) and Sulfur (Liu Huang); mix the powder with vinegar and apply directly to the gums for pain and periodontal swelling.

Pasta Acaciae seu Uncariae   Er Cha   (3)

Common Name: Acacia Catechu; it is also known as Gambir, but it should not be confused with Uncaria which is in the Rubiaceae family and is also popularly called gambir.

Family: Leguminosae (Acacia)

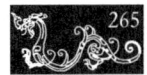

Part Used: The paste that is prepared from a dried concentrated decoction of the bark.

Energy and Flavors: bitter, astringent and neutral

Organ Meridians Affected: Lung and Heart

Actions: 1. Expectorant; 2. Clears Heat and drains Dampness; 3. Applied externally it stops bleeding.

Indications: 1. Cough associated with Heat and Phlegm. 2. Thirst; 3. Applied topically for bleeding of all kinds, cold sores, eczema and bleeding hemorrhoids.

Contraindications: This herb should not be used for symptoms of Cold and Dampness.

Dosage: .5 - 2 grams internally

Notes: The dried and powdered sap is made into a paste and topically applied for many conditions. The translation of the Chinese name literally means "childrens tea" which suggests its safety and overall beneficial effect for children. One study describes its being given to children for acute indigestion. It proved to be over 90% successful in one to seven days.

    For sore throat combine with Lonicera (Jin Yin Hua), Forsythia (Lian Qiao) and Arctium (Niu Bang Zi); for mouth and gum sores combine with Indigo (Qing Dai), Ox Gallstone (Niu Huang) and Borneol (Bing Pian); for excessive vaginal discharge combine with Alumen (Ming Fan) and Cnidium (She Chuang Zi) and use as a vaginal douche.

Camphora   Zhang Nao   (3)

Common Name: Camphor

Family: Lauraceae

Energy and Flavors: acrid, Hot and toxic

Organ Meridians Affected: Heart

Actions: 1. Moves the Blood and reduces inflammation; 2. Opens the Orfices and awakens the spirit; 3. Dispels Wind-Damp and kills parasites.

Indications: 1. Applied externally for Stagnation of Blood of all kinds including traumatic injury; 2. For Heat induced loss of consciousness and coma; 3. Applied topically for itching associated with sores or parasites.

Contraindications: This herb should not be used by pregnant women nor should it be used by those who are weak with Qi Deficiency or those with insomnia. This herb should be used with caution when taken internally.

Dosage: .05 - .15 grams internally

Notes: For scabies and lice apply topically as a wash or powder with Sulfur (Liu Huang) and Alumen (Ming Fan); for fainting and

unconsciousness combine with Musk (She Xiang) and Borneol (Bing Pian) and allow the patient to smell the preparation.

Hydnocarpi Anthelminticae   Da Feng Zi

Common Name: Hydnocarpi, Chaulmoogra seeds

Family: Flacourtiaceae

Energy and Flavors: pungent, Hot, toxic

Organ Meridians Affected: Kidney, Liver and Spleen

Actions: Used topically to expel Wind, dry Dampness and clear toxicity.

Indications: 1. Kills parasites; 2. Treats leprosy, scabies and tinea (fungi).

Contraindications: Avoid internal use as it is toxic and easily absorbed. Avoid or use carefully for Yin Deficiency with signs of inflammation.

Dosage: 0.3 - 0.9 g in decoctions or pills. Use more liberally externally in powders or pastes.

Notes: For scabies, apply topically as a wash or powder with Sulfur (Liu Huang), Camphor (Zhang Nao) and Alumen (Ming Fan).

Pseudobulbus Shancigu   Shan Ci Gu

Other Names: Cremastra variabilis, Tulipa edulis

Common Name: Chinese Tulip bulb

Family: Orchidaceae

Energy and Flavors: sweet, Cold, slightly toxic

Organ Meridians Affected: Liver and Stomach

Actions: 1. Clears Heat and toxicity; 2. Dissipates nodules.

Indications: Use for swollen glands, nodules, cancer and tumors, sores, ulcers, swellings and carbuncles.

Dosage: 3-9 grams in decoctions. Apply topically as a paste.

Notes: This herb has an antineoplastic effect probably due to the presence of colchicine. Avoid or use with great care internally. For nodules, tumors and cancers, the best application is as a paste externally applied with Nidus Vespae (Lu Feng Fang) and Manitis (Sang Piao Xiao); another combination for the same condition is applied topically as a poultice with Scorpion (Quan Xie) and Phytolacca (Shang Lu).

Nidus Vespae   Lu Feng Fang   (3)

Common Name: Hornet Nest

Family: Vespidae

Energy and Flavors: sweet, neutral and toxic

Organ Meridians Affected: Lung and Stomach

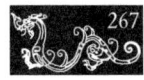

Actions: 1. Clears Heat, expels Wind, dries Damp and relieves pain.

Indications: 1. Applied topically as an ointment or a wash for a variety of skin ailments including rashes with itch, sores, scabies, carbuncles and Wind-Damp painful obstruction.

Contraindications: This herb should not be used by those with Qi or Blood Deficiency. This herb should not be used when there are open sores.

Dosage: 6 - 12 grams decocted; 1 - 3 grams as a powder internally.

Notes: For swollen glands take internally with Frankincense (Ru Xiang), Forsythia (Lian Qiao), Fritillary (Chuan Bei Mu) and Prunella (Xia Ku Cao); to relieve the itch of scabies or other rashes apply topically with Cicada Slough (Chan Tui) and Calomelas (Qing Fen); for urinary incontinence take internally with Manitis (Sang Piao Xiao).

Calomelas   Qing Fen   (3)

Common Name: Calomelas

Energy and Flavors: acrid, Cold, toxic

Organ Meridians Affected: Bladder, Kidney and Liver

Actions: 1. Relieves toxicity, kills parasites, used as an external wash for scabies and syphilitic sores; 2. Inhibits bleeding, diarrhea, dysentery with blood in the stools, abnormal uterine bleeding and leukorrhea. The powder can be applied topically for any type of bleeding; 3. Anti-inflammatory and expectorant for difficult-to-expectorate phlegm and Wind Phlegm conditions such as mania, coma and convulsions.

Contraindications: Not recommended for those with weak digestion.

Notes: For itch, ringworm, lice and scabies combine with Sulfur (Liu Huang), Camphor (Zhang Nao), Hydnocarpi (Da Feng Zi) and Realgar (Xiong Huang); for skin ulcers mix with powdered Gypsum (Shi Gao) and apply topically.

Realgar   Xiong Huang   (3)

Common Name: Realgar, arsenic sulfide

Energy and Flavors: bitter, acrid, Warm, poison

Organ Meridians Affected: Heart, Liver and Stomach

Actions: 1. Anti-toxic; 2. Kills parasites; 3. Relieves itch; 4. Heals snakebites and ulcerations; 5. Dries Dampness; 6. Treats malarial conditions.

Indications: 1. Relieves toxicity; 2. Abscesses and sores.

Preparations: 1. With Borneol and Phellodendron it is applied topically for scabies and eczema; 2. With Borneol it can be made into an alcoholic tincture and used topically for herpes zoster; 3. As a powder it is mixed with Alumen and it can be applied topically to treat nasal polyps; 4. As a powder combined with Excrementum trogopteri seu pteromi (Wu Ling Zhi) for poisonous snakebites and other venomous bites and stings.

Contraindications: Internally it is contraindicated during pregnancy and for Yin and Blood Deficiency. All toxic substances should be appropriately labeled and kept far out of reach of children.

Dosage: Internally 0.15 to 0.6 grams in pills or powders. A finely ground powder is applied topically to localized areas. Because its toxicity is absorbed through the skin, it should not be applied to a large area. Do not heat, as this generates an extremely toxic compound.

Notes: For scabies, lice, ringworm and eczema combine with Borneol (Bing Pian) and Phellodendron (Huang Bai); for herpes zoster, combine with Borneol (Bing Pian) as an alcoholic extract; for nasal polyps, tinea and Wind-Damp sores with itching, combine with Alumen (Ming Fan); for ulcerations of the mouth combine with Borax (Peng Sha) and Ox Gallstone (Niu Huang).

Sulfur   **Liu Huang**   (2)

Common Name: Flower of Sulfur

Energy and Flavors: pungent, Warm, mildly toxic

Organ Meridians Affected: Spleen and Kidneys

Actions: 1. Externally applied for the treatment of scabies, tinea infections (fungus infections); 2. Warms Kidney and Spleen Yang, treats impotence, frequent urination, chronic diarrhea and constipation caused by Coldness.

Contraindications: Not for symptoms of Yin Deficiency or Excess Yang.

Dosage: 1- 3 grams internally.

Notes: For scabies combine with Calomelas (Qing Fen) and Hydnocarpi (Da Feng Zi).

Minium   **Qian Dan**   (3)

Common Names: Lead Elixir (lead oxide red)

Energy and Flavors: acrid, Cool, toxic

Organ Meridians Affected: Heart, Liver, Spleen

Actions and Indications: 1. Apply topically as a paste to expel toxins, heal injuries, stop itching, expel pus; 2. Moves Phlegm downwards and suppresses spasms.

Contraindications: Not for Cold caused by Deficiency, not good to use for more than 3 days.

Dosage: 0.3 - 0.9 grams internally as a powder or pill.

Notes: To expel pus, promote healing, generate flesh and stop itching, mix as a paste and apply directly to the affected area; for burns, swelling and non-healing ulcers combine with Gypsum (Shi Gao) and apply topically.

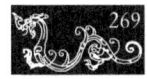

Strychni   **Ma Qian Zi**   (3)

Common Name: Nux Vomica Seeds
Part Used: Seed (Semen)
Family: Loganiaceae
Energy and Flavors: bitter, Cold, toxic
Organ Meridians Affected: Liver, Spleen

Actions and Indications: 1. Opens the meridians, reduces swelling, relieves pain, used for Wind-Damp conditions, trauma, abscesses, ulcers and Yin ulcers; 2. It is also useful for treating tumors.

Contraindications: Very toxic and should be used with great caution internally. Not to be used during pregnancy or for weak individuals.

Dosage: 0.3 -0.9 grams a day as a powder or in pills. Topically it can be applied as a powder locally.

Notes: For injuries, pain, swelling, fracture and sprains, combine with Olibanum (Ru Xiang), Myrrh (Mo Yao), Pyritum (Zi Ran Tong), Dipsacus (Xu Duan) and Drynaria (Gu Sui Bu) and apply topically as a paste or powder; for painful sores, abscesses, swellings, combine with Realgar (Xiong Huang), Olibanum (Ru Xiang) and Squama Manitis (Chuan Shan Jia); for Wind-Damp obstructions with spasm, weakness and numbness combine with Aconite (Fu Zi) and Clematis (Wei Ling Xian).

Discrimination:

Alumen (Ming Fan) – stops itch, relieves Damp-Heat, stops bleeding and diarrhea.

Borax (Peng Sha) – topically clears Heat and toxins, relieves vaginal sores, athlete's foot, clears Hot Phlegm from the Lungs.

Fructus Cnidii Monnieri (She Chuang Zi) – topically applied it is used for Damp-Heat, itch, parasites, as a douche for vaginal infections, internally it tonifies Kidney Yang.

Semen Momordicae Cochinchinensis (Mu Bie Zi) – apply topically for toxic swellings, breast abscesses, non-healing sores and swollen glands; it is also used to move Blood and relieve pain from injuries and contusions.

Pasta Acaciae seu Uncariae (Er Cha) – topically it can be used to drain Dampness, sores with purulent fluid, chronic non-healing sores.

Camphora (Zhang Nao) – applied externally for parasites, scabies, ringworm and itching; it also invigorates Blood, relieves pain from injuries and contusions.

Nidus Vespae (Lu Feng Fang) – applied externally as a wash for skin rash, itching, scabies, ringworm, sores and carbuncles.

Calomelas (Qing Fen) – relieves toxicity, relieves itch, kills parasites, dries Dampness, heals snakebites.

Realgar (Xiong Huang) – relieves toxicity, kills parasites, relieves itch, dries Dampness.

Sulfur (Liu Huang) – expels toxins, treats scabies and skin funguses, heals injuries, stops itching, expels pus.

Minium (Qian Dan) – expels toxins, heals injuries, stops itching, expels pus, moves Phlegm downwards and relieves spasms.

Semen Strychni (Ma Qian Zi) – opens the meridians, reduces swelling, relieves pain, treats rheumatic conditions, treats cancer and tumors.

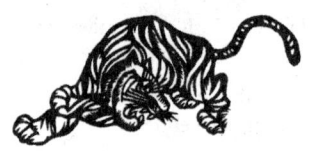

TWO
THE USE OF CHINESE HERBAL FORMULAS

Chinese herbalism is primarily based upon the use of compound herbal formulas, utilizing a combination of mostly herbs with minerals, insects, and animals. Students and most practitioners have come to rely on the classical corpus of medicinal formulations that have been evolved and passed down over the last 5000 years. It is the study and reliance on such tried and proven formulas that is at the heart of classical Chinese herbalism.

Why are formulas used over single herbs? Compound formulas are designed and intended to treat complex underlying imbalances, the sum of which eventually manifest as disease. While a simple imbalance may require only one or a few herbs, a complex imbalance involving more physiological dysfunctions requires the use of several herbs together in formula. Another reason is that through their combination, the complex biochemistry of herbs forms unique chemical compounds not naturally occurring in nature. In this sense, an herbal formula becomes synergistic, more than the mere sum of its parts.

Considering that each herb is, in itself, a factory of scores of biochemical components, that the interactions of these components vary according to the chemistry of the individual (expressed in TCM by the various diagnostic parameters), it is quite difficult, given the limits of contemporary scientific technology, to even track the effects of one or two herbs in a living body ("in vivo"). Therefore, unless one is content with evaluating mere statistical data as to a classical formula's effectiveness (as is documented in contemporary Chinese research), there is little hope in the foreseeable future for Western science being either willing or capable of tracking the labyrinthine physiological interactions of complex classical formulas that may range, on the average, from 3 to 20 or more herbs in a single formula.

At least in the early stages of study and practice, TCM students and practitioners are taught the individual herbs of the Materia Medica

and the various indications of time-honored classical formulas. This constitutes a formidable body of knowledge which must be absorbed before one is able to confront the even further complex enigma of practice, where students soon discover that despite years of training, patients seldom exactly fit the predefined molds of theory. An experienced practitioner must learn to add or subtract individual herbs according to each patient's condition, and even that may not be enough, as patients often respond better to the use of more than a single classical formula given alternately throughout each day. For instance, a woman with a complex menstrual irregularity may require the use of a Liver Qi regulating formula, such as Bupleurum and Peony Combination (Xiao yao san), taken twice daily after meals, with the more tonifying Blood tonic formula, Dang Gui Four Combination (Si wu tang), taken before meals.

Just knowing what herbs to prescribe is only one of the many obstacles to overcome in practice. The second, and often more daunting, is to achieve patient compliance, given the strange and unusual flavors of herbs. To facilitate this process, it becomes practical to not rely on a patient's ability to brew their own herbal formulas, which in many instances require several stages of preparation, but to use one of the various convenient preparations of concentrated dried extracts, liquid preparations, pills or premixed powders.

The admonition of my first Taoist Chinese herb teacher that "it takes more than one lifetime to become an herbalist" reflects a profound appreciation for the commitment to unceasing study of hundreds of herbs and formulas, along with the mastery of TCM diagnosis, that is necessary for effective practice. Given this, it is useful to outline both traditional and non-traditional approaches to study and practice.

The three basic parameters of study include, in order of importance: 1. traditional diagnosis, 2. Materia Medica and 3. traditional formulations. Formerly, and in many parts of China today, students are trained to first memorize some 250 to 300 herbs in their categories along with their energies, flavors and actions. Beginning with a small group of "base" formulas from which the majority of others are comprised or derived, a student of TCM must then commit to memory between 100 to 200 classical formulas, including their individual components, dosage, indications, contra-indications and, most important, standard methods of variation according to individual patient requirement.

Even to this day, traditional training of a Chinese herbalist in China or Taiwan involves chanting or reciting the formulas and their indications[1] aloud in the classroom. Upon graduation, many continue

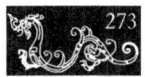

to chant the TCM formulas aloud in their respective clinical practices, earning the appellation, "singing doctors". Western students can modify this approach by developing a memorable phrase or rhyme based on the first letter of each herb in a formula.

Secondly, as a student will soon learn after the study of dozens of classical formulas, there are patterns of herbal combinations which frequently recur in many formulas. Usually these consist of two to four herbs at a time, such as the following:

Pinellia and Ginger for Phlegm conditions
Cinnamon and Prepared Aconite for Cold conditions
Oyster shell and Dragon bone for sedative effects
Coptis and Scutellaria for toxic conditions

Considering the vast number of formulas, students are advised to begin by mastering a few primary or "base" formulas. Some of the most successful practitioners often revolve their practice around the utilization and variation of 20 or 30 formulas, while others may have a repertoire of several hundred formulas to draw upon. On the average, a practitioner probably needs to know from 100 to 150 formulas which, in turn, can be modified to treat most presenting conditions.

In Japan, there is a distinction between a doctor's formula and a formula obtained directly from a pharmacy. The pharmacy may have literally thousands of "secret" formulas for specific disease conditions. In order to achieve maximum success, the goal of the pharmacy is to achieve a quick result based upon a limited objective of symptomatic relief. An herb doctor, on the other hand, may use only 150 or so formulas, but focuses more on the treatment of the whole person and the prevention of future disease.

Following is a short list of representative or "base" formulas with which one might begin:

Qi Tonic: Four Major Herbs (Si jun zi tang)
Blood Tonic: Dang Gui Four (Si wu tang)
Yin Tonic: Rehmannia Six (Liu wei di huang wan)
Yang Tonic: Rehmannia Eight (Ba wei di huang wan)
Warm Surface Relieving: Ephedra Combination (Ma huang tang) or Cinnamon Combination (Gui zhi tang)
Cold Surface Relieving: Lonicera and Forsythia Combination for Wind Heat (Yin qiao san)
Detoxifying: Coptis and Scutellaria Combination (Huang lian jie du tang) and Lonicera and Forsythia Combination (Yin qiao san)
Damp Heat: Gentiana Combination (Long dan xie gan tang) and Capillaris Formula (Yin chen hao tang)

Purgative: Major Rhubarb Combination (Da cheng qi tang) and Apricot Seed and Linum Formula (Ma zi ren wan)
Anti-parasitic: Mume Combination (Wu mei wan)
Diuretic: Poria Five Herb Combination (Wu ling san)
Digestive: Citrus and Crataegus Formula (Bao he wan)
Qi Regulation: Bupleurum and Peony Combination (Xiao yao wan)
Blood Regulation (circulatory stimulant): Cinnamon and Poria Combination (Gui zhi fu ling tang) and Dang Gui Four (Si wu tang)
Calming Sedative: Zizyphus Combination (Suan zao ren tang), Dragon Bone and Oyster Shell (Long gu mu li tang)
Dampness and Excess Mucus: Citrus and Pinellia Combination (Er chen tang)
Antirheumatic, Clearing Damp, Cold Wind: Du Huo and Loranthes Combination (Du huo ji sheng tang)

THE COMPUTER AND TCM

As with all studies in life, the computer represents a major step forward in the practice of TCM. The laborious process of recalling hundreds of TCM formulas with all their indications is easily facilitated by the use of a computer. The process of pattern recognition that is at the base of TCM at least in theory can figure into a computer program using artificial intelligence as a guide. What remains as constant is the ability of the practitioner to recognize and properly enter the data that will help the computer select one of a small number of appropriate formulas.

The computer can be used for a wide variety of other functions as well, to store data on patients for future recall and even through electronic mail to automatically place orders of herbs and prepared formulas to be sent to the patient. (See Sources and Resources in the Bibliography for herbal computer programs.)

DIFFERENCES BETWEEN CHINESE HERBALISM AND KANPO

Historically, one of the richest sources of classical formulas is Chang Chung Ching's *Shang Han Lun* and the companion book, *Formulas From the Golden Chamber*, first published during the Han dynasty in the 2nd century. These early texts were first brought to China by Buddhist monks and scholars and were adopted by the Japanese to form Japanese-Chinese herbal medicine, called "Kanpo". Because of the broad versatility of herbal formulas generally, many of these important classical TCM

formulas, set down over 1800 years ago, have lent themselves to uses often far exceeding those for which they were originally intended.

Because Kanpo is represented in the West simply as Chinese medicine, it is important to understand its differences with TCM. A major difference is the Kanpo herbalists' basing their diagnostic procedure more on abdominal diagnosis called 'fukushin', as opposed to the TCM herbalist who relies more on pulse, tongue and symptom-sign methods. Another important difference is that the average dose of a Kanpo formula is approximately one half to two thirds less than that used by the Chinese.

PRINCIPLES OF FORMULATION

Formulas consist of many herbs combined together according to their synergistic, antagonistic and harmonizing effects. Traditionally this is explained according to classical pharmaceutical concepts that organize formulas to mimic the organization of Confucian politics. Thus, the imperial herb(s) embodies the primary therapeutic intention of the formula, the ministerial herb(s) augments the primary action of the formula, the assistant herb(s) reduces any unwanted reactions of the formula and the servant herb(s) harmonizes and smoothes the action of the entire formula.

Considering that many formulas range from two to more than four herbs at a time, the above may only serve as an approximate guide. In applying the classical principle of formulation to actual formulas, we find that in those where there are less than two herbs, one herb may take up the role of more than one formulation principle. For instance, Licorice in many formulas can serve as both an assistant and servant. When there are more than four herbs, then two or more herbs can be used to fulfill a single formulation principle. For instance, the combination of Ginseng and Dang Gui may share the position of imperial herbs in a formula for Blood and Qi tonification.

Examples:
Ephedra Combination (Ma huang tang)
Ephedra – imperial herb to stimulate sweating
Cinnamon twig – ministerial herb that also causes sweating
Apricot seed – assistant herb with lubricating properties, which moderates the strong drying properties of Ephedra and Cinnamon twig
Licorice – servant herb that harmonizes the other ingredients in the formula

Major Four Herbs (Si jun zi tang)
Ginseng – imperial herb, Qi tonic
Atractylodes – ministerial herb, also tonifies Qi and aids digestion
Poria – assistant herb, clears Dampness
Licorice – servant, harmonizes

Dang Gui Four (Si wu tang)
Dang Gui – imperial herb, Blood tonic
Rehmannia – ministerial herb, Blood and Yin tonic
Peony alba – ministerial and assistant herb, Blood tonic, relaxes internal spasm and promotes circulation
Ligusticum – ministerial and servant, promotes Blood circulation

Ginseng and Astragalus Combination (Bu zhong yi qi tang)
Ginseng, Astragalus and Atractylodes – imperial herbs, Qi tonics
Dang gui – ministerial herb, tonifies Blood
Cimicifuga and Bupleurum – assistant herbs, raise the Qi and detoxify
Licorice, Citrus, Ginger and Jujube – servant herbs, harmonizing

Finally, the novice student of Chinese herbalism is encouraged to mainly use classical Chinese formulas whose therapeutic effects are well understood. Even advanced, so-called master herbalists primarily use a favored set of traditional formulas, varying each of them according to the individual symptoms of the patient. .

CHINESE FORMULAS

Note: All formulas accompanied with an asterisk are to be considered part of a basic set of representative formulas.

Aconite, Ginger and Licorice Combination (Si ni tang)*
Prepared Aconite (Fu Zi)   10-15gms Aconitum carmichaeli
Dry Ginger (Gan Jiang)   6-9gms Zingiberis officinalis
Honey Baked Licorice (Zhi Gan Cao) 10-15gms Glycyrrhiza uralensis
Properties and Actions:
a) Internal warming Yang stimulant

Indications: Reestablishes the Yang (vital function) and revives from collapse and shock. It is indicated for Internal Coldness of the Lesser Yin (Shao Yin) stage with cold extremities, chills with a strong feeling to curl up and lie down, lassitude, vomiting, lack of thirst, abdominal pain with a preference for warmth and pressure, diarrhea.

This condition can occur as a result of excessive sweating from an External Greater Yang (Tai Yang) syndrome. This condition can be the result of the course of the disease or mistreatment. If vomiting occurs after drinking the warm decoction, it may be taken cool. Down through the centuries it has come to be used for a variety of Deficient Yang conditions, including prostration and heart failure.

Tongue: white, damp coat or dark bluish purple

Pulse: deep, faint and thin

Contraindications: Not for Yin Deficient Heat.

Variations:

1. For chronic rheumatoid arthritis caused by Cold, add Cinnamon twig (Gui Zhi) and White Peony (Bai Shao).

2. For Deficient Qi add Ginseng (Ren Shen) or Codonopsis (Dang Shen).

3. For edema and fluid retention caused by Deficient Yang add Poria (Fu Ling) and Water Plantain (Ze Xie).

Achyranthes and Rehmannia Combination

(Restore the Left Pill - Zuo gui wan)

Prepared Rehmannia (Shu Di Huang)	15gms Rehmannia glutinosa
Dioscorea (Shan Yao)	9gms Dioscorea batata
Lycii berries (Gou Qi Zi)	9gms Lycium chinensis
Cornus berries (Shan Zhu Yu)	9gms Cornus officinalis
Cuscuta seed (Tu Si Zi)	9gms Cuscuta chinensis
Achyranthes (Niu Xi)	9gms Achyranthis bidentata
Antler Gelatin (Lu Jiao Jiao)	6gms Cervi Cornus Colla
Tortoise Shell Gelatin (Gui Ban Jiao)	6gms Colloid of turtle shell

Properties and Actions:

Nourishes the Yin of the Kidney and Liver.

Indications: For Yin Deficiency with symptoms of dizziness, night sweats, insomnia, thirst, dryness, weak memory, flushed face, infertility, uterine bleeding, amenorrhea, lower back pain, diabetes, addison's disease, TB, spermatorrhea.

Tongue: red

Pulse: thready and rapid

Aconite and Asarum combination (Ma huang fu zi xi xin tang)

Prepared Aconite (Fu Zi)	1-3gms Aconitum carmichaeli
Wild Ginger (Xi Xin)	3-6gms Asarum heterophylum

Ephedra (Ma Huang)   6-9gms Ephedra sinica

Properties and Actions:

a) Stimulating and warming diaphoretic, warms and disperses the surface

b) Internally warming

Indications: Weak and enfeebled individuals with the common cold, influenza or bronchitis, bronchial asthma, pneumonia, sinusitis, rhinitis, asthma, trigeminal neuralgia.

Tongue: pale and swollen with a white coat

Pulse: weak, thin and thready

Contraindications: Not for individuals with Excess Heat or Yin Deficiency.

Aconite, Ginseng and Ginger Combination (Fu zi li zhong wan) (see Ginseng and Ginger Combination)

Agastache Formula (Huo xiang zheng qi san)

Agastache (Huo Xiang)	6-9gms Agastache rugosa
Magnolia bark (Hou Po)	6-9gms Magnoliae officinalis
Perilla leaf (Zi Su Ye)	6-9gms Perillae frutescens
Angelica (Bai Zhi)	3-6gms Angelicae dahuricae
Citrus peel (Chen Pi)	3-6gms Citrus reticulata
Poria (Fu Ling)	6-9gms Poria cocos
White Atractylodes (Bai Zhu)	6-9gms Atractylodis alba
Areca peel (Da Fu Pi)	6-9gms Arecae catechu
Platycodon (Jie Geng)	6-9gms Platycodi grandiflorum
Pinellia (Ban Xia)	6-9gms Pinellia ternata
Baked Licorice (Zhi Gan Cao)	3-6gms Glycyrrhizae uralensis
Dried Ginger (Gan Jiang)	1-3gms Zingiberis officinalis
Jujube Dates (Da Zao)	3-5pcs Zizyphus jujuba

Properties and Actions:

a) Diuretic, carminative, clears Damp turbidity from the Spleen and Stomach

b) Diaphoretic for External conditions

Indications: For Internal Damp-Cold affecting the Spleen and digestion with External attack of Wind and Cold. Symptoms include fever, headache, cold phobia, chest fullness, abdominal discomfort, nausea and vomiting, rumbling with diarrhea. Can be used for summer diarrhea and gastritis.

Tongue: white body, greasy coat

Pulse: floating and tight

Contraindications: Not for Excess Heat conditions.

Antelope Horn and Uncaria Combination (Ling yang gou teng tang)

Antelope horn (Ling Yang Jiao)	1-3gms Saiga tatarica
Uncaria (Gou Teng)	9-12gms Uncaria spp.
Morus leaf (Sang Ye)	6-9gms Mori Alba
Fritillaria (Chuan Bei Mu)	9-12gms Fritillariae cirrhosae
Unprepared Rehmannia (Sheng Di Huang)	9-15gms Rehmanniae glutinosa
Chrysanthemum (Ju Hua)	9-12gms Chrysanthemi morifolii
White Peony (Bai Shao)	6-9gms Paeoniae alba
Licorice (Gan Cao)	1-3gms Glycyrrhizae uralensis
Poria (Fu Shen)	9-12gms Poria cocos
Bamboo shavings (Zhu Ru)	6-9gms Bambusa phyllostachys nigra

Properties and Actions:
a) Antispasmodic and anti-hypertensive, calms endogenous Liver Wind
b) Eliminates Heat

Indications: For Internal Heat and Liver Wind. Symptoms include high fever, hypertension, puerperal eclampsia, convulsions with mania, stiff neck, coma.

Tongue: red dry with prickles

Pulse: tight, wiry and rapid

Contraindications: Not for Internal Cold.

Variations:

1. With hypertension, headache and dizziness add Gentiana (Long Dan Cao), Prunella spike (Xia Ku Cao), Oyster shell (Mu Li), Gastrodia (Tian Ma).

2. With depleted body fluids add Donkey-Hide Gelatin (E Jiao), Ophiopogon (Mai Men Dong), Scrophularia (Xuan Shen).

Anemarrhena, Phellodendron and Rehmannia Formula
(Zhi bai di huang wan)

Anemarrhena (Zhi Mu)	6-9gms Anemarrhenae asphodeloides
Phellodendron (Huang Bai)	6-9gms Phellodendron amurense
Prepared Rehmannia (Shu Di Huang)	15-24gms Rehmannia glutinosa
Cornus (Shan Zhu Yu)	10-15gms Cornus officinalis
Dioscorea (Shan Yao)	10-15gms Dioscorea batatis
Water Plantain (Ze Xie)	9-12gms Alismatis plantago-aquatica
Moutan Peony (Mu Dan Pi)	9gms Paeonia suffruticosa
Poria (Fu Ling)	9gms Poria cocos

Properties and Actions:
a) Nutritive, nourishes Yin

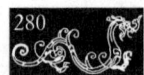

b) Alterative, clears Deficient Fire

Indications: For Yin Deficiency of the Kidney and Liver with symptoms of inflammation, night sweats, tinnitus, spermatorrhea, involuntary seminal emission, steaming feeling in the bones, loose teeth, swollen and inflamed gums. It can be used for gingivitis, diabetes, chronic urinary tract infections, sore throat.

Tongue: red body, little or no coat

Pulse: thin and rapid

Contraindications: Not for Yin (Cold-Damp) Excess.

Anemone Combination (Bai tou weng tang)*

Pulsatilla (Bai Tou Weng)	10-15gms Pulsatilla chinensis
Coptis (Huang Lian)	6-9gms Coptis chinensis
Phellodendron (Huang Bai)	9-12gms Phellodendron amurense
Fraxinus (Qin Pi)	10-15gms Fraxinus rhynchophyla

Properties and Actions:

Anti-dysenteric, dispels Excess Heat from the gastrointestinal tract

Indications: It is used to treat bacterial and amebic dysentery, leukorrhea with blood. Other symptoms include thirst.

Tongue: red with a yellow coat

Pulse: tight and rapid Pulse

Variation:

1. For Exterior-complex fever with an abhorrence to cold with Internal Heat add Honeysuckle (Jin Yin Hua) and Pueraria root (Ge Gen).

Apricot Seed and Perilla Formula (Xing su san)*

Apricot seed (Xing Ren)	6-9gms Prunus armeniacae
Perilla leaf (Zi Su Ye)	6-9gms Perilla frutescens
Citrus (Chen Pi)	3gms Citrus reticulata
Platycodon (Jie Geng)	3-6gms Platycodon grandiflorum
Peucedanum (Qian Hu)	6-9gms Peucedani praeruptorum
Bitter Orange (Zhi Ke)	6-9gms Citrus aurantium
Pinellia (Ban Xia)	6-9gms Pinellia ternata
Poria (Fu Ling)	9-12gms Poria cocos
Fresh Ginger (Sheng Jiang)	3-6gms Zingiberis officinalis
Jujube Dates (Da Zao)	3-5pcs Zizyphus jujuba
Licorice (Gan Cao)	3-6gms Glycyrrhiza uralensis

Properties and Actions:

a) Diaphoretic
b) Clears Wind-Cold
c) Soothes the Lung and relieves cough

Indications: For External Wind-Cold syndrome with Internal Phlegm and Dampness in the Lungs. Other symptoms include headache, lack of perspiration, cold intolerance, cough with thin white phlegm and nasal congestion. It can be used for common cold, bronchiectasis, pulmonary emphysema.

Tongue: white coating

Pulse: floating, slippery and slow

Variations:

1. If there is perspiration with a wiry and tight Pulse add Notopterygium (Qiang Huo).
2. If there is bloating and diarrhea add Black Atractylodes (Cang Zhu) and Magnolia bark (Hou Po).
3. If there is a headache above the eyes add Angelica dahurica (Bai Zhi).
4. If there is External Cold with Internal Heat add Scutellaria (Huang Qin).

Baked Licorice Combination (Zhi gan cao tang)

Licorice (Gan Cao)	9-12gms Glycyrrhiza uralensis
Ginseng (Ren Shen)	3-6gms Panax ginseng
Unprepared Rehmanni (Sheng Di Huang)	15-20gms Rehmannia glutinosa
Ophiopogon (Mai Men Dong)	6-9gms Ophiopogon japonicus
Cannabis seed (Huo Ma Ren)	9-12gms Cannabis sativa
Donkey-Hide Gelatin (E Jiao)	6-9gms Equus asini
Cinnamon twigs (Gui Zhi)	6-9gms Cinnamomum cassia
Fresh Ginger (Sheng Jiang)	6-9gms Zingiberis officinalis
Jujube Date (Da Zao)	3-5pcs Zizyphus jujuba

Properties and Actions:

a) Nutritive, replenishes Qi and Blood
b) Demulcent nutritive, nourishes the Yin and increases Pulse rate

Indications: Can be considered for coronary heart disease, rheumatic heart disease, myocarditis, arrhythmia, hyperthyroidism, neurasthenia.

Tongue: Pale, thin coat

Pulse: Thin, irregular heart beat

Variations:

1. For neurasthenia include Pinellia and Magnolia Combination (Ban xia hou po tang).
2. For arrhythmia with nervousness add Zizyphus (Suan Zao Ren).
3. For Lung Yin Deficiency with Dryness remove Cinnamon twigs (Gui Zhi) and Fresh Ginger (Sheng Jiang), add Lily bulb (Bai He) and Glehnia (Bei Sha Shen).

Bamboo and Poria Combination (Wen dan tang)
(Gallbladder Warming Decoction)

Pinellia (Ban Xia)	6-9gms Pinellia ternata
Citrus peel (Chen Pi)	6-9gms Citrus reticulata
Poria (Fu Ling)	9-12gms Poria cocos
Immature Bitter Orange (Zhi Shi)	6-9gms Citrus aurantium
Bamboo shavings (Zhu Ru)	6-9gms Bambusa phyllostachys nigra
Licorice root (Gan Cao)	1-3gms Glycyrrhiza uralensis
Jujube Dates (Da Zao)	3-5pcs Zizyphus jujuba

Properties and Actions:
a) It is expectorant, eliminates white, frothy mucus
b) Sedative for restlessness, insomnia, anxiety and nausea

Indications: For mucus conditions, pulmonary emphysema, restlessness, insomnia, anxiety, shyness and timidity, Liver and Stomach disharmony, nausea, dizziness, palpitations. It can be considered for upper respiratory conditions including bronchitis and emphysema. In addition. since the Gallbladder influences courage in the traditional sense, it is also useful for timidity and shyness as well as insomnia.

Tongue: white, greasy-looking coat
Pulse: gliding and slippery

Bezoar Resurrection Pills (An gong niu huang wan)*

Bos Calculus (Niu Huang)	30gms Bos Taurus Domesticus
Rhinoceros horn (Xi Jiao)	30gms Rhinoceros unicornis
(Substitute 4 times the amount with Water Buffalo horn)	
Musk (She Xiang)	7.5gms Moschus moschiferus
Coptis (Huang Lian)	30gms Coptis chinensis
Scutellaria (Huang Qin)	30gms Scutellaria baicalensis
Gardenia (Zhi Zi)	30gms Gardenia jasminoides
Curcuma (Yu Jin)	30gms Curcuma longa
Realgar (Xiong Huang)	30gms Arsenic disulfide

Borneol (Bing Pian)	7.5gms Dryobalanops aromatica
Cinnabar (Zhu Sha)	30gms Red Mercuric Sulfide
Pearl (Zhen Zhu)	15gms Pteria margaritifera
Gold leaf (Jin Bo)	three small sheets

Preparation: Grind to a fine powder. Mix with honey and make into 3 gram pills. Take 1 pill 2 or 3 times a day with warm water. Children should be given half the adult dose. If the patient is unconscious administer with a gastric tube.

Properties and Actions:

a) Clears Heat Toxin

b) Revives unconsciousness

Indications: High fever with coma, delirium, convulsions. It can be considered for encephalitis, meningitis, infantile convulsions, hepatic coma, cerebral vascular injury, stroke, dysentery and uremia.

Contraindications: Do not use long term or during pregnancy and do not subject to cooking or high heat.

Big Pearl for Internal Wind (Da ding feng zhu)

Egg yolk (Ji Zi Huang)	1-2pcs.
Unprepared Rehmannia (Sheng Di Huang)	9-15gms Rehmannia glutinosa
Donkey-Hide Gelatin (E Jiao)	6-9gms Equus asinus
Ophiopogon (Mai Men Dong)	10-15gms Ophiopogon japonicus
White Peony (Bai Shao)	9-12gms Paeonia alba
Tortoise Plastron (Gui Ban)	9-12gms Chinemys reevesii
Tortoise shell (Bie Jia)	9-12gms Amyda sinensis
Oyster shell (Mu Li)	9-12gms Ostrea spp.
Schisandra (Wu Wei Zi)	3-6gms Schisandra chinensis
Cannabis seed (Huo Ma Ren)	6-9gms Cannabis sativa
Baked Licorice (Zhi Gan Cao)	3-6gms Glycyrrhiza uralensis

Properties and Actions:

a) Nourish the Yin

b) Calms Internal Wind

Indications: For spasmodic convulsions caused by Deficiency of Yin with Internal Wind. Symptoms include fatigue, prostration, convulsions.

Tongue: dark red with thin coat

Pulse: weak and thin

Blood Replenishing Decoction (Ji chuan jian)

Cistanches (Rou Cong Rong)	6-9gms Cistanches salsa
Dang Gui (Dang Gui)	9-15gms Angelica sinensis
Achyranthes (Niu Xi)	6-9gms Achyranthis bidentatae
Water Plantain (Ze Xie)	6-9gms Alisma plantago-aquatica
Bitter Orange (Zhi Ke)	3-6gms Citrus aurantium
Cimicifuga (Sheng Ma)	3-6gms Cimicifuga foetida

Properties and Actions:

a) Demulcent laxative

b) Warms Kidney Yang

Indications: Chronic constipation, lower back pain, cold feeling in the lower back and anemia.

Tongue: pale with a thin white coat

Pulse: thready

Contraindications: Not for an individual with constipation caused by Excessive stagnant Fire and Heat.

Variations:

1. With Deficient Qi add Ginseng (Ren Shen).

2. With Kidney Deficiency add Prepared Rehmannia (Shu Di Huang).

3. For Chronic constipation add Cannabis seed (Huo Ma Ren) (or Flax seed) and Cynomorium (Suo Yang).

4. For severe lower back pains add Water Plantain (Ze Xie), Lycii berries (Gou Qi Zi) and Eucommia (Du Zhong).

5. For pains throughout the body add Angelica (Du Huo) and Loranthes (Sang Ji Sheng).

Blue Fairy Pills For Lower Back Pain (Qing e wan)

Psoralea (Bu Gu Zhi)	120gms Psoralea corylifolia
Eucommia bark (Du Zhong)	120gms Eucommia ulmoides
Walnut (Hu Tao Ren)	120gms Juglans regia
Garlic (Da Suan)	120gms Allium sativa

Properties and Actions:

a) Tonifies Kidney Yang

b) Treats lower back pain

Indications: For chronic lower back pain caused by Kidney Deficiency, weakness of the bones and muscles, spermatorrhea.

Tongue: pale and swollen with a white coat

Pulse: deep and slippery

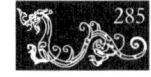

Bruise Relieving Powder (Qi li san)

Dragon's Blood (Xue Jie)	30gms Daemonorops draco
Musk (She Xiang)	.4gms Moschus moschiferus
Borneol (Bing Pian)	.4gms Dryobalanops aromatica
Mastic (Ru Xiang)	5gms Boswellia carterii
Safflower (Hong Hua)	5gms Carthamus tinctorius
Cinnabar (Zhu Sha)	4gms Red mercuric sulfide
Catechu (Er Cha)	7.5gms Acacia catechu
Myrrh (Mo Yao)	5gms Commiphora myrrha

Properties and Actions:

a) Promotes blood circulation, removes Stagnation

b) Relieves pain and stops bleeding

Indications: Mix the powder with wine and apply topically for external or internal injuries, wounds, burns, cuts and injuries of all kinds.

Tongue: dark red or blue-purple

Pulse: knotted

Bupleurum and Zhi Shi Formula (Si ni san or Frigid Extremities Powder)*

Bupleurum (Chai Hu)	9-12gms Bupleurum falcatum
Immature Bitter Orange (Zhi Shi)	6-9gms Citrus aurantium
White Peony (Bai Shao)	9-12gms Paeonia alba
Licorice (Gan Cao)	3-6gms Glycyrrhiza uralensis

Properties and Actions:

a) Regulates Liver and Spleen

b) Eliminates Internal Heat

Indications: Loss of consciousness caused by heat exposure, chronic hepatitis, nervous stomach, chest neuralgia, worms in the liver and bile duct, hernia, inflammation of the pancreas or the appendix.

Tongue: pale with white coat

Pulse: tight and bowstring

Explanation of the formula:

This formula is characterized by herbs that have opposite directional influences in the body. Bupleurum is an upward rising herb that enters the Liver, Immature Bitter Orange is descending and also enters the Liver, Peony is Internal and Licorice harmonizes the center. The effect of the different directions is to disentangle Heat in the Liver, Stomach and Spleen territories. This Heat locked Internally is the cause of frigid extremities in this case. By releasing the Internal Heat, the external limbs are warmed.

Symptoms of Liver and Stomach disharmony that are relieved with this formula include painful fullness in the hypochondrium and Stomach, acid regurgitation, belching, nausea, vomiting. There will be a thin yellowish coat on the Tongue and the Pulse tends to be wiry.

Bupleurum and Cinnamon Combination (Chai hu gui zhi tang)

Bupleurum (Chai hu)	15gms Bupleurum falcatum
Pinellia (Ban Xia)	12gms Pinellia ternata
Ginseng (Ren Shen)	6gms Panax ginseng
White Peony (Bai Shao)	6gms Paeonia alba
Scutellaria (Huang Qin)	6gms Scutellaria baicalensis
Cinnamon twigs (Gui Zhi)	6gms Cinnamomum cassia
Fresh Ginger (Sheng Jiang)	3gms Zingiberis officinalis
Licorice (Gan Cao)	3gms Glycyrrhiza uralensis
Jujube Dates (Da Zao)	3-5pcs Zizyphus jujuba

One of the most frequently indicated formulas useful for hundreds of conditions. This is because it harmonizes Internal and External symptoms, Cold and Heat, Excess and Deficiency. It is a combination of both Minor Bupleurum and Cinnamon Combination (Xiao chai hu tang and Gui zhi tang).

Properties and Actions:

a) Antipyretic, treats upper respiratory problems

b) Carminative and hepatic

c) Neuromuscular: intercostal neuralgia, headache, arthralgia, nephritis, pyelitis

d) Nervine tonic

Indications: For the common cold, influenza, pneumonia, TB, pleuritis, indigestion, gas, hepatitis, neurosis, nervous exhaustion, headache, irritability, insomnia, female disorders, hysteria, epilepsy and cardiac disorders.

Tongue: thin, white coat

Pulse: wiry and bowstring

Bupleurum and Dang Gui Formula (Xiao yao san or Rambling Powder)*

Bupleurum (Chai Hu)	6-9gms Bupleurum falcatum
Angelica (Dang Gui)	6-9gms Angelica sinensis
White Peony (Bai Shao)	8-12gms Paeoniae alba
Poria (Fu Ling)	9-15gms Poria cocos
Mentha (Bo He)	1-3gms Mentha haplocalyx

Fresh Ginger (Sheng Jiang)	1-3gms Zingiberis officinalis
Baked Licorice (Zhi Gan Cao)	3-6gms Glycyrrhiza uralensis

Properties and Actions:

a) Harmonizes the function of Liver and Spleen

b) Relieves Liver Qi stagnation

c) Nourishes the Blood

Indications: Used for Blood Deficiency with disharmony of Liver and Spleen. Symptoms include chest fullness and pain, anemia, dizziness, headache, dry mouth and throat, tiredness, loss of appetite, irregular menstruation, leukorrhea, tiredness, breast distention, malarial symptoms with alternate chills and fever. It can also be given for chronic hepatitis.

Tongue: pale red

Pulse: thready, tight and weak

Bupleurum and Dragon Bone Combination

(Chai hu jia long gu mu li tang)

Bupleurum (Chai Hu)	9-12gms Bupleurum falcatum
Poria (Fu Ling)	4.5gms Poria cocos
Dragon Bone (Long Gu)	4.5gms Stegodon orientalis
Oyster shell (Mu Li)	4.5gms Ostrea testa
Pinellia (Ban Xia)	6-9gms Pinellia ternata
Rhubarb (Da Huang)	6gms Rheum palmatum
Cinnamon twigs (Gui Zhi)	4.5gms Cinnamomum cassia
Scutellaria (Huang Qin)	4.5gms Scutellaria baicalensis
Ginseng (Ren Shen)	4.5gms Panax ginseng
Fresh Ginger (Sheng Jiang)	4.5gms Zingiberis officinalis
Jujube Dates (Da Zao)	4-5pcs Zizyphus jujuba

Properties and Actions:

a) Harmonizes Interior and Exterior

b) Relieves Stagnation

c) Sedative

Indications: The Qi is not transforming and therefore floats upward. This causes symptoms of anxiety, nervousness, and palpitations. Symptoms of all three Yang stages are present. These may include chest fullness, irritability with palpitations, urinary difficulty, constipation, nervous anxiety, hysteria, body heaviness and stiffness, and epilepsy.

This formula was originally prescribed to remedy the adverse reaction resulting from the use of Rhubarb (Da Huang: a purgative), inappropriately given during the early stages of colds and flu. It would weaken the outer defenses further and drive the External pathogenic influence deeper, causing Heat to concentrate itself in the chest. Bupleurum (Chai Hu) is the principal herb for resolving chest oppression caused by Stagnant Liver Qi. Because the Yang is driven inward with the inappropriate use of purgatives, it is unable to maintain the Exterior, causing a feeling of stiffness and heaviness.

Tongue: red with a moist coat

Pulse: wiry and rapid

Bupleurum and Peony Combination (Jia wei xiao yao san)

Bupleurum (Chai Hu)	6-9gms Bupleurum falcatum
Dang Gui (Dang Gui)	6-9gms Angelica sinensis
White Peony (Bai Shao)	8-12gms Paeoniae alba
Poria (Fu Ling)	9-15gms Poria cocos
Dry-fried Atractylodes (Zhi Bai Zhu)	3gms Atractylodis alba
Moutan Peony (Mu Dan Pi)	1.5gms Paeonia suffruticosa
Gardenia fruit (Zhi Zi)	1.5gms Gardeniae jasminoidis
Baked Licorice (Zhi Gan Cao)	3-6gms Glycyrrhiza uralensis
Mentha (Bo He)	1-3gms Mentha haplocalycis

Properties and Actions:

a) Harmonizes Liver and Spleen

b) Digestive, tonifies Spleen

c) Alterative, clears Deficient Heat

Indications: Spleen Qi Deficiency with Liver Qi Stagnation changes to Heat causing increased irritability, short temper, tidal fever, sweating, blood shot eyes, palpitations, increased menstrual flow, uterine bleeding, dry mouth, lower abdominal pressure and painful urination. This formula is taken with a small amount of Fresh Ginger (Sheng Jiang) and Mint (Bo He). For difficult and painful urination add Plantain seeds (Che Qian Zi). Compare with Bupleurum and Dan Gui Formula (Xiao yao san) which is less tonifying and less detoxifying.

Bupleurum and Schizonepeta Formula (Shi wei bai du tang)

Bupleurum (Chai Hu)	9gms Bupleurum falcatum
Fresh Ginger (Sheng Jiang)	3gms Zingiberis officinalis
Siler (Fang Feng)	6gms Siler seseloides
Angelica Du Huo (Du Huo)	6gms Angelica pubescens
Poria (Fu Ling)	6gms Poria cocos

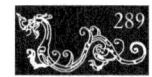

Platycodon (Jie Geng)	9gms Platycodon grandiflorum
Schizonepeta (Jing Jie)	3gms Schizonepeta tenuifolium
Ligusticum (Chuan Xiong)	9gms Ligusticum wallichii
Licorice (Gan Cao)	3gms Glycyrrhiza uralensis
Cherry Bark	9gms Prunus yedoemisis

Properties and Actions:
a) Detoxifying, aids Liver detoxifying function
b) Clears the skin

Indications: For lymphadenitis, carbuncles, furuncles, boils, mastitis, skin diseases such as dermatitis, urticaria, eczema, acne, ophthalmia, nasal congestion, external and middle ear infection.

Tongue: red with a yellow coat
Pulse: rapid

Bupleurum, Cinnamon Twig and Ginger Combination
(Chai hu gui zhi gan jiang tang)

Bupleurum (Chai Hu)	24gms Bupleurum falcatum
Cinnamon twigs (Gui Zhi)	9gms Cinnamomum cassia
Ginger (Gan Jiang)	6gms Zingiberis officinalis
Trichosanthes (Tian Hua Fen)	12gms Trichosanthis kirilowii
Scutellaria (Huang Qin)	9gms Scutellaria baicalensis
Oyster shell (Mu Li)	6gms Ostrea testa
Honey-Baked Licorice (Zhi Gan Cao)	6gms Glycyrrhiza uralensis

Properties and Actions:
a) Treats recurring fevers and chills
b) Resolves phlegm and relieves chest fullness and congestion
c) Warms the extremities

Indications: This formula is used for more sensitive type individuals with intermittent fever, with chills, chest fullness, stress and anxiety, heart palpitations, thirst, cold hands and feet, loose stool or diarrhea. It can be considered for the common cold, TB, pneumonia, bronchitis, pleurisy, peritonitis, insomnia, hepatitis and inflammation of the Gallbladder.

Bupleurum Formula (Yi gan san)

Atractylodes (Bai Zhu)	3gms Atractylodes alba
Poria (Fu Ling)	3gms Poria cocos
Angelica (Dang Gui)	3gms Angelica sinensis
Ligusticum (Chuan Xiong)	3gms Ligusticum wallichii

Gambir (Gou Teng)	3gms Uncaria spp.
Bupleurum (Chai Hu)	1.5gms Bupleurum falcatum
Licorice (Gan Cao)	1.5gms Glycyrrhiza uralensis

Properties and Actions:
a) Antispasmodic, calms Liver Wind
b) Tonifies Liver Blood and Qi

Indications: Used for many types of spasmodic conditions including Liver Wind problems with symptoms of nervousness, irritability, insomnia caused by over-excitement, seizure disorders, hysteria, night fears, spasms, feverishness, abdominal swelling, reduced appetite, restless sleep caused by Wood over dominating Spleen-Earth.

Note: To aid assimilation, it is usually taken with 2 1/2 grams of Citrus peel (Chen Pi).

Capillaris Combination (Yin chen hao tang)*

Capillaris (Yin Chen Hao)	9gms Artemisia capillaris
Gardenia fruit (Zhi Zi)	6gms Gardenia jasminoides
Rhubarb (Da Huang)	6-9gms Rheum palmatum

Properties and Actions:
Clears Internal Damp-Heat

Indications: For Internal Damp Heat with symptoms of jaundice and yellowish eyes, abdominal fullness and discomfort, thirst, decreased urination. It is indicated for acute infectious hepatitis, cholecystitis and cholelithiasis (gallstones).

Tongue: red body with a thick yellow coat

Pulse: slippery and rapid

Variations:

1. For fullness and discomfort in the chest and abdomen add Turmeric tuber (Yu Jin) and Immature Bitter Orange (Zhi Shi).

2. With intermittent fever, malaria, headache, bitter mouth taste add Bupleurum (Chai Hu), Scutellaria (Huang Qin) and Coptis (Huang Lian).

3. For accompanying nausea, vomiting and indigestion add Black Bamboo shavings (Zhu Ru) and Medicated Leaven (Massa Fermentata Medicinalis: Shen Qu).

Cannabis Seed Pills (Ma zi ren wan)*

Cannabis (crushed) (Ma Zi Ren)	25gms Cannabis sativa
(Flax seed is sometimes substituted for Cannabis seed)	
White Peony (Bai Shao)	12gms Paeonia alba

Apricot seed (Xing Ren)	9gms Prunus armeniaca
Immature Bitter Orange (Zhi Shi)	9gms Citrus aurantium
Rhubarb (Da Huang)	6-9gms Rheum officinalis
Magnolia Bark (Hou Po)	9gms Magnolia officinalis

Properties and Actions:

Lubricating laxative

Indications: Dry stool, chronic constipation in the weak and elderly, frequent urination, hemorrhoids.

Contraindication: Not to be used for constipation during pregnancy.

Tongue: dry and red with little or no coat

Variation: For bleeding hemorrhoids add Sophora flower (Huai Hua) and Sanguisorba root (Di Yu).

Cinnabar Sedative Pills (Zhu sha an shen wan)*

Cinnabar (Zhu Sha)	3-6gms Mercuric oxide
Coptis (Huang Lian)	6-9gms Coptis chinensis
Angelica (Dang Gui)	6-9gms Angelica sinensis
Fresh Rehmannia (Sheng Di Huang)	6-9gms Rehmannia glutinosa
Licorice (Gan Cao)	3-6gms Glycyrrhiza uralensis

Properties and Actions:

a) Sedative and tranquilizing

b) Clears Heart Fire

c) Nourishes the Blood

d) Nourishes the Yin

Indications: It can be used for insomnia, anxiety, palpitations, poor memory, palpitations, shortness of breath, neurosis, hysteria, depression, psychosis, schizophrenia.

Tongue: red

Pulse: thready and rapid

Contraindications: Because cinnabar is toxic, avoid overdosing (not more than 2 grams at a time) and not for more than one week at a time. It is contraindicated during pregnancy.

Cinnamon and Dragon Bone Combination

(Gui zhi long gu mu li tang)

Cinnamon twig (Gui Zhi)	4gms Cinnamomum cassia
Peony (Bai Shao)	4gms Paeoniae alba
Fresh Ginger (Sheng Jiang)	4gms Zingiberis officinalis

Dragon Bone (Long Gu) 3gms Stegodon orientalis
Oyster shell (Mu Li) 3gms Ostreae testa
Licorice (Gan Cao) 2gms Glycyrrhiza uralensis
Jujube Dates (Da Zao) 6pcs Zizyphus jujubae

Properties and Actions:

a) Nerve tonic

b) Warming stimulant, tonifies Yang

Indications: For nervous exhaustion, nervousness, palpitations, exhaustion caused by sexual excess, impotence, insomnia, enuresis and nighttime urination. It is also for abdominal spasms and pains. Commonly there will be umbilical palpitations as a result of the extreme exhaustion. It is also indicated for symptoms of Heart Yang Deficiency.

Cinnamon and Poria Combination (Gui zhi fu ling wan)
Cinnamon twig (Gui Zhi) 6-9gms Cinnamomum cassia
Poria (Fu Ling) 6-9gms Poria cocos
Moutan Peony (Mu Dan Pi) 6-9gms Paeonia suffruticosa
Persica seed (Tao Ren) 6-9gms Prunus persica
Red Peony (Chi Shao Yao) 6-9gms Paeonia lactiflora

Properties and Actions:

a) Promotes blood and lymphatic circulation, thus removing Stagnant Blood.

b) Softens and resolves hard lumps such as cysts and fibroids.

Indications: It is used for Blood and Fluid Stagnation especially of the female reproductive organs. Symptoms may include fibroids and cysts in the lower abdomen, painful, spasmodic and irregular menstruation characteristic of endometriosis. It is used for infertility, dysmenorrhea, post-partum bleeding, retention of the placenta.

Cinnamon Combination (Gui zhi tang)*
Cinnamon twig (Gui Zhi) 6-9gms Cinnamomum cassia
White Peony (Bai Shao Yao) 6-9gms Paeonia alba
Fresh Ginger (Sheng Jiang) 3-6gms Zingiberis officinalis
Prepared Licorice (Zhi Gan Cao) 3-6gms Glycyrrhiza uralensis
Jujube Dates (Da Zao) 3-6pcs Zizyphus jujuba

Rice congee (porridge), one bowl a half hour after perspiring.

Properties and Actions:

a) Warming diaphoretic

b) Tonic, regulating the constructive or nutritive energy (Ying) and the immune system (Wei).

Indications: For Deficient Wind-Cold Exterior condition. The symptoms are: colds, flus, fever, headache, intolerance to Wind and Cold, spontaneous and involuntary perspiration, decreased body resistance, postpartum care, morning sickness, skin diseases (eczema, frostbite, tinea, etc.). The involuntary sweating that occurs with this formula is an indication of Internal weakness.

This is a surface relieving formula. However, because the patient is weak, there may already be involuntary perspiration. This type of sweating is not effective, however, in overcoming the pathogenic influence. The sweating that will occur after taking this formula will help the body to overcome the pathogenic influence. The rice congee taken a half hour after sweating is to replenish whatever Qi may have been lost in the process.

Tongue: thin, white coat

Pulse: floating and slow

Notes: Compare the indications for this formula which is External Cold Deficiency, with Ephedra Combination, External Cold Excess, and Pueraria Combination which is for individuals with average constitution.

Variations:

1. For arthritis caused by Wind-Cold-Damp add: Turmeric rhizome (Jiang Huang) 6-9gms, Wild Ginger (Xi Xin) 3-6gms, Clematis (Wei Ling Xian) 3-6gms.

2. With stiff neck add Pueraria (Ge Gen) 6-9gms. This is called Gui Zhi Jia Ge Gen Tang.

3. With nocturnal emission, excessive dreams, lower part of the body Coldness, dizziness, loss of hair, add: Dragon Bone (Long Gu) and Oyster shell (Mu Li) 10-15gms of each.

4. With dyspnea, asthma and phlegm add: Magnolia bark (Hou Po) 6-9 grams, Apricot Seed (Xing Ren) 6-9gms. This is called Cinnamon, Magnolia and Apricot Seed Combination (Gui zhi hou po xing ren tang).

Cinnamon Twig Paeonia and Anemarrhena Decoction

(Gui zhi shao yao zhi mu tang)

Cinnamon twig (Gui Zhi)	6-9gms Cinnamomum cassia
White Peony (Shao Yao)	6-9gms Paeonia alba
Anemarrhena (Zhi Mu)	6-9gms Anemarrhena asphodeloides
Ephedra (Ma Huang)	6-9gms Ephedra sinica
Siler (Fang Feng)	6-9gms Siler seseloides
Atractylodes (Bai Zhu)	6-9gms Atractylodes alba
Prepared Aconite (Fu Zi)	6-9 Aconitum carmichaeli
Baked Licorice (Zhi Gan Cao)	3-6gms Glycyrrhiza uralensis
Fresh Ginger (Sheng Jiang)	3-5pcs Zingiberis officinalis

Properties and Indications:

a) Clears Wind and Damp

b) Clears Heat and inflammation and relieves pain

Indications: For rheumatic and arthritic conditions caused by Wind-Cold-Damp. Symptoms include joint pains with inflammation and swelling, no increase of body temperature, edema.

Tongue: yellow coat

Pulse: slippery and rapid

Circuligo and Epimedium Combination (Er xian tang)*

Circuligo (Xian Mao)	6-15gms Circuligo orchioides
Epimedium (Yin Yang Huo)	9-15gms Epimedium macranthum
Morinda (Ba Ji Tian)	6-9gms Morinda officinalis
Angelica (Dang Gui)	6-9gms Angelica sinensis
Phellodendron (Huang Bai)	4-9gms Phellodendrum amurense
Anemarrhena (Zhi Mu)	4-9gms Anemarrhena asphodeloides

Properties and Actions:

a) Nourishes Yin and tonifies Yang of the Kidney.

b) Clears Deficient Fire

c) Regulates the Chong (vital reproductive energy) and the Ren (conception vessel) meridians.

Indications: It is a good alternative tonic for those who might need Rehmannia Eight Formula (Ba Wei Di Huang wan) but it is too Hot and Damp. It is the most representative formula for all menopausal imbalances. It can also be used for irregular menstruation, tinnitus, flaccid muscles, coldness of the feet and lower back, dizziness, headache. Some conditions for which it may be considered are menopause, amenorrhea, hypertension and hypotension, nephritis and chronic urinary tract infections.

Tongue: pale

Pulse: thin and rapid

For menopausal hot flashes add Sprouted Rice (Nuo Dao Gen Mai), Oyster shell (Mu Li) and White peony (Bai Shao Yao)

For menopausal insomnia add Biota (Bai Zi Ren), Zizyphus seeds (Suan Zao Ren), Prepared Licorice (Zhi Gan Cao), Sprouted Rice (Nuo Dao Gen Mai), Oyster shell (Mu Li) and Jujube Dates (Da Zao).

For menopausal low back pain and knee weakness add Loranthes (Sang Ji Sheng), Eucommia bark (Du Zhong) and Dipsacus (Xu Duan)

For fatigue add Ginseng (Ren Shen) and Astragalus (Huang Qi)

For Yin Deficiency remove Curculigo and add Eclipta (Han Lian Cao), Asparagus root (Tian Men Dong) and Ligustrum seed (Nu Zhen Zi)

For Yang Deficiency with Dampness remove Anemarrhena, Phellodendron and Morinda and add Lycii berries (Gou Qi Zi), Dioscorea (Shan Yao), Codonopsis (Dang Shen), Poria (Fu Ling), Rubi fruit (Fu Pen Zi) and Atractylodes (Bai Zhu).

For fluid Dryness with constipation add Cannabis seed (Huo Ma Ren), Cistanches (Rou Cong Rong), Achyranthis root (Niu Xi), Polygonum multiflorum root (He Shou Wu), Angelica (Dang Gui) and Immature citrus (Zhi Shi).

Citrus and Crataegus Formula (Preserve Harmony Pill or Bao he wan)*

Hawthorn berries(Shan Zha)	9-15gms Crataegus pinnatifida
Medicated Leaven (Shen Qu)	9-12gms Massa Fermentata Medicinalis
Radish seed (Lai Fu Zi)	6-9gms Raphani sativi
Citrus peel (Chen Pi)	6-9gms Citri reticulatae
Pinellia (Ban Xia)	9-12gms Pinelliae ternatae
Poria (Fu Ling)	9-12gms Poria cocos
Forsythia (Lian Qiao)	3-6gms Forsythia suspensa

Properties and Actions:

a) Digestive

b) Reduces Food Stagnation

c) Harmonizes the Stomach

Indications: It is used for food poisoning and overindulgence in rich foods, alcohol, meat or greasy foods. There may be symptoms of abdominal distention with fullness of the stomach, epigastrium and chest, occasional pain, belching, acid regurgitation, nausea and vomiting, aversion to food, diarrhea or constipation.

Tongue: yellow, greasy coated

Pulse: slippery

Variations: For more severe abdominal distention, add Green Citrus (Zhi Shi) and Magnolia bark (Hou Po).

For constipation add Rhubarb (Da Huang) and Betel Nut (Bing Lang).

Citrus and Pinellia Combination (Er chen tang or Two Cured Decoction)*

Pinellia (Ban Xia)	15gms Pinellia ternata
Citrus peel (Chen Pi)	15gms Citri reticulatus
Poria (Fu Ling)	9gms Poria cocos
Baked Licorice (Zhi Gan Cao)	4gms Glycyrrhizae uralensis

Preparation: Prepare as a decoction adding 3gms of Fresh Ginger (Sheng Jiang) and 1pc of Umeboshi Plum (dried or salt preserved).

Properties and Actions:
a) Dries Damp and dispels Phlegm
b) Regulates Qi and harmonizes the Middle Warmer (Stomach and Spleen).
Indications: Cough with Damp-Cold Phlegm caused by Cold-Damp of the Spleen and Stomach. Symptoms may include chest and epigastric fullness, nausea, vomiting, lassitude, feeling of heaviness (from excess mucus), possibly vertigo and palpitations in extreme cases. May be considered for upper respiratory tract infection, chronic bronchitis, cough, goiter, chronic gastritis, peptic ulcer and Meniere's disease.
Tongue: moist, greasy white coat
Pulse: slippery

Variations:
1. For Damp-Heat of the Upper Warmer add Scutellaria (Huang Qin), Gardenia (Zhi Zi), Apricot seed (Xing Ren) and Platycodon (Jie Geng).
2. For Damp-Heat in the Lower Warmer add Sophorae (Ku Shen), Phellodendron (Huang Bai) and Talcum (Hua Shi).
3. For Wind-Dampness add Clematis (Wei Ling Xian), Gentiana (Qin Jiao), Xanthium (Cang Er Zi) and Cinnamon twigs (Gui Zhi).
4. For cough with copious sputum caused by External Cold in the Lungs add Ephedra (Ma Huang) and Apricot seed (Xing Ren).
5. For vomiting caused by a Cold Stomach add Dried Ginger (Gan Jiang) and Cardamon (Sha Ren).
6. For vomiting of clear fluids add Black Atractylodes (Cang Zhu) and White Atractylodes (Bai Zhu).
7. For chronic Phlegm in the channels and flesh leading to rubbery nodules add Oyster shell (Mu Li), Scrophularia (Xuan Shen), Laminaria (Kun Bu) and Sargassi (Hai Zao).
8. For Spleen and Kidney Yang Deficiency characterized by coughing of thin, watery sputum, deep pulse and urinary problems, add Cinnamon bark (Rou Gui) and Prepared Aconite (Fu Zi).
9. For insomnia and sleepiness after meals add White Atractylodes (Bai Zhu) and Sweet Flag (Shi Chang Pu).
10. For severe coughing at night caused by Phlegm and Blood Deficiency add Angelica (Dang Gui).
11. For Damp-Phlegm obstructing the womb with irregular menstruation and copious leukorrhea add Ligusticum (Chuan Xiong) and Angelica (Dang Gui).
12. For Phlegm and Dryness together, substitute Trichosanthis (Gua Lou) and Fritillary Bulb (Chuan Bei Mu) for Pinellia (Ban Xia).

13. For dizziness or vertigo, headache, full, stifling feeling in the chest, nausea, vomiting, headache; Tongue: white greasy coat; Pulse: slippery, wiry or bowstring, add: Gastrodia (Tian Ma) and 1 slice of Fresh Ginger (Sheng Jiang) and 3-4 pcs of Jujube Date (Da Zao). This becomes Pinellia and Gastrodia Combination (Ban xia bai zhu tian ma tang)*. It is used to dry and dissolve Phlegm and smooth the Liver and quiet Liver-Wind (antispasmodic).

This formula forms the basis for countless other combinations that deal with Phlegm and fluid accumulation or what in Ayurvedic medicine is called 'kapha', or mucus humour.

For instance Six Gentlemen Decoction (Liu jun zi tang) combines Pinellia, Poria, Licorice and Citrus with Ginseng and White Atractylodes as a Spleen tonic. This reflects the relationship of the Spleen Qi to fluid metabolism.

Another variation is Pinellia and Gastrodia Combination that combines Gastrodia (Tian Ma) and Atractylodes (Bai Zhu) to calm Liver-Wind and dissolve Dampness. It is used for symptoms associated with dizziness, vertigo, heaviness of the head, headache, and other central neurological symptoms caused by Wind and Phlegm.

Bamboo and Poria Combination (Wen dan tang) adds Bamboo Shavings (Zhu Ru) 6gms, Green Citrus (Zhi Shi) 6gms and Fresh Ginger (Sheng Jiang) 3-6gms to clear Hot-Phlegm with symptoms of coughing of copious thick, yellow sputum that is difficult to expectorate.

Artemisia Annua and Scutellaria Decoction to Clear the Gallbladder (Hao qin qing dan tang) is another formula variation that adds Sweet Annie (Qing Hao) 6-9gms, Scutellaria (Huang Qin) 6-9gms, Bamboo Shavings (Zhu Ru) 9g and Bi Yu San 9-12gms (a combination of equal parts Talcum, Indigo and Licorice). It is used to clear Heat from the Gallbladder, relieve acute conditions of the Gallbladder as well as symptoms of acute hepatitis, acute gastritis, pneumonia, hypertension, coronary artery disease, pyelonephritis, and Meniere's disease, all associated with acute Damp Heat syndromes.

Apricot Kernel and Perilla Leaf Powder (Xing su san) adds Perilla leaf (Zi Su Ye), Peucedani (Qian Hu), Apricot seed (Xing Ren), 3pcs of Jujube Date (Da Zao) and 3gms of Licorice (Gan Cao). It is used to disperse and lubricate Dryness to treat deep coughs with associated symptoms of watery sputum, stuffy nose, slight headache, chills without sweating, but a dry throat and a dry tongue with a white coating and a wiry pulse.

Clear the Nutritive Decoction (Qing ying tang)
Rhinoceros horn (Xi Jiao)   6-9gms Rhinoceros unicornis

Fresh Rehmannia (Di Huang)	9-15gms Rehmannia glutinosa
Scrophularia (Xuan Shen)	6-9gms Scrophularia ningpoensis
Ophiopogon (Mai Men Dong)	6-9gms Ophiopogon japonicus
Bamboo leaf (Zhu Ye)	3-6gms Phylostachys nigra
Coptis (Huang Lian)	1-3gms Coptis chinensis
Lonicera flowers (Jin Yin Hua)	6-9gms Lonicerae japonicae
Forsythia (Lian Qiao)	6-9gms Forsythia suspensa
Red Sage (Dan Shen)	3-6gms Salvia miltiorrhiza

Properties and Actions:
a) Clears Heat from the Nutritive Ying level.
b) Nourishes Yin and Vital Essence

Indications: For Heat that penetrates the Nutritive Ying level with symptoms of nighttime fever, either Excessive thirst or lack of thirst, restlessness, delirium, insomnia.

Tongue: deep crimson and dry

Pulse: thin and rapid

It can be considered for epidemic meningitis, encephalitis B and septicemia.
Contraindications: Not for conditions of Cold Dampness

Clear the Stomach Powder (Qing wei san)

Coptis (Huang Lian)	2-6gms Coptis chinensis
Cimicifugae (Sheng Ma)	3-6gms Cimicifuga foetida
Moutan Peony (Mu Dan Pi)	2-9gms Paeonia suffruticosa
Unprepared Rehmannia (Sheng Di Huang)	1-12gms Rehmannia glutinosa
Angelica sinensis (Dang Gui)	1-12gms Angelica sinensis

Preparation: Grind to a powder and add one tablespoon to a cup of boiling water. Increase or decrease the dose as indicated and needed.

Properties and Indications: Specific for Heat in the Stomach with symptoms of toothache, sore gums, lips and Tongue, mouth sores, facial swelling, pain in the head, bad breath, dry mouth.

Tongue: red with little or no coat

Pulse: rapid, slippery and full

Clematis and Stephania Combination (Shu jing huo xue tang)
(Decoction to Dredge the Meridians & Vitalize Blood)

Angelica (Dang Gui)	5gms Angelicae sinensis
White Peony (Bai Shao)	4gms Paeoniae alba
Rehmannia, raw (Sheng Di Huang)	4gms Rehmannia glutinosa

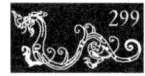

Ligusticum (Chuan Xiong)	3gms Ligustici wallichii
Persica seed (Tao Ren)	4gms Prunus persica
Poria (Fu Ling)	4gms Poria cocos
Atractylodes (Cang Zhu)	4gms Atractylodes lancea
Citrus peel (Chen Pi)	4gms Citri reticulatae
Notopterygium (Qiang Huo)	3gms Notopterygium incisium
Angelica (Bai Zhi)	3gms Angelicae dahuricae
Clematidis (Wei Ling Xian)	4gms Clematidis chinensis
Stephania (Fang Ji)	3gms Stephaniae tetrandrae
Sileris (Fang Feng)	3gms Siler divaricata
Gentiana (Long Dan Cao)	3gms Gentiana macrophyllae
Achyranthes (Niu Xi)	4gms Achyranthis Bidentatae
Licorice (Gan Cao)	2gms Glycyrrhizae uralensis
Fresh Ginger (Sheng Jiang)	3-6gms Zingiberis officinalis

Preparation: Decoct the above herbs with three slices of fresh Ginger root.

Properties and Actions:

a) Opens circulation of the channels and collaterals, stimulates blood circulation, removes Blood stagnation.

b) Antirheumatic, removes Damp stagnation.

Indications: Body aches, muscle aches and joint pains caused by External factors of Wind, Cold, Heat and Damp with Internal Deficiency.

Clove and Persimmon Calyx Combination (Shi di tang)

Clove (Ding Xiang)	6gms Eugenia caryophyllata
Persimmon Calyx (Shi Di)	6-9gms Diospyros kaki
Fresh Ginger (Sheng Jiang)	6-9gms Zingiberis officinalis
Ginseng (Ren Shen)	3-6gms Panax ginseng

Properties and Actions:

a) Directs Qi downward (hiccups and belching)

b) Warms the Middle Warmer

Indications: hiccups, belching or vomiting.

Tongue: pale Tongue, white coat

Pulse: deep, slow Pulse

Variation: For Deficient Qi add Ginseng (Ren Shen)

Cnidium and Green Tea Combination (Chuan xiong cha tiao san)*

Ligusticum (Chuan Xiong)	6-9gms Ligusticum wallichii

Notopterygium (Qiang Huo)	6-9gms Notopterygium incisium
Angelica (Bai Zhi)	6-9gms Angelica dahuricae
Asarum (Xi Xin)	3-6gms Asarum heterophylii
Schizonepetae (Jing Jie)	6-9gms Schizonepatae tenuifoliae
Siler (Fang Feng)	6-9gms Siler seseloides
Mentha (Bo He)	3-6gms Mentha haplocalyx
Licorice (Gan Cao)	3-6gms Glycyrrhiza uralensis

Preparation: Grind all the ingredients into a powder and take with a cup of green tea.

Properties and Actions:

a) Analgesic, relieves Wind

Indications: For headache (bilateral, frontal, occipital, vertical and migraine) caused by tension, spasm and Wind. There may also be symptoms of chills, vertigo, dizziness, nasal congestion and fever. It is useful for all kinds of headaches caused by Wind and Cold. It is also useful for rhinitis, common cold and sinusitis.

Contraindications: Not for headaches caused by Wind-Heat.

Variations:

1. For headache caused by Wind-Heat add Chrysanthemum flowers (Ju Hua), White-Stiff Silkworm (Jiang Can), Baked Licorice (Zhi Gan Cao). This is called Ju hua cha tiao san.

Coix Combination (Yi yi ren tang)

Ephedra (Ma Huang)	6gms Ephedra sinica
Angelica sinensis (Dang Gui)	6-9gms Angelica sinensis
White Atractylodes (Bai Zhu) or Atractylodes lancea (Cang Zhu)	9gms Atractylodes alba
Coix (Yi Yi Ren)	24-30gms Coix lachryma-jobi
Cinnamon twigs	6gms Cinnamomum cassia
White Peony (Bai Shao)	9gms Paeonia alba
Prepared Licorice (Zhi Gan Cao)	3gms Glycyrrhiza uralensis

Properties and Indications: Removes Dampness, inflammation and promotes blood circulation in the joints. Relieves arthritic and rheumatic conditions.

Conduct the Heart Fire Downward (Dao chi san)*

Unprepared Rehmannia (Sheng Di Huang)	10-15gms Rehmannia glutinosa
Akebia (Mu Tong)	9-12gms Akebia trifoliata
Bamboo leaf (Zhu Ye)	6-9gms Phylostachys nigra
Licorice (Gan Cao)	3-6gms Glycyrrhiza uralensis

Properties and Indications: Directs the Heat from the Heart down to the Small Intestine and opens urination. It is associated with conditions of acute urinary tract infection, heat sensation in the chest, mouth sores, dark red urine with a short difficult stream.

Tongue: red

Pulse: rapid

Contraindications: Avoid using with patients with diarrhea

Variations:

1. For excessive Heart Fire add Coptis (Huang Lian)

2. For blood in the urine add Eclipta (Han Lian Cao), Cephalanoplos and Imperatae (Bai Mao Gen)

3. For Yin Deficiency add Anemarrhena (Zhi Mu) and Dendrobium (Shi Hu).

Coptis and Cinnamon Formula (Jiao tai wan)

(Grand Communication Pill)

Coptis (Huang Lian)	6-9gms Coptis chinensis
Cinnamon bark (Rou Gui)	3-6gms Cinnamomum cassia

Properties and Indications: Restores the functional communication between the Heart and the Kidneys. It is useful for treating nervousness, anxiety and insomnia with cold extremities caused by Kidney Yang Deficiency. Coptis is used to clear evil Heat from the Heart and thereby calm the mind. By so doing, the ability of the Kidneys to foster a sense of inner rootedness and strength is facilitated so the normal functional relationship between Fire and Water is restored. With the anxiety of the Heart and mind quelled, the Yin is no longer threatened, Kidney Yin is able to ascend and Heart Yin is nourished.

Coptis and Scutellaria Combination (Huang lian jie du tang)*

Coptis (Huang Lian)	9-12gms Coptis chinensis
Baikal Skullcap (Huang Qin)	9-12gms Scutellaria baicalensis
Phellodendron (Huang Bai)	9-12gms Philodendron amurense
Gardenia fruit (Zhi Zi)	3-6gms Gardenia jasminoides

Properties and Actions:

a) Detoxifies, anti-inflammatory, alterative, antibiotic

Indications: It can be applied for infections and inflammations, high fever, irritability, boils, dryness of the mouth and throat, insomnia, spitting of blood, nosebleeds caused by Excess Heat, cancer.

Tongue: red body and yellow coat

Pulse: strong and rapid

Contraindications: Not for a person with no Tongue fur on the Tongue which indicates Stomach Yin Deficiency.

Pueraria, Scute and Coptis Combination (Ge gen huang qin huang lian tang)
Pueraria (Ge Gen)   10-15gms Pueraria lobata
Baikal Skullcap (Huang Qin)   6-9gms Scutellaria baicalensis
Coptis (Huang Lian)   3-6gms Coptis chinensis
Honey Baked Licorice (Zhi Gan Cao)   3-6gms Glycyrrhiza uralensis
Properties and Actions:
a) Clears both External and Internal acute inflammations
b) Relieves muscle aches of the neck
Indications: An individual with an External condition with Internal Heat in the gastrointestinal tract with symptoms of fever, feeling of Heat in the chest, diarrhea, bacterial and amebic dysentery, acute colitis.

Symptoms may include fever, diarrhea, a sensation of Heat in the chest, dry mouth, Heat in the epigastric area, dry mouth and thirst.

Tongue: red with a yellow coat

Pulse: rapid.

Contraindications: Not for an individual with diarrhea caused by Coldness.
Variations:
1. For diarrhea and vomiting add Pinellia (Ban Xia)
2. For abdominal pain add Saussurea root (Mu Xiang) and White Peony (Bai Shao).
3. For acute colitis add Honeysuckle (Jin Yin Hua) and Plantago seed (Che Qian Zi)
4. For mastitis add Dandelion root (Pu Gong Ying) and Honeysuckle (Jin Yin Hua)

Dang Gui and Arctium Combination (Xiao feng san)
Schizonepeta (Jing Jie)   3gms Schizonepetae tenuifoliae
Siler (Fang Feng)   3gms Siler divaricatae
Arctii (Niu Bang Zi)   3gms Arctii lappae
Cicada periostracum (Chan Tui)   3gms Periostracum cicadae
Black Atractylodes (Cang Zhu)   3gms Atractylodes lancea
Sophora (Ku Shen)   3gms Sophorae flavescentis
Akebia (Mu Tong)   3-6gms Akebia quinata
Moutan peony (Mu Dan Pi)   1.5gms Paeonia suffruticosa
Anemarrhena (Zhi Mu)   3gms Anemarrhenae asphodeloides

Raw rehmannia (Sheng Di Huang)	3gms Rehmannia glutinosa
Angelica (Dang Gui)	3gms Angelica sinensis
Black Sesame seeds (Hei Zhi Ma)	3gms Sesame indici
Licorice (Gan Cao)	1.5gms Glycyrrhiza uralensis

Properties and Actions:
a) Disperses Wind
b) Dispels Dampness
c) Cools the Blood and clears Heat

Indications: Used for chronic skin conditions associated with weeping (moist) and redness. It can be considered for a variety of skin problems including eczema, psoriasis, urticaria, dermatitis, purpura, tinea or fungus infections and skin rashes (including baby's diaper rash).

Tongue: yellow or white coat

Pulse: rapid

Dang Gui and Peony Formula (Dang gui shao yao san)

Angelica (Dang Gui)	6-9gms Angelica sinensis
White Peony (Bai Shao)	6-9gms Paeonia alba
Ligusticum (Chuan Xiong)	6-9gms Ligusticum wallichii
Atractylodes (Bai Zhu)	6-9gms Atractylodes alba
Poria (Fu Ling)	6-9gms Poria cocos
Alisma (Ze Xie)	6-9gms Alisma plantago-aquatica

Properties and Actions:
a) Nourishes the Blood
b) Tonifies Qi
c) Removes Damp

Indications: Anemia with continuous abdominal pains caused by Spleen and Kidney Deficiency. There may be urinary problems with lower limb edema. Symptoms include pale complexion, fatigue, anemia, mild abdominal pains, feeling of heaviness, edema, tinnitus, lower back pain, palpitations. It is mostly used for weaker women, with possible symptoms of anemia, lower back pain, painful menstruation, pelvic inflammatory disease, chronic nephritis, edema, beriberi, habitual and threatened miscarriage, menopause.

Tongue: pale with a thin coat

Pulse: deep, thready and weak

Variations:

1. For threatened miscarriage add Eucommia (Du Zhong), Dipsacus (Xu Duan), Cardamon (Sha Ren), Artemisiae argyii (Ai Ye), Scutellaria (Huang Qin).
2. For enlarged liver add Saussureae (Mu Xiang), Turmeric tuber (Yu Jin) and Immature Citrus (Zhi Shi).
3. For severe Dampness take with Poria Five Herb Combination (Wu ling san).
4. With Cold conditions add Cinnamon bark (Rou Gui) and Evodia (Wu Zhu Yu).
5. For Hot conditions add Moutan Peony (Mu Dan Pi) and Gardenia (Zhi Zi).

Dang Gui and Evodia Combination (Wen jing tang)

Evodia fruit (Wu Zhu Yu)	6gms Evodia rutaecarpa
Cinnamon twigs (Gui Zhi)	6gms Cinnamomi cassiae
Angelica (Dang Gui)	9gms Angelica sinensis
Ligusticum (Chuan Xiong)	9gms Ligusticum wallichii
White Peony (Bai Shao)	9gms Paeonia alba
Donkey-Hide Gelatin (E Jiao)	9gms Equus asinus
Ophiopogon (Mai Men Dong)	9gms Ophiopogon japonicus
Moutan Bark (Mu Dan Pi)	9gms Paeonia suffruticosa
Ginseng (Ren Shen)	6gms Panax ginseng
Pinellia (Ban Xia)	9gms Pinellia ternata
Fresh Ginger (Sheng Jiang)	9gms Zingiberis officinalis
Licorice (Gan Cao)	3gms Glycyrrhiza uralensis

Properties and Actions:
a) Warms channels and menses and disperses Cold
b) Nourishes and promotes the circulation of Blood

Indications: Uterine bleeding, irregular menstruation, prolonged menstruation, breakthrough bleeding between menses, infertility, cold and swollen lower abdomen, dry lips, low grade fever, increased feverishness in the evening caused by Deficient Blood, chronic pelvic inflammation.

Variations:
1. For Qi Deficiency add Astragalus (Huang Qi).
2. For incessant uterine bleeding with light colored blood omit Moutan Peony (Mu Dan Pi), add Fried Ginger (Pao Jiang), Mugwort (Ai Ye), Prepared Rehmannia (Shu Di Huang).
3. For severe Cold abdominal pains omit Moutan Peony (Mu Dan Pi) and add Mugwort (Ai Ye), Cinnamon bark (Rou gui).

4. For infertility caused by Blood Deficiency and Cold add Cyperus (Xiang Fu) and Green Citrus (Qing Pi) to be taken daily only during the menstrual flow.

5. For severe Qi stagnation add Cyperus (Xiang Fu) and Lindera (Wu Yao).

6. For chronic endometritis add Frankincense (Ru Xiang) and Tian Qi Ginseng (San Qi).

Coptis and Rhubarb Combination (San huang xie xin tang)

Rhubarb (Da Huang)	3-6gms Rheum palmatum
Scutellaria (Huang Qin)	3-6gms Scutellaria baicalensis
Coptis (Huang Lian)	3-6gms Coptis chinensis

Properties and Actions:
a) Detoxifies and clears Heat from the gastro-intestinal tract
b) Opens the Gallbladder

Indications: It can be used for toxicity, habitual constipation, anxiety, gastritis, peptic ulcer, gastrorrhagia, hemorrhoids, hemorrhoidal bleeding, arteriosclerosis, liver disorders, hypertension and recovery from stroke.

Tongue: red with a greasy yellow coat

Pulse: full and possibly wiry and rapid

Contraindications: Not suitable for individuals lacking in true Heat or with Qi Deficiency.

Dang Gui and Gelatin Combination (Jiao ai tang)

Prepared Rehmannia (Shu Di Huang)	12gms Rehmannia glutinosa
Angelica (Dang Gui)	9gms Angelica sinensis
Ligusticum (Chuan Xiong)	6gms Ligusticum wallichii
White Peony (Bai Shao)	9gms Paeonia alba
Donkey-Hide Gelatin (E Jiao)	9gms Equus asinus
Mugwort (Ai Ye)	9gms Artemisia argyii
Licorice (Gan Cao)	3gms Glycyrrhiza uralensis

Properties and Actions:
a) Nourishes the Blood
b) Stops bleeding
c) Prevents miscarriage

Indications: For menstrual bleeding caused by Deficiency and Cold of the Chong (vital) and Ren (Conception vessel) channels, abdominal pain, constant spotting, post partum bleeding, bleeding during pregnancy and threatened miscarriage. There will be light colored blood without clots, weakness and sore, aching back, menorrhagia.

Tongue: pale
Pulse: thin, thready Pulse
Contraindications: Not for bleeding conditions caused by Heat.
Variations:
1. With lower back pain add Eucommia bark (Du Zhong) and Loranthus (Sang Ji Sheng)
2. With Deficient Qi add Codonopsis (Dang Shen) and Astragalus (Huang Qi) or with Ginseng and Longan Combination (Gui pi tang).
3. For threatened miscarriage, bleeding during pregnancy and lower back pain omit Ligusticum (Chuan Xiong) and add Atractylodes (Bai Zhu), Eucommia (Du Zhong) and Loranthus (Sang Ji Sheng).

Dang Gui and Jujube Combination (Dang gui si ni tang)
Angelica (Dang Gui)	9-12gms Angelica sinensis
Cinnamon twig (Gui Zhi)	9-12gms Cinnamomum cassia
White Peony (Bai Shao)	10-15gms Paeonia alba
Wild Ginger (Xi Xin)	3-6gms Asarum heterotropoides
Akebia (Mu Tong)	6-9gms Akebia trifoliata
Baked Licorice (Zhi Gan Cao)	3-6gms Glycyrrhiza uralensis
Jujube Dates (Da Zao)	3-5pcs Ziziphus jujube

Properties and Indications:
a) Warms the meridians and disperses Cold
b) Promotes blood circulation and nourishes the Blood
Indications: It can be used for anemia, frostbite, dysmenorrhea, hernia caused by Coldness, thromboangiitis obliterans.
Tongue: pale with a white coat
Pulse: thin and slow Pulse

Dang Gui, Dipsacus and Tian Qi Ginseng Combination (Shu jin san)
Angelica (Dang Gui)	9-12gms Angelica sinensis
Achyranthes (Niu Xi)	9-15gms Achyranthis bidentatae
Gambir (Gou Teng)	9-12gms Uncariae spp.
Chaenomeles (Mu Gua)	9-15gms Chaenomeles lagenaria
Notopterygium (Qiang Huo)	6-9gms Notopterygium incisium
Ligusticum (Chuan Xiong)	9-12gms Ligusticum wallichii
Lycii berries (Gou Qi Zi)	6-9gms Lycium chinensis
Siler (Fang Feng)	9-12gms Siler seseloides
Dipsacus (Xu Duan)	9-12gms Dipsacus japanicus

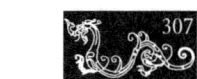

Tian Qi Ginseng (San Qi)   9-12gms Panax pseudoginseng

Actions and Indications: It soothes the muscles and tendons and benefits blood circulation. It is a good tonic for the Liver and Kidneys, relieving numbness, arthritis and lower back and leg pains.

Dose: About 9gms of the powder or two tablespoons of the alcoholic extract are taken twice a day until the condition improves.

Dang Gui Four Combination (Si wu tang)*

Prepared Rehmannia (Shu Di Huang)	10-15gms Rehmannia glutinosa
Angelica (Dang Gui)	9-12gms Angelica sinensis
Ligusticum (Chuan Xiong)	6-9gms Ligusticum wallichii
White Peony (Bai Shao)	9-12gms Paeonia lactiflora

Actions and Indications:

a) Restores and nourishes Blood

b) Stimulates blood circulation

Indications: Anemia, pale, sallow complexion and fingernails, dizziness, vertigo, irregular menstruation, ringing in the ears, stopped menstruation, threatened miscarriage, post-partum anemia.

Tongue: pale

Pulse: thready and weak

Note: This is the mother formula for all Blood Deficiency disorders.

Variations:

1. For increased Blood Stagnation add Peach seeds (Tao Ren) and Carthamus flowers (Hong Hua); this becomes Tao hong si wu tang.

2. For uterine bleeding add Donkey-Hide Gelatin (E Jiao) and Mugwort (Ai Ye). A version of this is commercially available as Tang Kwei Gin.

3. For painful menstruation with anemia and Stagnation, add Blood and Qi moving herbs including Motherwort (Yi Mu Cao), Cyperus (Xiang Fu), Corydalis (Yan Hu Suo).

Dang Gui, Gentiana and Aloe (Dang gui long hui wan)

Angelica (Dang Gui)	6-9gms Angelica sinensis
Aloe (Lu Hui)	6-9gms Aloe vera
Gentiana (Long Dan Cao)	6-9gms Gentiana scabra
Coptis (Huang Lian)	9-12gms Coptis chinensis
Scutellaria (Huang Qin)	9-12gms Scutellaria baicalensis
Phellodendron (Huang Bai)	9-12gms Phellodendron amurense
Gardenia (Zhi Zi)	3-6gms Gardenia jasminoides
Rhubarb (Da Huang)	3-6gms Rheum palmatum

Indigo (Qing Dai)	3-6gms Isatis tinctoria
Saussurea (Mu Xiang)	6-9gms Saussurea lappa
Musk (She Xiang)	.3-.5gms Moschus moschiferus

Properties and Actions: Purge fire from the Liver and Gallbladder

Indications: For conditions of Excessive Liver and/or Gallbladder Heat or Fire. Symptoms include headache, dizziness, vertigo, red face and eyes, mania, irritable and easily angered, bitter taste in the mouth, dry throat, tinnitis, chest pains, heavy fullness of the abdomen, constipation, urine is yellow or red. It can be considered for hypertension, mania, chest pains, convulsions, leukemia.

Pulse: bowstring, and rapid

Tongue: red with a yellow coat

Dang Gui Decoction for Frigid Extremities (Dang gui si ni tang)

Angelica (Dang Gui)	9-12gms Angelica sinensis
White Peony (Bai Shao Yao)	9-12gms Paeonia alba
Cinnamon twigs (Gui Zhi)	9gms Cinnamomum cassia
Asarum (Xi Xin)	3-6gms Asarum heterophylii
Akebia (Mu Tang)	6-9gms Akebia quinata
Prepared Licorice (Zhi Gan Cao)	3-6gms Glycyrrhiza uralensis
Jujube Dates (Da Zao)	12-15 pcs. Zizyphus jujuba

Properties And Actions:

a) Warms the channels and dispels Cold

b) Tonifies Blood

Indications: For Yang Deficiency with Blood Deficiency and Cold invasion. It can be used for a wide variety of Cold disorders ranging from general poor circulation, dysmenorrhea, Raynaud's disease, fibromyalgia, sciatica, chillblains, frostbite, gangrene, hernia, calluses and corns, thromboangiitis obliterans, varicose veins, peptic ulcer and testicular pains.

Contraindications: Do not use for conditions of Yin Deficiency. Use with caution during warm weather.

Variations:

1. For painful menstruation add Cyperus (Xiang Fu), Fennel (Xiao Hui Xiang), Lindera (Wu Yao), Alpinia (Gao Liang Jiang).

2. For painful menstruation with Yin Deficiency remove Akebia (Mu Tong) and add Prepared Rehmannia (Shu Di Huang).

3. For hernia and testicular pains add Fennel seeds (Xiao Hui Xiang).

4. For chronic sciatica add Prepared Aconite (Fu Zi), Dipsacus (Xu Duan), Eucommia (Du Zhong), Cibotii (Gou Ji) and Rhubarb (Da Huang).

Dianthus Formula (Ba zheng san) *

Akebia stem (Mu Tong)	10gms Akebia trifoliata
Dianthus (Qu Mai)	10gms Dianthus superbus
Polygonum (Bian Xu)	10gms Polygonum aviculare
Talcum (Hua Shi)	15gms Talcum
Juncus (Deng Xin Cao)	10gms Juncus effusus
Plantain seed (Che Qian Zi)	10gms Plantago asiatica
Gardenia (Zhi Zi)	6gms Gardenia jasminoides
Rhubarb (Da Huang)	9gms Rheum palmatum
Baked Licorice (Zhi Gan Cao)	4gms Glycyrrhiza uralensis

Properties and Actions:

a) Diuretic

b) Clears Damp-Heat from the Urinary Bladder

Indications: It is useful for frequent and painful urination, scanty or obstructed flow, kidney stones, cystitis, urethritis, stones in the urinary tract, acute prostatitis.

Contraindications: For Deficient patterns or for pregnant women.

Disperse Vital Energy in the Liver Powder (Chai hu su gan san)

Bupleurum (Chai Hu)	6gms Bupleurum falcatum
White Peony (Bai Shao)	4gms Paeonia alba
Bitter Orange (Zhi Ke)	4gms Citrus aurantium
Cyperus (Xiang Fu)	4gms Cyperus rotundus
Ligusticum (Chuan Xiong)	4gms Ligusticum wallichii
Prepared Licorice (Zhi Gan Cao)	1.5gms Glycyrrhiza uralensis

Properties and Actions: Disperses Stagnant Liver Qi and Blood.

Indications: Chest pains, hypertension, dysmenorrhea, irregular menstruation, breast distention, hysteria.

Tongue: thin white coat

Pulse: tight and/or bowstring

Variations:

1. For severe abdominal pain add Corydalis (Yan Hu Suo) and Sichuan Chinaberry (Chuan Lian Zi).

2. For bitter taste in the mouth add Coptis (Huang Lian) and Scutellaria (Huang Qin)

3. For acid regurgitation add Cuttlefish Bone (Hai Piao Xiao).

Dragon Bone and Oyster Shell Combination (Long gu mu li tang)*
Dragon Bone (Long Gu)   6-9gms Stegodon orientalis
Oyster shell (Mu Li)   6-9gms Ostrea spp.
Properties and Actions: Calms spirit, anchors the Yang, calms the Yin and lubricates Dryness.
Indications: Sedative, calms spirit, aphrodisiac, astringent, night sweats, palpitations, chest discomfort, acid indigestion.

Du Huo and Loranthes Combination (Du huo ji sheng tang)*
Angelica Du Huo (Du Huo)   6-9gms Angelica pubescens
Large Leaf Gentian (Qin Jiao)   3-6gms Gentiana macrophylla
Siler (Fang Feng)   3-6gms Siler seseloides
Wild Ginger (Xi Xin)   1-3gms Asarum heterophylii
Loranthus (Sang Ji Sheng)   6-9gms Loranthi parasiticus
Eucommia (Du Zhong)   3-6gms Eucommia ulmoides
Achyranthes (Niu Xi)   3-6gms Achyranthis bidentatae
Cinnamon Bark (Rou Gui)   1-3gms Cinnamomum cassia
Angelica (Dang Gui)   3-6gms Angelica sinensis
Ligusticum (Chuang Xiong)   3-6gms Ligusticum wallichii
Prepared Rehmannia (Shu Di Huang)   6-9gms Rehmannia glutinosa
White Peony (Bai Shao)   3-6gms Paeonia alba
Ginseng (Ren Shen)   3-6gms Panax ginseng
Poria (Fu Ling)   9-12gms Poria cocos
Licorice (Gan Cao)   3-6gms Glycyrrhiza uralensis
Properties and Actions:
a) Anti-rheumatic, clears Wind, Cold and Damp Stagnation
b) Strengthens the function of the Liver and Kidney
c) Tonifies Qi and Blood
Indications: It is indicated for chronic lower back pain, sciatica and other rheumatic and arthritic conditions caused by Deficient Qi and Blood with Deficiency of the Liver and Kidney. Symptoms are aggravated by Cold, Damp conditions, with numbness and pain in the joints and knees.
Tongue: pale with white coat
Pulse: weak and thready
Contraindication: Because it is a heating formula it should not be used for acute inflammatory stages of lumbago, sciatica and arthritic conditions.
Variations:

1. For severe pain add Prepared Aconite (Fu Zi) (actually Unprepared Aconite, called Chuan Wu Tou, is used; but no more than 1 to 3 grams to begin and cooked for at least one hour to lessen its toxicity).

2. For Blood and Qi Stagnation add Persica seed (Tao Ren), Carthamus flowers (Hong Hua) and Cyperus (Xiang Fu).

Modified Du Huo and Loranthes Combination (Du huo ji sheng tang)

Gypsum (Shi Gao)	30gms Gypsum
Dioscorea (Shan yao)	12gms Dioscorea batata
Polygonum cuspidati (Hu xiang)	12gms Polygonum cuspidati
Honeysuckle stem (Ren dong teng)	30gms Lonicera japonica
Anemarrhena (Zhi mu)	10gms Anemarrhena asphodeloidis
Notopterygium (Qiang huo)	10gms Notopterygium incisum

For lupus with arthritic symptoms. If these are more prominent with Heat, pain and swelling of the affected joint, the treatment should aim at clearing Dampness, Wind and Heat and opening the meridians.

Eight Precious Herbs (Ba zhen tang)

Ginseng (Ren Shen)	6-9gms Panax ginseng
White Atractylodes (Bai Zhu)	9-12gms Atractylodes alba
Poria (Fu Ling)	9-12gms Poria cocos
Baked Licorice (Zhi Gan Cao)	3-6gms Glycyrrhiza uralensis
Angelica (Dang Gui)	9-12gms Angelica sinensis
Ligusticum (Chuan Xiong)	6-9gms Ligusticum wallichii
Prepared Rehmannia (Shu Di Huang)	9-12gms Rehmannia glutinosa
White Peony (Bai Shao)	6-9gms Paeoniae alba
Fresh Ginger (Sheng Jiang)	1-3gms Zingiberis officinalis
Jujube Dates (Da Zao)	3-5 pcs Zizyphus jujuba

Properties and Actions:

a) Tonifies Qi and Blood.

Indications: Symptoms are fatigue, pallor, dizziness, shortness of breath, palpitations, anorexia. It is indicated for conditions such as anemia, weakness, tiredness, irregular menses caused by exhaustion, postpartum recovery, chronic Deficiency conditions.

Tongue: pale, thin white coat.

Pulse: thready and weak or artificially inflated or big and soft

Contraindications: Not for Excess conditions with acute inflammatory symptoms.

Note: This is a combination of Dang Gui Four and Major Four Herbs.

Variations:

1. For Deficient Qi, Blood and Yang with Coldness add Astragalus (Huang Qi) and Cinnamon bark (Rou Gui).

2. For irregular menstruation with fatigue, clear or whitish discharge add Motherwort (Yi Mu Cao)

Ephedra and Ginkgo Combination (Ding chuan tang)
(Treat Asthma Decoction)

Ginkgo seed (Bai Guo)	3-7pcs Ginkgo biloba
Ephedra (Ma Huang)	6-9gms Ephedra sinica
Perilla seed (Zi Su Zi)	9-12gms Perilla frutescens
Tussilago (Kuan Dong Hua)	9-12gms Tussilago farfara
Apricot seed (Xing Ren)	9-12gms Prunus armeniaca
Mulberry bark (Sang Bai Pi)	9-12gms Morus alba
Scutellaria (Huang Qin)	6-9gms Scutellaria baicalensis
Pinellia (Ban Xia)	9-12gms Pinellia ternata
Licorice (Gan Cao)	3-6gms Glycyrrhiza uralensis

Properties and Actions:
a) Clears Lung Heat
b) Expectorant for asthma

Indications: Asthma caused by Heat in the Lung, chronic bronchitis, bronchial asthma, pulmonary emphysema possibly with accompanying thirst, restlessness, fever, headache, spontaneous perspiration.

Tongue: red with yellow coat
Pulse: slippery and rapid

Ephedra, Apricot, Gypsum and Licorice Decoction (Ma xing shi gan tang)

Ephedra (Ma Huang)	6-9gms Ephedra sinica
Apricot seed (Xing Ren)	6-9 Prunus armeniaca
Gypsum (Shi Gao)	15-30 Calcium sulfate
Baked Licorice (Zhi Gan Cao)	3-6 Glycyrrhiza uralensis

Properties and Actions:
a) Clears External conditions
b) anti-asthmatic

Indications: For External Wind Heat and Interior Lung Heat. Symptoms include fever, with or without perspiration, asthma, thirst and Dryness.

Tongue: either a thin white or yellow coat
Pulse: floating, rapid and slippery

Contraindication: Not for asthma caused by Wind Cold.

Ephedra Decoction (Ma huang tang)*

Ephedra(Ma Huang)	6-9gms Ephedra sinica
Cinnamon twig (Gui Zhi)	6-9gms Cinnamomum cassia
Apricot seed (Xing Ren)	6-9gms Prunus armeniaca
Prepared Licorice (Zhi Gan Cao)	3-6gms Glycyrrhiza Uralensis

Properties and Actions:
a) Warm stimulating diaphoretic
b) Dispels External Wind-Cold
c) Anti-asthmatic.

Indications: It is used for Greater Yang (Tai Yang) conditions, with Excess conformation, fever, chills with intolerance of cold, lack of perspiration, general aching feeling throughout the body, headache, asthma. With appropriate presentation it can be considered for a wide variety of upper respiratory conditions including the common cold, asthma, cough and bronchitis.

Tongue: thin white coat

Pulse: floating and slow

Contraindications: It is a warming and stimulating formula and not suitable for those with Internal weakness and Deficiency or for those with the common cold caused by External Wind-Heat attack.

Variations:

1. For arthritic Wind-Cold-Damp condition add White Atractylodes (Bai Zhu); this is called Ma huang jia zhu tang.

2. For common cold with perspiration, headache, nasal obstruction, cough with phlegm, eliminate Cinnamon twig (Gui Zhi). This is called San ao tang.

3. Ma Huang and Apricot Seed Combination (Ma xing shi gan tang); this contains Ephedra (Ma Huang), Apricot seed (Xing Ren), Licorice (Gan Cao) and Gypsum (Shi Gao) 10-20gms. Because of the addition of Gypsum (Shi Gao) it relieves Internal Heat and thirst. It is useful for common cold with fever, pneumonia, bronchitis, bronchial asthma, cardiac asthma, whooping cough, measles and hemorrhoids.

4. Ma Huang and Coix Combination (Ma xing yi gan tang) is comprised of Ephedra (Ma Huang), Apricot seed (Xing Ren), Licorice (Gan Cao) and Coix (Yi Yi Ren) 10-20gms. It is for superficial neuralgic, rheumatic and arthritic symptoms caused by an accumulation of Dampness in the muscles. It is also useful for frostbite, eczema, dandruff, calluses and corns.

5. Major Blue Dragon (Da qing long tang) adds 10-20gms of Gypsum (Shi Gao) to help reduce Internal fever and Heat and 3-6gms of Fresh Ginger (Sheng Jiang) to eliminate External Wind and Cold. It is for more severe fever with restless irritability, intolerance of cold, headache, muscle-aches, lack of perspiration, asthma, thirst and edema. The Pulse is floating, tight and possibly rapid. The Tongue has a thin white or yellow coat. This contrasts with the indications of Minor Blue Dragon (Xiao qing long tang) with symptoms of less severe fever with watery phlegm, allergic rhinitis, labored asthmatic breathing.

Ephedra, Aconite and Asarum Combination (Ma huang fu zi xi xin tang)

Ephedra (Ma Huang)	6-9gms Ephedra sinica
Prepared Aconite (Fu Zi)	3-6gms Aconitum carmichaeli
Wild Ginger (Xi Xin)	1-3gms Asarum heterotropoides

Properties and Actions:
a) Clears External Wind-Cold and induces diaphoresis
b) Tonifies Yang

Indications: For External Wind-Cold (common cold and influenza) with Yang Deficiency. This formula is indicated when there is Cold and Deficiency and may be tried when other formulas seem to be not strong enough. Symptoms include fever, severe cold intolerance, pale complexion, weakness and cold extremities.

Contraindication: Not for individuals with Yin Deficiency.

Eriobotrya and Ophiopogon Combination (Qing zao jiu fei tang)

Mulberry leaf (Sang Ye)	3gms Mori alba
Gypsum (Shi Gao)	10gms Gypsum fibrosum
Gelatin (E Jiao)	2.4gms Asini gelatinum corii
Ophiopogon (Mai Men Dong)	3.6gms Ophiopogonis japonicus
Black Sesame seeds (Hei Zhi Ma)	2.4gms Sesami indica
Ginseng (Ren Shen)	2gms Panax Ginseng
Apricot seed (Xing Ren)	2gms Pruni Armeniacae
Loquat (Pi Pa Ye)	3gms Eriobotryae japonicae
Licorice (Gan Cao)	2gms Glycyrrhizae uralensis

Properties and Actions:
a) Moistens the Lung and treats Dryness
b) Tonifies Qi
c) Lubricates, cools and nourishes Essence of the Lung

Indications: Symptoms include dry cough with no phlegm, fever, headache, dry throat and nostrils. May be considered for symptoms of upper respiratory infections, hemoptysis, cough with influenza, asthma.

Tongue: red and dry with a thin white coat

Pulse: weak, thin and thready

Eucommia and Rehmannia Combination (Restore the Right; You gui wan)

Cooked Rehmannia (Shu Di Huang)	20-30gms Rehmannia glutinosa
Cornus berries (Shan Zhu Yu)	10-15gms Cornus officinalis
Dioscorea (Shan Yao)	15-20gms Dioscorea batatas
Eucommia bark (Du Zhong)	10-15gms Eucommia ulmoides
Lycii berries (Gou Qi Zi)	10-15gms Lycium chinensis
Cuscuta seeds (Tu Si Zi)	10-15gms Cuscuta chinensis
Angelica (Dang Gui)	10-15gms Angelica sinensis
Antler Gelatin (Lu Jiao Jiao)	15-20gms Cervus nippon
Prepared Aconite (Fu Zi)	6-9gms Aconitum carmichaeli
Cinnamon bark (Rou Gui)	6-9gms Cinnamomum cassia

Properties and Actions:

a) Tonifies Kidney Yang and treats spermatorrhea.

Indications: Symptoms include Coldness, pale complexion, spontaneous perspiration, premature ejaculation, impotence, lower back and joint pains, dizziness, spermatorrhea, enuresis. It may be considered for symptoms of spermatorrhea, chronic nephritis, diabetes, impotence and infertility.

Tongue: pale

Pulse: deep, slow and weak

Evodia Combination (Wu zhu yu tang)

Evodia (Wu Zhu Yu)	9-12gms Evodia rutaecarpa
Ginseng (Ren Shen)	9-12gms Panax ginseng
Fresh Ginger (Sheng Jiang)	15-20gms Zingiber officinale
Jujube Dates (Da Zao)	5-6pcs Zizyphus jujuba

Properties and Actions:

a) Warms the Liver and Stomach

b) Anti-emetic

Indications: For Cold Deficiency of the Stomach and Liver with symptoms of retching, vomiting, headache after eating, acid regurgitation, stomach pains, fullness and hardness in the epigastric area. It can be considered for acute and chronic gastritis, cholecystitis, morning sickness, nervous

headaches, migraine headache, hypertension, trigeminal neuralgia and Meniere's disease.

Tongue: swollen and pale with a white coat

Pulse: deep and slow

Note: Acute symptoms should be relieved after a half hour. It there is difficulty keeping it down try taking it cool.

Variations:

1. For extreme vomiting and morning sickness add Pinellia (Ban Xia) and Cardamon (Sha Ren).

2. For hernial problems caused by Cold add Prepared Aconite (Fu Zi).

3. For severe headache add Ligusticum (Gao Ben), Angelica dahurica (Bai Zhi), Ligusticum (Chuan Xiong) and Angelica (Dang Gui).

4. For severe stomach pains add Saussurea (Mu Xiang).

5. For severe Coldness add Dry Ginger (Gan Jiang) and Galangal (Gao Liang Jiang).

Five Peel Decoction (Wu pi yin)

Poria (Fu Ling)	9-12gms Poria cocos
Mulberry bark (Sang Bai Pi)	9-12gms Mori alba
Ginger peel (Sheng Jiang Pi)	6-9gms Zingiberis officinalis
Areca peel (Da Fu Pi)	9-12gms Areca catechu
Citrus peel (Chen Pi)	6-9gms Citrus reticulata

Properties and Indications:

a) Reduces edema, diuretic

b) Regulates and strengthens Spleen Qi

Indications: Used for general edema and heaviness throughout the entire body, with abdominal and chest discomfort and rapid breathing. It can be considered for cardiac and nephritic edema, edema associated with pregnancy, edema and swelling in hot weather.

Tongue: white and greasy

Pulse: thin or moderate and greasy

Contraindications: Not for individuals without symptoms of edema

Forsythia and Rhubarb Combination (Liang ge san)

Rhubarb (Da Huang)	6-9gms Rheum Officinale
Mirabilitum (Mang Xiao)	6-9gms Natrum sulphate
Gardenia fruit (Zhi Zi)	3-6gms Gardenia jasminoides
Scutellaria (Huang Qin)	3-6gms Scutellaria baicalensis

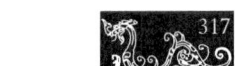

Forsythia (Lian Qiao)	12-15gms Forsythia suspensa
Mentha (Bo He)	3-6gms Mentha haplocalyx
Licorice (Gan Cao)	3-6gms Glycyrrhiza uralensis
Bamboo leaves (Zhu Ye)	3gms Lophatheri gracilis
Honey (Mix with tea) (Mel)	

Properties and Actions:

a) Febrifuge, clears Heat from the Upper Warmer

b) Clears Heat from the Middle and Lower Warmers and promotes bowel movement.

Indications: Fever, thirst, burning feeling over the chest and diaphragm, constipation, dark, concentrated urine, rashes caused by Stomach Heat, irritability and mania, red complexion, mouth sores, toothache, sore throat, nosebleed. It may be considered for acute fevers and inflammations such as epidemic meningitis, encephalitis B, acute cholecystitis (Gallbladder inflammation), cholelithiasis (gallstones), measles and other eruptive diseases

Tongue: red with a yellow coat

Pulse: rapid and slippery

Variations:

a) For gallstones add Lysimachia (Jin Qian Cao).

2. For accompanying jaundice add Capillaris (Yin Chen Hao) and Turmeric tuber (Yu Jin).

3. For eruptive skin rashes remove Mirabilitum (Mang Xiao) and add Lithospermum (Zi Cao) and Carthamus flowers (Hong Hua).

4. For sore throat remove Mirabilitum (Mang Xiao) and Rhubarb (Da Huang) and add Indigo (Da Qing Ye) and Honeysuckle Flowers (Jin Yin Hua).

Four Major Herbs Decoction (Si jun zi tang)*

Ginseng (Ren Shen)	6-9gms Panax ginseng
White Atractylodes (Bai Zhu)	6-9gms Atractylodes alba
Poria (Fu Ling)	6-9gms Poria cocos
Honey Baked Licorice (Zhi Gan Cao)	3-6gms Glycyrrhiza uralensis

Properties and Actions:

a) Tonifies Qi

b) Strengthens the Spleen and Stomach

Indications: For individuals with low energy and weak digestion with symptoms of pallor, timidity and soft spoken voice, muscular weakness, loss of appetite, abdominal distention, nausea and vomiting, boborygmus,

loose stool. It can be used for chronic gastrointestinal conditions in individuals with low energy and weak digestion.

Tongue: pale with thin white coat

Pulse: thin and weak

Note: This is the father formula for all Qi tonics.

Contraindications: Not for Excess conditions.

Variations:

1. With Qi Stagnation add Citrus peel (Chen Pi).

2. With phlegm and mucus add Citrus peel (Chen Pi) and Pinellia (Ban Xia) (Six Major Herbs – Liu jun zi tang).

3. With Deficiency of both Qi and Blood add Dang Gui Four (Ba zhen tang).

Frigid Extremities Decoction (Si ni tang) *

Prepared Aconite (Fu Zi)	6-9gms Aconitum carmichaeli
Dry Ginger (Gan Jiang)	4.5gms Zingiber officinale
Honey Baked Licorice (Zhi Gan Cao)	6gms Glycyrrhiza uralensis

Properties and Actions:

a) Metabolic stimulant, stimulates Yang

b) Warms and counteracts Internal Cold

Indications: Aversion to Cold, with Coldness in the Stomach and Spleen, vomiting, diarrhea, lethargy, abdominal pain, lack of thirst.

Tongue: white moist coat

Pulse: thin, deep and faint

Variation: By adding 6-9gms of Ginseng (Ren Shen), the formula has wider tonic properties, tonifying Yin, Blood and Qi. Both these formulas are appropriate for both the Shao Yin and Jue Yin Stages as well.

Note: This is the basic metabolic stimulant formula.

Contraindications: Not for individuals with Excess Heat.

Gardenia and Poria Combination (Wei wu lin san)

Poria (Fu Ling)	12gms Poria cocos
Angelica (Dang Gui)	9gms Angelica sinensis
White Peony (Bai Shao)	6gms Paeonia alba
Gardenia Buds (Zhi Zi)	6gms Gardenia jasminoides
Licorice (Gan Cao)	3gms Glycyrrhiza uralensis

Properties and Actions:

a) Diuretic

b) Clears Damp-Heat

Indications: It is used for Damp-Heat in the Lower Warmer. Conditions for which this formula may be considered are: cystitis, urethritis, urinary stones and venereal infections. It is most applicable for chronic cystitis with Internal Heat in the Urinary Bladder, painful urination, fatigue, urinary calculus, hematuria.

Tongue: red with a thick yellow coat

Pulse: rapid and full

Gardenia and Prepared Soybean Decoction (Zhi zi dou chi tang)

Gardenia fruit (Zhi Zi) 9gms Gardeniae jasminoidis
Prepared Black Soybean (Dan Dou Chi) 9gms Glycine max

Properties and Actions:

a) Anti-inflammatory, clears Heat, relieves fever and irritability

b) Mild sedative, relieves insomnia and restlessness, full sensation in the chest.

Indications: With the appropriate symptoms it may be considered for conditions of catarrhal jaundice, cancer of the esophagus, constriction of the esophagus, inflammation of the stomach, pharyngitis, nervous exhaustion, exhaustion and fatigue from sweating or vomiting and hemoptysis.

Tongue: slightly yellow tongue coat

Pulse: slightly rapid pulse

Gasping Formula (Xiang sheng po tai luen)

Forsythia (Lian Qiao)	2.5gms Forsythia suspensa
Platycodon (Jie Geng)	2.5gms Platycodon grandiflorum
Licorice (Gan Cao)	2.5gms Glycyrrhiza uralensis
Rhubarb (Da Huang)	1.0gms Rheum palmatum
Cardamon (Sha Ren)	1.0gms Amomum villosum
Ligusticum (Chuang Xiong)	1.0gms Ligusticum wallichii
Terminalia (He Zi)	1.0gms Terminalia chebulae
Catechu (Er Cha)	2.0gms Acaciae seu uncariae
Mint (Bo He)	4.0gms Mentha haplocalyx

Properties and Actions:

a) Clears Heat and relieves irritation of the throat

Indications: Relieves hoarseness and sore throat

Gastrodia and Uncaria Combination (Tian ma gou teng yin)*

Gastrodia (Tian Ma)	3gms Gastrodia elata
Uncaria (Gou Teng)	3gms Uncariae spp.
Abalone shell (Shi Jue Ming)	10gms Haliotidis concha
Gardenia fruit (Zhi Zi)	3gms Gardenia jasminoides
Scutellaria (Huang Qin)	3gms Scutellaria baicalensis
Eucommia (Du Zhong)	3gms Eucommiae ulmoides
Loranthus (Sang Ji Sheng)	3gms Loranthus parasiticus
Motherwort (Yi Mu Cao)	3gms Leonurus heterophyllus
Fleece Flower stem (Ye Jiao Teng)	3gms Polygonum multiflorum
Achyranthes (Niu Xi)	3gms Achyranthis bidentatae
Poria (Fu Shen)	3gms Poria cocos

Properties and Actions:
a) Anti-hypertensive
b) Clears Heat

Indications: Calms the Liver, clears Heat, nourishes Yin, treats headache, vertigo, treats paralysis and convulsions, spasms, trembling, insomnia, coma, Bell's palsy, hemiplegia, hypertension, trigeminal neuralgia.

Tongue: red with a yellow coat
Pulse: rapid

Generate the Pulse Powder (Sheng mai san)*

Ginseng (Ren Shen)	6-9gms Panax ginseng
Ophiopogon (Mai Men Dong)	6-9gms Ophiopogon japonicus
Schisandra (Wu Wei Zi)	6-9gms Schisandra chinensis

Properties and Actions:
a) Tonifies Qi and nourishes Yin
b) Inhibits Excessive perspiration

Indications: It counteracts symptoms associated with Hot climates and helps to promote the secretion of body fluids and alleviate thirst. It is useful for symptoms of exhaustion and fatigue with shortness of breath, excessive perspiration and thirst.

Some of the medical conditions it can be considered for include chronic coughs, pulmonary wasting diseases such as TB and general lung weakness. Various cardio-pulmonary conditions may also be considered such as cardiac weaknesses including coronary heart disease, angina, arrhythmia, cardio-pulmonary disease, myocardial infarction, strokes.

Tongue: little or no coat, pale, possibly with a red tip
Pulse: thin and thready

Contraindications: Should not be used during External diseases with high fever. One should always first treat the acute symptoms before treating the underlying chronic conditions for which most tonic formulas are indicated. If given prematurely, such tonic formulas, instead of imparting strength to the patient, strengthen and prolong the course of the disease.

Gentiana Combination (Long dan xie gan tang)*

Gentiana (Long Dan Cao)	3-6gms Gentiana macrophyllae
Scutellaria (Huang Qin)	9-12gms Scutellaria baicalensis
Gardenia (Zhi Zi)	6-9gms Gardenia jasminoides
Alisma (Ze Xie)	6-9gms Alisma plantago-aquatica
Akebia (Mu tong)	6-9gms Akebia trifoliata
Unprepared Rehmannia (Sheng Di Huang)	9-12gms Rehmannia glutinosa
Dang Gui tails (Dang Gui Wei)	6-9gms Angelica sinensis
Bupleurum (Chai Hu)	6-9gms Bupleurum falcatum
Licorice (Gan Cao)	1-3gms Glycyrrhiza uralensis

Properties and Actions:

a) Clears Heat and Fire from the Liver and Gallbladder

b) Clears Heat from the Triple Warmer

Indications: One of the major formulas for clearing Damp-Heat and Fire (inflammation) throughout the body. Some of its many uses are as follows: urethritis, cystitis, endometritis, vaginal inflammation, leukorrhea, genital itch, herpes zoster, pelvic inflammatory disease (PID), venereal ulcer, swollen glands in the groin (lymphadenitis), testicle pain (orchitis), acute prostatitis, acute conjunctivitis, acute otitis media, boils and carbuncles, hypertension, hepatitis, acute cholecystitis, acute pyelitis.

Tongue: red with a yellow coat

Pulse: rapid, full

Contraindications: Not for individuals who have a weak, delicate conformation.

Ginseng and Longan Combination (Gui pi tang)*

Ginseng (Ren Shen)	6-9gms Panax ginseng
Astragalus (Huang Qi)	9-12gms Astragalus membranaceus
Angelica (Dang Gui)	6-9gms Angelica sinensis
Longan berries (Long Yan Rou)	6-9gms Euphoria longan
White Atractylodes (Bai Zhu)	6-9gms Atractylodes alba
Saussurea (Mu Xiang)	3-6gms Saussurea lappa
Poria (Fu Ling)	9-12gms Poria cocos

Polygala (Yuan Zhi)	3-6gms Polygala tenuifolia
Zizyphus seeds (Suan Zao Ren)	9-12gms Zizyphus spinosa
Fresh Ginger (Sheng Jiang)	1-3gms Zingiber officinalis
Jujube Dates (Da Zao)	3-6pcs Zizyphus jujuba

Properties and Actions:
a) Tonify and nourish Qi and Blood
b) Tonify Heart and Spleen

Indications: For Heart and Spleen Deficiency with symptoms of forgetfulness, palpitation, insomnia, nightmares, fatigue, decreased intake of food, pale complexion, uterine bleeding or menorrhagia.

This formula has broad applications including symptoms of hypoglycemia, nervous weakness (neurasthenia), gastric and duodenal ulcers, functional uterine bleeding, aplastic anemia, general anemia, chronic bleeding, menorrhagia, uterine bleeding.

Tongue: pale, white, swollen with thin white coat

Pulse: thready and weak

Note: Saussurea (Mu Xiang) should not be boiled for a long time; put in towards the end of preparing the other herbs in the formula.

Variations:

1. For irregular menstruation with increased discharge of light blood add Donkey-Hide Gelatin (E Jiao), Loranthus (Sang Ji Sheng), Fleece Flower (He Shou Wu)

2. To tonify Blood, add Prepared Rehmannia (Shu Di Huang)

Modified Ginseng and Longan Combination (Gui pi tang) with Eclipta (Han Lian Cao) 12gms, Donkey-skin gelatin (E jiao) 10gms. Use for thrombocytopenic purpura from Deficient Spleen Qi with lighter or more pinkish purpuras that appear and disappear intermittently and fatigue, dizziness, palpitations, lack of appetite and a pale Tongue with little fur, weak Pulse.

Ginseng, Poria and Atractylodes Powder (Shen ling bai zhu san)

Ginseng (Ren Shen)	9-12gms Panax ginseng
Lotus seed (Lian Zi Rou)	15-20gms Nelumbo nucifera
Dioscorea (Shan Yao)	10-15gms Dioscorea opposita
White Atractylodes (Bai Zhu)	9-12gms Atractylodes alba
Poria (Fu Ling)	10-15gms Poria cocos
Dolichos (Bai Bian Dou)	15-20gms Dolichos lablab
Coix (Yi Yi Ren)	20-30gms Coix lachryma-jobi
Cardamon (Sha Ren)	3-6gms Amomum villosum

Platycodon (Jie Geng)　　　　　6-9gms Platycodon grandiflorum
Baked Licorice (Zhi Gan Cao)　　3-6gms Glycyrrhiza uralensis

Properties and Actions:

a) Tonify Qi

b) Tonify Spleen and Stomach

c) Clear Spleen Dampness

Indications: For Dampness of the Spleen and Stomach with Qi Deficiency. Symptoms include: weakness, fatigue, abdominal swelling, indigestion, nausea, vomiting, loose stool and diarrhea. It can be used for chronic gastro-enteritis, infantile diarrhea, edema and fluid retention, anemia, pulmonary tuberculosis, chronic nephritis.

Tongue: wet

Pulse: weak and slippery

Contraindication: Not for an individual with a strong conformation and Excess.

Variation: For Qi Stagnation add Citrus peel (Chen Pi) and Saussurea (Mu Xiang)

Ginseng and Astragalus Combination (Bu zhong yi qi tang)*

Astragalus (Huang Qi)　　　　　6-15gms Astragalus membranaceus
Ginseng (Ren Shen)　　　　　　6-9gms Panax ginseng
White Atractylodes (Bai Zhu)　　9-12gms Atractylodes alba
Licorice (Gan Cao)　　　　　　 3-6gms Glycyrrhiza uralensis
Angelica (Dang Gui)　　　　　　6-9gms Angelica sinensis
Black Cohosh (Sheng Ma)　　　　3-6gms Cimicifuga foetida
Bupleurum (Chai Hu)　　　　　　6-9gms Bupleurum falcatum
Citrus peel (Chen Pi)　　　　　　3-6gms Citrus reticulata

Properties and Actions:

a) Tonifies Qi of the Spleen and Stomach

b) Raises the Yang

c) Detoxifies

Indications: It may be considered for chronic fatigue and weakness where sub-acute feverish or inflammatory symptoms arise as a result of physical exertion or stress. Symptoms include aversion to cold, poor appetite, preference for warmth including warm food and drink, general tiredness and weakness, shortness of breath, spontaneous perspiration, slow speech, a tendency to huddle up, thirst, loose stool. The complexion tends to be shiny and pale, the Tongue light with a thin white coat and the Pulse weak and inflated.

This is traditionally considered the supreme tonic of Chinese herbalism. Besides tonifying Qi and Blood, the addition of Bupleurum (Chai Hu) and Cimicifuga (Sheng Ma) combine both anti-inflammatory properties with ascending qualities, which assists the Yang. The formula is designed to treat a condition of exhaustion where the Yang of the Middle and Upper Warmer collapses down into the Yin of the Lower Warmer. The result is a weakening of the immune system where energetically the Yang is unable to circulate and ascend so that it is unable to adequately protect itself from External pathogenic influences. The formula is therefore indicated for intermittent fevers and prolapse and perhaps bleeding of the internal organs because of weakness and exhaustion.

Tongue: pale, scalloped on the edges
Pulse: thin and weak

Ginseng and Dang Gui Ten Combination (Shi quan da bu tang)

Ginseng (Ren Shen)	6-9gms Panax ginseng
White Atractylodes (Bai Zhu)	9-12gms Atractylodes alba
Poria (Fu Ling)	12-15gms Poria cocos
Baked Licorice (Zhi Gan Cao)	3-6gms Glycyrrhiza uralensis
Prepared Rehmannia (Shu Di Huang)	9-12gms Rehmannia glutinosa
White Peony (Bai Shao)	12-15gms Paeoniae lactiflorae
Angelica (Dang gui)	12-15gms Angelicae sinensis
Ligusticum (Chuan Xiong)	6-9gms Ligusticum wallichii
Cinnamon bark (Rou Gui)	6-9gms Cinnamomum cassia
Astragalus (Huang Qi)	6-9gms Astragalus membranaceus

Preparation:

Grind all together and take 6 grams as a single dose in boiled hot water to which has been added three slices of Fresh Ginger (Sheng Jiang) and 2 pieces of Jujube Dates (Da Zao).

Properties and Actions:

a) Warms and tonifies Qi and Blood.

b) Tonifies Yang

Indications: It is a warmer Yang tonic than Eight Precious Herbs (Ba zhen wan) and tonifies Qi and Yang of the Spleen and Kidney. It also nourishes the Blood. It can be used for consumptive disorders with cough and reduced appetite, spermatorrhea and weakness of the lower extremities. Often a slower capacity to heal is caused by Deficient Qi and Blood so that this formula is particularly useful to promote healing caused by Deficiency. It can also be used for gynecological conditions where there is continuous spotting from uterine bleeding. Two or three times the amount of Codonopsis (Dang Shen) is commonly substituted for Ginseng (Ren Shen).

Tongue: pale with a thin white coat
Pulse: weak and thready

Ginseng and Ginger Combination or **Regulate the Middle Pill** (Li zhong wan)*

Dry Ginger (Gan Jiang)	9gms Zingiber officinalis
Ginseng (Ren Shen)	9gms Panax ginseng
White Atractylodes (Bai Zhu)	9gms Atractylodes alba
Baked Licorice (Zhi Gan Cao)	9gms Glycyrrhiza uralensis

Preparation: Grind the ingredients into a powder. Heat honey without burning. Stir the herb powder into the honey until it is a thick doughy consistency. Roll into balls about half the size of a lime. Take two or three daily before meals. The pills should equal about 6-9 grams of the powdered herb for a single dose. It can also be taken as a decoction. The pill is often taken with rice congee. Unless it is an acute case, Codonopsis (Dang Shen) can be doubled in amount and substituted for Ginseng (Ren Shen).

Properties and Actions:

a) Tonic, warms and tonifies Spleen and Stomach Yang

b) Strengthens digestion and raises digestive metabolism

Indications: It may be considered for symptoms of Deficiency exhibited as diarrhea with watery stool, nausea and vomiting, no particular thirst, loss of appetite, abdominal pain.

Tongue: pale tongue with white coat

Pulse: deep and thin

Note: When Spleen Yang is injured (Middle Warmer) the clear Yang cannot ascend. This causes diarrhea with loose watery stool. When the Stomach loses its ability to make the turbid Yin descend, nausea and vomiting ensue.

This formula is often combined with either or both Cinnamon (Rou Gui) 6gms and Prepared Aconite (Fu Zi) 6gms to make it stronger and warmer; this is Aconite, Ginger and Ginseng Combination (Fu zi li zhong wan). It is particularly useful for vegetarians, who through eating too much cold, raw food, have injured the Spleen Yang and seriously weakened their digestive metabolism.

Contraindications: Not for conditions of Excess Heat.

Ginseng and Zizyphus Combination
(Tian wang bu xin tang - Emperor of Heaven's Tonic Pill for the Mind)

Unprepared Rehmannia (Sheng Di Huang)	10-15gms Rehmannia glutinosa
Asparagus root (Tian Men Dong)	9-12gms Asparagus cochinchinensis
Ophiopogon (Mai Men Dong)	9-12gms Ophiopogon japonicus
Ginseng (Ren Shen)	6-9gms Panax ginseng (or 9-12gms of Radix Codonopsis - Dang Shen)

Biota seed (Bai Zi Ren)	9-12gms Biotae orientalis
Zizyphus seeds (Suan Zao Ren)	9-12gms Zizyphus spinosa
Salvia Root (Dan Shen)	9-12gms Salvia miltiorrhiza
Angelica (Dang Gui)	6-9gms Angelica sinensis
Poria (Fu Ling)	9-12gms Poria cocos
Scrophularia (Xuan Shen)	9-12gms Scrophularia ningpoensis
Schisandra fruit (Wu Wei Zi)	9-12gms Schisandra chinensis
Polygala (Yuan Zhi)	6-9gms Polygala tenuifolia
Platycodon (Jie Geng)	3gms Platycodon grandiflorum
Cinnabar (Zhu Sha)	0.5-1gm Cinnabaris

(Pills were traditionally dusted with cinnabar that contributed to the action of the formula)

Properties and Actions:

a) Nutritive tonic, Nourishes Yin, Blood and Vital Essence of the Heart and Kidney

b) Clears away evil Heat, clears Deficient Heat

c) Sedative

Indications: For Deficient Yin and Blood, flaming up of Deficient Fire (inflammation from stress, especially mental stress) manifested with palpitations, insomnia, amnesia, tiredness, nocturnal emission, mouth sores, dry feces. It can be considered for nervousness, palpitations, tachycardia, insomnia, hypertension, hyperthyroidism caused by Deficient Yin and Blood, menopausal syndrome. This formula is sometimes called the "scholar's or student's formula" as it is very useful for symptoms that are caused by excessive mental activity.

Tongue: reddish body with little or no fur

Pulse: thin and rapid

Contraindications: Not for Spleen and Stomach weakness with tendency to bloat, loose stools, edema and fluid retention.

Goiter Pills (Xiao lei wan)

Fritillary (Zhe Bei Mu)	10-15gms Fritillaria thunbergii
Oyster shell (Mu Li)	15-20gms Ostreae spp.
Scrophularia (Xuan Shen)	10-15gms Scrophularia ningpoensis

Properties and Actions:

a) Clears Heat and eliminates Phlegm

b) Softens hard lumps and nodules

Indications: It is indicated for goiter, swollen glands, scrofula and subcutaneous lumps caused by Stagnation of Heat and Phlegm. Besides its

obvious use for goiter, it can be used for accompanying hyperthyroidism, thyroiditis and lymphadenitis.

Variations:

a) For large swellings and goiter add Laminaria Seaweed (Kun Bu), Sargassum Seaweed (Hai Zao) and Prunella (Xia Ku Cao).

2. For more Fire and Phlegm add Anemarrhena (Zhi Mu) and Moutan Peony (Mu Dan Pi).

3. For Stagnant Liver Qi add Bupleurum (Chai Hu), Cyperus (Xiang Fu) and Green Tangerine peel (Qing Pi).

Gypsum Combination (Shi gao tang)

Gypsum (Shi Gao)	15-30gms Calcium sulfate
Ephedra (Ma Huang)	6-9gms Ephedra sinica
Prepared Soybean (Dan Dou Chi)	6-9gms Glycine max
Coptis (Huang Lian)	3-6gms Coptis chinensis
Scutellaria (Huang Qin)	3-6gms Scutellaria baicalensis
Phellodendron (Huang Bai)	3-6gms Phellodendron amurense
Gardenia fruit (Zhi Zi)	6-9gms Gardenia jasminoides

Properties and Actions:

a) Antipyretic, lowers high fever

b) Diaphoretic, induces perspiration

c) Clears Heat

Indications: For high fevers with chills but without sweating. There is accompanying irritability, sleeplessness, possible mania, headache, thirst, nosebleeds, and coughing up blood, acute skin rashes.

It is a Greater Yang (Tai Yang) stage condition where External Cold persists with accompanying Internal Heat. It can be considered for acute infections, severe acute skin rashes, inflammation of the gallbladder, pancreas, appendix and for acute pelvic inflammatory disease.

Tongue: yellow with a dry coat

Pulse: forceful, large or slippery and rapid

Variation: By the addition of Fresh Ginger (Sheng Jiang), Jujube Dates (Da Zao) and green tea this formula becomes suitable for Heat and inflammation in all three Warmers and is called Gypsum, Coptis and Scutellaria Combination (Huang lian jie du tang)

Increase Body Fluids Decoction (Zhen yi tang)

Scrophularia (Xuan Shen)	10-15gms Scrophularia ningpoensis
Ophiopogon (Mai Men Dong)	10-15gms Ophiopogon japonicus
Fresh Rehmannia (Sheng Di Huang)	15-20gms Rehmannia glutinosa

Properties and Actions: Moisten and increase fluids

Indications: It is indicated for Sunlight Stage (Yang Ming) conditions with symptoms of Yin Deficiency including constipation, dryness and thirst. It may be used for a variety of wasting and inflammatory conditions including shrunken dry colon, hemorrhoids, irritable bowel syndrome, pancreatitis and inflamed skin conditions such as erysipelas.

Tongue: crimson with a yellow coat

Pulse: deep and weak

Contraindication: Not for an individual who has Yin Deficiency with no constipation.

Variations: For severe constipation add Rhubarb (Da Huang) and Mirabilitum (Mang Xiao).

Inula Flower and Hematite Decoction (Xuan fu dai zhe tang)

Inula flower (Xuan Fu Hua)	6-9 gms Inula japonica
Hematite (Dai Zhe Shi)	10-15 gms Hematite
Pinellia (Ban Xia)	6-9gms Pinellia Ternata
Ginseng (Ren Shen)	3-6 gms Panax ginseng
Fresh Ginger (Sheng Jiang)	9-12 gms Zingiberis officinalis
Prepared Licorice (Zhi Gan Cao)	3-6 gms Glycyrrhiza uralensis
Jujube Dates (Da Zao)	3-5pcs Ziziphus jujuba

Properties and Actions:

a) Regulates the downward flow of Stomach Qi

b) Expectorant, treats hiccups

Indications: Used for hiccup, nausea, vomiting, belching, abdominal blockage and distention.

Tongue: slippery and greasy

Pulse: wiry, bowstring and weak

Contraindications: Not for morning sickness

Jade Screen Powder (Yu ping feng san)

Astragalus (Huang Qi)	10-15gms Astragalus membranaceus
White Atractylodes (Bai Zhu)	9-12gms Atractylodes alba
Ledebouriella (Fang Feng)	9-12gms Ledebouriella seseloides

Properties and Actions:

a) Tonifies Qi, strengthens the Wei Qi

b) Internal Cold and Deficiency

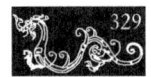

Indications: For lowered body resistance to colds and flu, spontaneous and involuntary perspiration, pale complexion. It can be considered for common colds, influenza, allergic and chronic rhinitis.

Tongue: light red with a thin white coat

Pulse: weak and floating

Variations:

1. For chronic or allergic rhinitis add Magnolia flower (Xin Yi Hua) and Xanthium fruit (Cang Er Zi).

2. For spontaneous perspiration add Ephedra root (Ma Huang Gen) and Light Wheat (Fu Xiao Mai: Triticum aestivum).

Kaki Combination (Ding xiang shi di tang)

Cloves (Ding Xiang)	1.5gms Syzygium aromaticum
Persimmon calyx (Shi Di)	5.0gms Diospyros kaki
Fresh Ginger (Sheng Jiang)	6-9gms Zingiberis officinalis
Ginseng (Ren Shen)	3-6gms Panax ginseng

Properties and Actions:

a) Tonifies Qi

b) Warms the center (Spleen and Stomach)

c) Directs rebellious Qi downward

Indications: Primarily used to treat belching and hiccup. Can also be used for morning sickness, postoperative spasms of the diaphragm.

Kaki Combination (Shi Di Tang) Omits Ginseng (Ren Shen) when there is chest fullness with incessant belching and hiccup.

Ledebouriella and Platycodon Formula (Fang feng tong sheng; also commonly known as Siler and Platycodon Formula)

Ledebouriella (Fang Feng)	3gms Ledebouriella seseloides
Schizonepetae (Jing Jie)	3gms Schizonepeta tenuifolia
Ephedra (Ma Huang)	1.5gms Ephedra sinica
Platycodon (Jie Geng)	2gms Platycodon grandiflorum
Field Mint (Bo He)	1.5gms Mentha
Forsythia (Lian Qiao)	1.5gms Forsythia suspensa
Scutellaria (Huang Qin)	2gms Scutellaria baicalensis
Gardenia fruit (Zhi Zi)	1.5gms Gardenia jasminoides
Rhubarb (Da Huang)	1.5gms Rheum palmatum
Gypsum (Shi Gao)	2gms Calcium sulfate
Talcum (Hua Shi)	3gms Talcum

Mirabilitum (Mang Xiao)	1.5gms Sodium sulfate
Angelica (Dang Gui)	1.5gms Angelica sinensis
Ligusticum (Chuan Xiong)	1.5gms Ligusticum wallichii
White Atractylodes (Bai Zhu)	2gms Atractylodes alba
White Peony (Bai Shao)	1.5gms Paeonia alba
Licorice (Gan Cao)	2gms Glycyrrhiza uralensis
Dry Ginger (Gan Jiang)	1.5gms Zingiberis officinalis

Properties and Actions: Removes Internal and External Heat.

Indications: Gradually eliminates all Excesses, increases stool and urine output, counteracts obesity, especially with Stephania and Astragalus Combination (Fang ji huang qi tang), treats gastro-intestinal ulcers, constipation, irregular pulse, palpitations, angina, valvular diseases, cardiac asthma, arteriosclerosis, hypertension, nephrosis, urinary calculi, nocturnal emission, impotence, stiff shoulders, arthritis, neuralgia, lymphatic swellings, skin problems including psoriasis, eczema, hives, urticaria, rosaceae, athlete's foot, hair loss, inflammation of the eyes, conjunctivitis, gum disease.

Tongue: red with a yellow coat
Pulse: bounding and rapid

Licorice, Sprouted Wheat and Jujube Date Decoction (Gan mai da zao tang)

Licorice (Gan Cao)	9-12gms Glycyrrhiza uralensis
Sprouted Wheat (Fu Xiao Mai)	30-50gms Triticum aestivum
Jujube Dates (Da Zao)	10-15pcs Zizyphus jujuba

Properties and Actions:
a) Sedative and antispasmodic
b) Nourishing tonic

Indications: It is indicated as a tranquilizing sedative, with antispasmodic and Spleen tonifying properties. It can be used by itself or added to any formula when there are symptoms of stress, anxiety, mania, insomnia and convulsions.

Tongue: thin white coat
Pulse: thin and thready

Variations:
1. To increase its sedative action add Zizyphus (Suan Zao Ren), Biota seeds (Bai Zi Ren), Poria (Fu Shen) and Albizzia flower (He Huan Hua).

Lily Bulb Decoction to Consolidate the Lungs (Bai he gu jin tang)*

Lily bulb (Bai He)	6-9gms Lilium brownii
Prepared Rehmannia (Shu Di Huang)	6-9 gms Rehmannia glutinosa

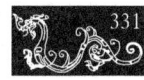

Unprepared Rehmannia (Sheng Di Huang)	6-9 gms Rehmannia glutinosa
Ophiopogon (Mai Men Dong)	6-9 gms Ophiopogon japonicus
White Peony, stir fried (Bai Shao Yao)	6-9 gms Paeonia alba
Angelica (Dang Gui)	6-9 gms Angelica sinensis
Scrophularia (Xuan Shen)	6-9 gms Scrophularia ningpoensis
Platycodon (Jie Geng)	3-6 gms Platycodon grandiflorum
Fritillaria (Chuan Bei Mu)	6-9 gms Fritillaria cirrhosa
Licorice (Gan Cao)	3 gms Glycyrrhiza uralensis

Properties and Actions:

a) Nourishes Lung and Kidney Yin

b) Lubricates the Lung and clears phlegm

Indications: For Lung and Kidney Yin Deficiency with symptoms of mild Fire. For chronic bronchitis, bronchiectasis, asthma, hemoptysis, chronic pharyngitis, laryngitis, vocal polyps, pneumothorax, cor pulmonale, silicosis and pulmonary TB.

Contraindications: Avoid for conditions of Deficient Spleen or Food Stagnation.

Variations:

1. For excessive phlegm add Fructus Trichosanthis (Gua Lou) and Cortex Mori (Sang Bai Pi).

2. For fever with Heat in the Lungs with signs of yellow or green phlegm add Anemarrhena (Zhi Mu) and Houttuyniae (Yu Xing Cao).

3. For Pulmonary TB with Heat, shortness of breath, night sweats, malar flushing, irritability, insomnia add Carapax Amydae (Bie Jia). Use with Western medicine.

4. For constipation add Semen Trichosanthis Kirlowii (Gua Lou Ren).

5. For coughing of blood remove Platycodon and add Imperata (Bai Mao Gen) and agrimony (Xian He Cao).

6. For Lung cancer with Yin Deficiency add Houttuyniae (Yu Xing Cao), Red Peony (Chi Shao), Scutellariae barbatae (Ban Zhi Lian) and Oldenlandia (Bai Hua She She Cao).

Liver Strengthening Decoction (Yi guan jian)

Unprepared Rehmannia (Sheng Di Huang)	10-15gms Rehmannia glutinosa
Glehnia (Bei Sha Shen)	6-9gms Glehnia littoralis
Ophiopogon (Mai Men Dong)	6-9gms Ophiopogon japonicus
Angelica (Dang Gui)	6-9gms Angelica sinensis
Lycii Berries (Gou Qi Zi)	6-9gms Lycium chinensis
Chinaberry (Chuan Lian Zi)	3-6gms Melia toosendan

Properties and Actions:
a) Tonifies Liver and Kidney Yin
b) Regulates Qi

Indications: Liver and Kidney Yin Deficiency with Liver Qi Stagnation. Symptoms include chest fullness and pains, acid regurgitation, dryness of the throat and mouth and bitter taste. It can be used for chronic hepatitis, nervous gastrointestinal tract, gastric and duodenal ulcers.

Contraindication: Not for an individual with phlegm congestion in the chest.

Variations:
1. For increased phlegm add Fritillary (Chuan Bei Mu).
2. For bitter and dry mouth taste add Coptis (Huang Lian).
3. For severe abdominal pains add White Peony (Bai Shao) and Licorice (Gan Cao).

Lindera Decoction (Jia wei wu yao tang; Augmented Lindera Decoction)

Lindera (Wu Yao)	3gms Linderae strychnifoliae
Cardamon (Sha Ren)	3gms Amomum villosum
Saussureae (Mu Xiang)	3gms Saussurea lappa
Corydalis (Yan Hu Suo)	3gms Corydalis yanhusuo
Cyperus (Xiang Fu)	3gms Cyperus rotundus
Licorice (Gan Cao)	3gms Glycyrrhiza uralensis
Arecae Nut (Bing Lang)	3gms Areca catechu

Properties and Actions:
a) Regulates and moves Qi
b) Regulates Blood
c) Relieves pain

Indications: Take as a powder with Fresh Ginger (Sheng Jiang) tea. It is used for Stagnation of Qi and Blood. For delayed menstruation, with scanty, dark blood clots, swollen lower abdomen before menstruation, swollen, sensitive breasts.

Tongue: normal

Pulse: wiry or choppy

Lindera Formula for Regulating Qi (Wu yao shun qi wan)

Lindera (Wu Yao)	9-15gms Lindera strychnifolia
Stiff Silkworm (Jiang Can)	3-6gms Bombyx mori
Ligusticum (Chuan Xiong)	6-9gms Ligusticum wallichii

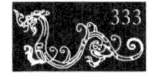

Angelica (Bai Zhi)	6-9gms Angelica dahurica
Ephedra (Ma Huang)	6-9gms Ephedra sinica
Platycodon (Jie Geng)	6-9gms Platycodon grandiflorum
Bitter Orange (Zhi Ke)	3-6gms Citrus aurantium
Citrus Peel (Chen Pi)	3-6gms Citrus reticulata
Dry Ginger (Gan Jiang)	3-6gms Zingiberis officinalis
Licorice (Gan Cao)	3-6gms Glycyrrhiza uralensis

Properties and Actions:
a) Regulates Qi and relieves Wind (antispasmodic)
b) Clears Cold Phlegm

Indications: For sequellae of stroke with symptoms of paralysis, hemiplegia, trigeminal neuralgia, Bell's palsy, deviation of the eyes and mouth, difficult speech, dyspnea, muscle aches, painful arms and shoulders.

Pulse: Full and tight

Lonicera and Forsythia Combination (Yin qiao san) *
Honeysuckle and Forsythia Powder (Yin Qiao San)
Source: Systematic Differentiation of Warm diseases (Wen bing tiao bian)

Honeysuckle (Jin Yin Hua)	9-15gms Lonicera japonicae
Forsythiae (Lian Qiao)	9-15gms Forsythia suspensae
Platycodon (Jie Geng)	3-6gms Platycodon grandiflori
Burdock seed (Niu Bang Zi)	9-12gms Arctii lappa
Field Mint (Bo He)	3-6gms Mentha haplocalycis
Schizonepetae (Jing Jie)	6-9gms Schizonepetae tenuifoliae
Prepared Soybeans (Dan Dou Chi)	3-6gms Glycine max
Black Bamboo leaf (Dan Zhu Ye)	3-6gms Lophatheri gracilis
Phragmitis (Lu Gen)	15-30gms Phragmitis communis
Licorice (Gan Cao)	3-6 gms Glycyrrhizae uralensis

Preparation: Originally it was prepared by first cooking the Phragmitis (Lu Gen) long enough for the aroma to become strong. The other herbs are ground into a powder and taken in 9gm doses with the decoction. Today the entire formula is taken in decoction, or more commonly it is taken in patent pill form. If cooking, only add Bo He Mint (Bo He) for the last five minutes.

Properties and Actions:
a) Diaphoretic, disperses External Wind-Heat
b) Alterative, antibiotic and antiviral, clears Internal Heat and relieves toxicity

Indications: It can be used for upper respiratory tract infections, colds, influenza with fever with slight or no chills, headache, thirst, cough, sore throat, acute bronchitis, measles, epidemic parotitis, acute endometritis, and early stage encephalitis or meningitis.

Tongue: red tipped with a thin, white or yellow coat

Pulse: rapid and floating

Note: This is a cooling formula with some mild nourishing properties. One practitioner favors its use along with or in place of antibiotic drugs when they are to be taken long term as in the treatment of certain venereal diseases and Lyme's disease.

Contraindications: It is contraindicated for colds and influenza caused by Wind-Cold. For this condition, one should consider using Nine Ingredients with Notopterygium (Jiu wei qiang huo tang). It is also not effective for Damp-Heat syndromes for which one would consider Gentiana Combination (Long dan xie gan tang).

Variation: For severe colds and flu add 9-12 grams of Notopterygium (Qiang Huo) and 20-30gms of Isatis (Ban Lan Gen).

Lotus Stem and Ginseng Combination (Qing shu yi qi tang)

Watermelon rind (Xi Gua Cui Yi)	10gms Citrulli lanatus
American Ginseng (Xi Yang Shen)	2gms Panax quinquefolium
Lotus stem (He Geng)	3gms Nelumbinis nucifera
Dendrobium (Shi Hu)	4gms Dendrobii nobile
Ophiopogon (Mai Men Dong)	3gms Ophiopogon japonicus
Coptis (Huang Lian)	0.5gms Coptis chinensis
Anemarrhena (Zhi Mu)	2gms Anemarrhena asphodeloides
Black Bamboo leaf (Dan Zhu Ye)	2gms Phylostachys nigra
Licorice (Gan Cao)	3gms Glycyrrhizae uralensis
Rice sprouts(Jing Mi)	5gms Oryzae sativa

Properties and Actions:

a) Clears Summer-Heat and nourishes the Qi

b) Demulcent and cooling, replenishes body fluids

Indications: For Summer-Heat, heat stroke, dehydration, high fever with excessive perspiration, thirst, nervousness and restlessness, exhaustion. It can be used to treat summer colds and flu, heat stroke and sun stroke.

Tongue: red or pale

Pulse: thin and rapid

Contraindications: Not for individuals with conditions that are not caused by excessive heat exposure.

Lycium, Chrysanthemum and Rehmannia Combination (Qi ju di huang wan)

This is Rehmannia Six Formula (Liu wei di huang wan) with the addition of Lycii Berries (Gou Qi Zi) and Chrysanthemum (Ju Hua).

Properties and Actions:

a) Nourishes Kidney and Liver Yin

b) Improves vision

Indications: Blurred vision, eyes are dry, itchy and painful, dizziness, thirst, high blood pressure. It can be considered for a number of symptoms associated with Liver and Kidney Yin Deficiency including glaucoma, opthalmalgia, diabetes, and cataracts.

Magnetite and Cinnabar Sedative (Ci zhu wan)

Magnetite (Ci Shi)	20-30gms Magnetitum
Cinnabar (Zhu Sha)	3-6gms Red mercuris oxide
Medicated Leaven (Shen Qu)	9-12gms Massa Fermentata

Properties and Actions:

a) Quiets Heart Fire

b) Clears vision

Indications: For Deficient Kidney Essence with Heart Fire. Symptoms include palpitations, insomnia, deafness, tinnitus, blurred vision, dizziness and headache. It may be considered for many eye problems including cataract, retinitis, glaucoma, as well as ear problems such as deafness, tinnitus and emotional problems including schizophrenia, mania and epilepsy.

Variations:

1. For epilepsy with profuse phlegm add Arisaema (Dan Nan Xing), Pinellia (Ban Xia) and Stiff Silkworm (Jiang Can).

2. To increase sedative action and to treat mania and schizophrenia add Coptis (Huang Lian), Gardenia (Zhi Zi) and Arisaema (Dan Nan Xing).

3. For Kidney Essence Deficiency add Lycii Berries (Gou Qi Zi), Ligustrum Fruit (Nu Zhen Zi), Cuscuta (Tu Si Zi) and Prepared Rehmannia (Shu Di Huang).

Magnolia and Ginger Formula (Ping wei san)*

Black Atractylodes (Cang Zhu)	6-9gms Atractylodes lancea
Magnolia bark (Hou Po)	3-6gms Magnolia officinalis
Citrus peel (Chen Pi)	3-6gms Citrus reticulata
Fresh Ginger (Sheng Jiang)	1.3gms Zingiberis officinalis
Licorice (Gan Cao)	1.3gms Glycyrrhizae uralensis
Jujube Dates (Da Zao)	3-5pcs Zizyphus jujuba

Properties and Actions:
a) Carminative, relieves bloating and clears Spleen Dampness
b) Promotes the function of the Stomach and digestion

Indications: Bloated abdomen, lack of appetite, nausea and vomiting, belching with acid regurgitation, loose stool and diarrhea, dull, heavy feeling. It can be used for chronic stomach problems including gastritis and nervous stomach.

Tongue: greasy, white and swollen

Pulse: slippery

Variations:

1. To further augment the properties of the formula add Pinellia (Ban Xia) and Agastache (Huo Xiang).

2. For indigestion add Medicated Leaven (Shen Qu) and Sprouted Barley (Mai Ya).

3. For bloated abdomen with constipation add Areca seed (Bing Lang) and Radish seeds (Lai Fu Zi).

4. For abdominal bloating caused by Cold-Damp with a preference for warmth add Dry Ginger (Gan Jiang), Cinnamon bark (Rou Gui) and Cardamon seed (Cao Dou Kou).

Magnolia and Hoelen Combination (Wei ling tang)

Alisma (Ze Xie)	2.5gms Alisma plantago-aquatica
Poria (Fu Ling)	2.5gms Poria cocos
Polyporus (Zhu Ling)	2.5gms Polyporus umbellatus
Cinnamon twig (Gui Zhi)	2.0gms Cinnamomum cassia
White Atractylodes (Bai Zhu)	2.5gms Atractylodes alba
Black Atractylodes (Cang Zhu)	2.5gms Atractylodes lancea
Magnolia bark (Hou Po)	2.5gms Magnolia officinalis
Citrus peel (Chen Pi)	2.5gms Citrus reticulata
Licorice (Gan Cao)	1.0gms Glycyrrhizae uralensis
Fresh Ginger (Sheng Jiang)	1.5gms Zingiberis officinale
Jujube Dates (Da Zao)	3-5pcs Zizyphus jujuba

Properties and Actions:
a) Eliminates Dampness of the Spleen (relieves bloating)
b) Carminative, restores the function of the Stomach and assists digestion.

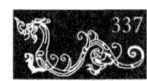

Indications: Abdominal bloating and fullness, loss of appetite, dull heavy feeling in the head and body, watery diarrhea, decreased urination. It is more diuretic and generally for a more chronic condition than Magnolia and Ginger Combination (Ping wei san) but has similar uses in that it can be used for chronic gastritis, nervous stomach, ascites, edema caused by Heart or Kidney malfunction, gastro-enteritis, swollen testicles and urinary retention.

Tongue: white with a greasy coat

Pulse: slippery and thready

Major Bupleurum Combination (Da chai hu tang)

Bupleurum (Chai Hu)	9-12gms Bupleurum falcatum
Scutellaria (Huang Qin)	9-12gms Scutellaria baicalensis
Bitter Orange (Zhi Shi)	6-9gms Citrus aurantium
Rhubarb (Da Huang)	6-9gms Rheum officinalis
Pinellia (Ban Xia)	6-9gms Pinellia ternata
White Peony (Bai Shao)	6-9gms Paeonia officinale
Fresh Ginger (Sheng Jiang)	3-6gms Zingiberis officinalis
Jujube Dates (Da Zao)	3-5pcs Zizyphus jujuba

Properties and Actions:

a) Treats Lesser Yang (Shao Yang: Gallbladder) Excess conditions

b) Laxative, purges Internal Heat

Indications: For Lesser Yang (Shao Yang) and Sunlight Yang (Yang Ming) conditions with symptoms of alternating fever and chills, constipation or diarrhea, bitter taste in the mouth, nausea and vomiting, a blocked, full feeling in the abdomen with spasmodic pain. It can be considered for constipation, acute pancreatitis, acute cholecystitis, biliary calculus (gallstones).

Tongue: yellow coat

Pulse: wiry/tight and forceful

Variations:

1. With jaundice and hepatitis, add Capillaris (Yin Chen Hao), Gardenia fruit (Zhi Zi) and Phellodendron (Huang Bai).

2. For vomiting and nausea, add Coptis (Huang Lian) and Evodia fruit (Wu Zhu Yu).

3. With more severe constipation add Mirabilitum (Mang Xiao).

Major Rhubarb Combination (Da cheng qi tang)*

Rhubarb (Da Huang)	9-12gms Rheum officinale
Mirabilitum (Mang Xiao)	6-9gms Natrum sulphuricum

Magnolia bark (Hou Po)   9-12gms Magnolia officinalis
Immature Bitter Orange (Zhi Shi)   9-12gms Citrus aurantium

Preparation: First cook the Magnolia bark (Hou Po) and Bitter Orange (Zhi Shi), then add the Rhubarb (Da Huang) and finally dissolve the Mirabilitum.

Actions and Properties: This formula is used to purge Heat from the Stomach and Intestines and relieve constipation.

Indications: For Sunlight Yang (Yang Ming) disorders with symptoms of constipation, fever, fullness of the abdomen, irritability, which can exacerbate to mania and delirium. It is used for a variety of Excess Internal conditions including constipation, intestinal obstruction, gallbladder inflammation, acute appendicitis, coma and seizures.

Tongue: yellow coated, possibly with raised prickles

Pulse: slippery, full and rapid

Mantis Egg-case Powder (Sang piao xiao san)*

Mantis Egg-Case (Sang Piao Xiao)   9-12gms Paratendodera sinensis
Dragon Bone (Long Gu)   10-20gms Stegodon orientalis
Ginseng (Ren Shen)   6-9gms Panax ginseng
Poria (Fu Shen)   6-9gms Poria cocos
Acorus (Chang Pu)   6-9gms Acorus gramineus
Polygala (Yuan Zhi)   3-6gms Polygala tenuifolia
Angelica (Dang Gui)   6-9gms Angelica sinensis
Tortoise Plastron (Gui Ban)   10-15gms Chinemys reevesii

Properties and Actions:

a) Regulates Kidney and Heart

b) Consolidates Essence

Indications: Frequent urination, enuresis, spermatorrhea, forgetfulness, diabetes mellitus.

Tongue: pink with a white coat

Pulse: deep and weak

Contraindications: Not for frequent urination associated with inflammation and with burning sensation.

Variations:

1. For spermatorrhea add Cornus (Shan Zhu Yu) and Astragalus seed (Sha Yuan Zi).

2. For Enuresis add: Raspberry fruit (Fu Pen Zi) and Black Cardamon seed (Yi Zhi Ren).

3. For forgetfulness, palpitations and insomnia add Schisandra (Wu Wei Zi) and Zizyphus (Suan Zao Ren).

Minor Bluegreen Dragon Decoction (Xiao qing long tang)

The legendary Eastern wood spirit is depicted as the spirit of the ocean waves which generate clouds and stimulate rainfall.

Ephedra (Ma Huang)	6-9gms Ephedra sinica
Cinnamon twigs (Gui Zhi)	9-12gms Cinnamomum cassia
Dried Ginger (Gan Jiang)	9-12gms Zingiberis officinale
Wild Ginger (Xi Xin)	3-6gms Asarum heterotropoides
Schisandra (Wu Wei Zi)	3-6gms Schisandra chinensis
White Peony (Bai Shao)	9-12gms Paeonia alba
Pinellia (Ban Xia)	9-12gms Pinellia ternata
Prepared Licorice (Zhi Gan Cao)	3-6gms Glycyrrhiza uralensis

Properties and Actions:

a) Diaphoretic, stimulant, diuretic, astringent

b) Warms, astringes and eliminates Fluid Stagnation (white mucus)

c) Warms the Lungs

d) Adjusts the direction of Qi downwards.

Preparation: This decoction should ideally be taken as a hot decoction. If taken in pill form, it should be accompanied with hot water or Fresh Ginger (Sheng Jiang) tea.

Indications: It is indicated for exterior Wind-Cold-Damp. It is useful for all acute upper respiratory infections including colds, coughs, influenza, bronchitis, emphysema, bronchial and chronic asthma, upper respiratory allergies. Symptoms may include fever, chills, lack of perspiration, clear mucus discharges, cough, shortness of breath, full and heavy feeling in the chest.

Tongue: white with a greasy coat

Pulse: floating, slippery

Contraindications: It should not be used long term nor for Heat conditions with coughing of blood or coughing caused by Yin Deficiency. It should also be used with caution for hypertension.

Variations:

1. For severe exterior Wind-Cold increase Ephedra (Ma Huang) and Cinnamon twigs (Gui Zhi).

2. For coughs add Apricot seed (Xing Ren).

3. For marked congestion, copious phlegm, difficulty breathing while laying down, a slippery and wet **Tongue** coat and a wiry and tight or wiry and slippery **Pulse**, increase the dosage of Wild Ginger (Xi Xin) and Pinellia (Ban Xia) and add Fresh Ginger (Sheng Jiang).

4. For pronounced nasal congestion, runny nose and headache, substitute Fresh Ginger (Sheng Jiang) for Dried Ginger (Gan Jiang) and Red Peony (Chi Shao) for White Peony (Bai Shao) and add Ledebouriella (Fang Feng) and Schizonepeta (Jing Jie).

5. For Internal Heat add Gypsum (Shi Gao).

Minor Bupleurum (Xiao chai hu tang)*

Bupleurum (Chai Hu)	12-15gms Bupleurum falcatum
Scutellaria (Huang Qin)	9-12gms Scutellaria baicalensis
Pinellia (Ban Xia)	9-12gms Pinellia ternata
Fresh Ginger (Sheng Jiang)	3-6gms Zingiberis officinalis
Ginseng (Ren Shen)	6-9gms Panax ginseng
Licorice (Gan Cao)	3-6gms Glycyrrhiza uralensis
Jujube Dates (Da Zao)	3-5pcs Zizyphus jujuba

Properties and Actions:

a) Treats the Lesser Yang (Shao Yang) channel (Gallbladder and Triple Warmer)

b) Harmonizing: regulates the Liver and Spleen functions, addresses combined Yin-Yang symptoms of External and Internal, Excess and Deficiency, and Hot and Cold.

Indications: Treats symptoms that may have begun with acute-External complex and have penetrated to an intermediate, lingering stage. Thus there may be alternating fever and chills, stuffy full feeling in the chest, bitter flavor in the mouth, dizziness, lack of appetite, fatigue and nausea. It can be used for lingering colds, coughs, bronchitis and asthma. Because of its broad action it can also be considered for conditions such as malaria, cholecystitis, hepatitis, jaundice and irregular menstruation. Recently it is being viewed as a good general immune tonic and has been studied and beneficially employed for the treatment of HIV and AIDS conditions.

Tongue: thin white coat

Pulse: wiry and tight

Variations:
1. To strengthen immunity add Astragalus (Huang Qi) 9-12 gms, Schisandra (Wu Wei Zi) 6-9gms, Ligustrum (Nu Zhen Zi) 6-9gms.
2. For malaria add Dichroa Root (Chang Shan) and Cardamon seed (Cao Guo).

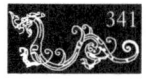

3. For Yin Deficiency add Tortoise shell (Bie Jia) and Wormwood (Qing Hao).

4. For bloating with abdominal pain add Corydalis (Yan Hu Suo), Cyperus (Xiang Fu) and Immature Bitter Orange (Zhi Shi).

Minor Cinnamon and Paeonia Combination (Xiao jian zhong tang)

Cinnamon twigs (Gui Zhi)	12gms Cinnamomum cassia
Jujube Dates (Da Zao)	3-5pcs Zizyphus jujuba
Fresh Ginger (Sheng Jiang)	12gms Zingiberis officinalis
Baked Licorice (Zhi Can Cao)	6gms Glycyrrhiza uralensis
White Peony (Bai Shao)	12gms Paeoniae alba
Barley Malt (Yi Tang)	40gms Maltose

Properties and Actions:
a) Warms and tonifies the Spleen and Stomach
b) Tonifies Qi
c) Relieves spasmodic pain

Indications: For delicate malnourished individuals with a tendency towards fatigue, including thin weak children who are slow in developing and maturing. It is also indicated for wasting conditions. It can be used for gastric and duodenal ulcers, chronic hepatitis, aplastic anemia, postpartum fever, nervous collapse, abdominal spasms.

Minor Pinellia and Poria Combination (Xiao ban xia jia fu ling tang)

Pinellia (Ban Xia)	6-9gms Pinellia ternata
Fresh Ginger (Sheng Jiang)	6gms Zingiberis officinalis
Poria (Fu Ling)	6-9gms Poria cocos

Properties and Actions:
a) Expectorant
b) Antiemetic

Indications: It may be considered for vomiting, acute gastroenteritis, beriberi, pleurisy.

Minor Rhubarb Combination (Xiao Cheng Qi Tang)

Rhubarb (Da Huang)	9-12gms Rheum palmatum
Magnolia bark (Hou Po)	6-9gms Magnolia officinalis
Immature Bitter Orange (Zhi Shi)	6-9 Citrus aurantium

Properties and Action: Similar purgative to Major Rhubarb Combination (Da Cheng Qi Tang) but milder.

Morus and Chrysanthemum Combination (Sang ju yin)*

Mulberry leaf (Sang Ye)	6-9gms Morus Alba
Chrysanthemum (Ju Hua)	3-6gms Chrysanthemum morifolium
Mentha (Bo He)	3-6gms Mentha arvensis
Apricot seed (Xing Ren)	6-9gms Prunus armeniaca
Platycodon (Jie Geng)	6-9gms Platycodon grandiflorum
Forsythia (Lian Qiao)	6-9gms Forsythia suspensa
Phragmites (Lu Gen)	6-9gms Phragmites communis
Licorice (Gan Cao)	3-6gms Glycyrrhiza uralensis

Properties and Actions:
a) Cooling diaphoretic
b) Dispels Wind-Heat
c) Antitussive, relieves cough

Indications: Wind-Heat conditions with symptoms of the common cold, influenza, coughs, acute stages of bronchitis and throat infections, conjunctivitis.

Tongue: thin white coat

Pulse: floating and rapid

Contraindications: Not for upper respiratory conditions associated with Wind-Cold.

Morus and Lycium Formula (Xie bai san)

Lycium bark (Di Gu Pi)	9-15gms Lycium chinensis
Mulberry bark (Sang Bai Pi)	9-15gms Mori alba
Prepared Licorice (Zhi Gan Cao)	3-5gms Glycyrrhiza uralensis
Rice (Jing Mi)	15gms Oryza sativa

Properties and actions:
a) Clear Heat from the Lungs
b) Stop cough and treat asthma

Indications: Shortness of breath, dryness of the mouth and throat, hemoptysis, fever in the afternoon. It can also be used for measles and pneumonia.

Tongue: red with a yellow coat

Pulse: thin and rapid

Mume Formula (Wu mei wan) *

Mume plum (Wu Mei)	10-15gms Prunus mume

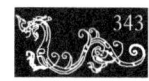

Wild Ginger (Xi Xin)	1-3gms Asarum heterotropoides
Dried Ginger (Gan Jiang)	6-9gms Zingiberis officinalis
Zanthoxylum (Hua Jiao)	1-3gms Zanthoxylum bungeanum
Cinnamon twig (Gui Zhi)	6-9gms Cinnamomum cassia
Prepared Aconite (Fu Zi)	6-9gms Aconitum carmichaeli
Coptis (Huang Lian)	3-6gms Coptis chinensis
Phellodendron (Huang Bai)	6-9gms Phellodendron amurense
Ginseng (Ren Shen)	6-9gms Panax ginseng
Angelica (Dang Gui)	6-9gms Angelicae sinensis

Properties and Actions:

a) Warming stimulant and tonic for the Internal Organs

b) Tonifies Qi

c) Anthelmintic, removes parasites.

Indications: It is indicated for symptoms of cold extremities caused by infestation of worms with intestinal pains, nausea and vomiting, diarrhea. It is effective for chronic dysentery, roundworms, tape worms, roundworms in the bile duct, chronic gastroenteritis, post-gastrectomy syndrome and colitis.

Tongue: red with map-like peeled looking coat

Pulse: deep (hidden), wiry and tight

Contraindications: Not for diarrhea caused by Excess and Damp-Heat. Diarrhea caused by Cold tends to be thin loose stools and slower to complete. That which is caused by Excess Damp-Heat tends to be more explosive.

Variations:

1. For amebic dysentery, tapeworm, pinworms and other internal parasites eliminate Prepared Aconite (Fu Zi) and Cinnamon (Rou Gui) and add 6-9gms Rhubarb (Da Huang) and take with 10-30gms crushed Brucea seeds (Ya Dan Zi).

2. To increase the anthelmintic effect, add 6-9gms each of Quisqualis fruit (Shi Jun Zi), Betel nut (Bing Lang) and Melia bark (Ku Lian Pi).

3. To eliminate the parasite through the stools, add 6-9 gms Rhubarb (Da Huang).

4. If there is no Coldness in the extremities, eliminate Cinnamon twigs (Gui Zhi) and Prepared Aconite (Fu Zi).

5. If there is severe vomiting, add 3-6gms Evodia (Wu Zhu Yu) and 6-9gms Pinellia (Ban Xia).

Nine Herbs with Notopterygii Decoction (Jiu wei qiang huo tang)

Notopterygium (Qiang Huo)	9gms Notopterygium incisium
Ledebouriella (Fang Feng)	9gms Ledebouriella seseloides

Black Atractylodes (Cang Zhu)	9gms Atractylodes lancea
Ligusticum (Chuan Xiong)	6gms Ligusticum wallichii
Angelicae dahurica (Bai Zhi)	6gms Angelicae dahurica
Unprepared Rehmannia (Sheng Di Huang)	6gms Rehmannia glutinosa
Scutellaria (Huang Qin)	6gms Scutellaria baicalensis
Wild Ginger (Xi Xin)	3gms Asarum heterophylii
Licorice (Gan Cao)	3gms Glycyrrhiza uralensis

Properties and Actions:
a) Promotes perspiration, expels Cold and Heat evils
b) Eliminates Wind-Damp evil

Indications: Primarily for External Wind-Cold-Damp invasion with symptoms of chills, fever, lack of perspiration, headache and general aches, bitter mouth taste and thirst.

Tongue: white tongue fur

Pulse: floating pulse

Variations:
1. To clear Internal Heat evil more, omit Angelica dahurica (Bai Zhi) and add Angelica pubescentis (Du Huo), Stephania (Fang Ji), Coptis (Huang Lian), Anemarrhena (Zhi Mu), White Atractylodes (Bai Zhu). This formula clears both External Wind and Cold but has stronger ability to remove Internal Heat evil.
2. Combine with Lonicera and Forsythia Combination (Yin Qiao San) for greater effectiveness in treating influenza and pneumonia.

Notopterygium and Turmeric Combination (Chuan bi tang)

Notopterygium (Qiang Huo)	6-9gms Notopterygium incisium
Turmeric (Jiang Huang)	6-9gms Curcuma longa
Astragalus (Huang Qi)	9-12gms Astragalus membranaceus
Angelica (Dang Gui)	6-9gms Angelica sinensis
Red Peony (Chi Shao)	6-9gms Paeonia lactiflora
Ledebouriella (Fang Feng)	6-9gms Ledebouriellae seseloides
Fresh Ginger (Sheng Jiang)	3-6gms Zingiberis officinalis
Licorice (Gan Cao)	3-6gms Glycyrrhiza uralensis
Jujube Dates (Da Zao)	3-6 pcs Zizyphus jujuba

Properties and Actions:
a) Counteracts Wind and Cold
b) Anti-rheumatic

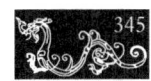

Indications: For muscular pains, "50-years-old shoulder pain", "40-years-old wrist pain" (carpal tunnel), lumbago, neck spasms, limited mobility and muscular spasms of the limbs and headaches caused by Cold and spasms.

Tongue: greasy white coat

Pulse: floating and/or tight

Ophiopogon Combination (Mai men dong tang)

Ophiopogon (Mai Men Dong)	15-20gms Ophiopogon japonicus
Pinellia (Ban Xia)	6-9gms Pinellia ternata
Ginseng (Ren Shen)	3-6gms Panax ginseng
Rice (Jing Mi)	15-20gms Oryza sativa
Licorice (Gan Cao)	3-6gms Glycyrrhiza uralensis
Jujube Dates (Da Zao)	3-5pcs Zizyphus spinosa

Properties and Actions:

a) Nourishes Stomach and Lung Yin

b) Antitussive, lowers the Qi

Indications: Cough with little or no phlegm, hiccup, thirst, dry throat. It can be considered for TB, wasting lung diseases with accompanying dryness, bronchitis.

Tongue: red tip

Pulse: weak and rapid

Variations:

1. For Lung Yin Deficiency add Glehnia (Bei Sha Shen), Solomon's Seal (Yu Zhu), Asparagus root (Tian Men Dong).
2. For Stomach Yin Deficiency add Dendrobium (Shi Hu) and Trichosanthes root (Tian Hua Fen).

Ophiopogon and Trichosanthes Combination (Mai men dong yin si)

Ophiopogon (Mai Men Dong)	7gms Ophiopogon japonicus
Pueraria (Ge Gen)	3gms Pueraria lobata
Licorice (Gan Cao)	1gm Glycyrrhiza uralensis
Ginseng (Ren Shen)	2gms Panax ginseng
Unprepared Rehmannia (Sheng Di Huang)	4gms Rehmannia glutinosa
Trichosanthes root (Tian hua fen)	2gms Trichosanthes kirilowii
Poria (Fu Ling)	6gms Poria cocos
Bamboo leaf (Zhu Ye)	1gms Phylostachys nigra
Anemarrhena (Zhi Mu)	3gms Anemarrhena asphodeloides

Schisandra (Wu Wei Zi)　　　　1gms Schisandra chinensis

Properties and Actions:

a) Expectorant

b) Tonifies the Yin of the Lung

Indications: It clears evil Phlegm and moistens Dryness of the Lung. It can be used for chronic bronchitis, tuberculosis, chronic coughing, and coarse skin caused by diabetes.

Tongue: dry **Tongue** with thin yellow coat

Pulse: rapid and thin

Persica and Rhubarb Combination (Tao he cheng qi tang)

Persica seed (Tao Ren)	6-9gms Prunus persica
Cinnamon twigs (Gui Zhi)	3-6gms Cinnamomum cassia
Rhubarb (Da Huang)	6-9gms Rheum palmatum
Mirabilitum (Mang Xiao)	3-6gms Sodium sulphate
Baked Licorice (Zhi Gan Cao)	3-6gms Glycyrrhiza Uralensis

Properties and Actions:

a) Dispels Heat and Blood Stagnation in the Lower Warmer (especially indicated for symptoms of the lower left abdomen while Rhubarb and Moutan Combination (Da Huang Mu Dan Tang) is for the lower right abdomen)

Indications: Sharp lower abdominal pains, nervousness and anxiety, delirium, thirst, hard stool, difficult urination, elevated temperature at night. It may be considered for irregular menstruation, dysmenorrhea, amenorrhea, retained placenta, acute pelvic inflammation, intestinal obstruction and constipation.

Tongue: red and dry

Pulse: deep, strong

Variations:

1. For severe Blood Stagnation add Dang Gui and Carthamus (Hong Hua).

2. For Stagnation of Qi add Green Citrus (Qing Pi) and Cyperus (Xiang Fu).

3. For retention of the placenta add Trogopterus feces (Wu Ling Zhi) and Cattail Pollen (Pu Huang).

Pinellia and Magnolia Combination (Ban xia hou po tang)*

Pinellia (Ban Xia)	6-9gms Pinellia ternata
Magnolia bark (Hou Po)	6-9gms Magnolia officinalis
Perilla leaf (Zi Su Ye)	6-9gms Perilla frutescens

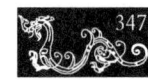

Poria (Fu Ling)	9-12gms Poria cocos
Fresh Ginger (Sheng Jiang)	10-15gms Zingiberis officinalis

Properties and Actions:

a) Regulates the flow of Qi, treats esophageal spasm

b) Clears Phlegm

Indications: It is specific for plum pit throat (globus hystericus). Symptoms include a feeling of blockage of the throat, difficulty swallowing, nausea, cough with phlegm. It may be considered for neurotic globus hystericus, gastrointestinal neurosis (nervous stomach), spasms of the esophagus, chronic bronchitis, laryngitis and tracheitis.

Tongue: white and moist or moist and greasy

Pulse: wiry and tight or wiry and slippery

Variations:

1. For deficient Qi add Ginseng (Ren Shen), Areca seed (Bing Lang), Lindera (Wu Yao) and Aquilaria (Chen Xiang).

2. If there is simply vomiting with complete lack of thirst only use Pinellia (Ban Xia) and Fresh Ginger (Sheng Jiang). This is called Minor Pinellia Combination (Xiao Ban Xia Tang).

3. For more extreme Qi congestion add: Bupleurum (Chai Hu), Turmeric tuber (Yu Jin), Cyperus (Xiang Fu), Green Tangerine peel (Qing Pi).

Pinellia Combination (Ban xia xie xin tang)*

Pinellia (Ban Xia)	9gms Pinellia ternata
Coptis (Huang Lian)	3gms Coptis chinensis
Scutellaria (Huang Qin)	9gms Scutellaria baicalensis
Dry Ginger (Gan Jiang)	9gms Zingiberis officinalis
Ginseng (Ren Shen)	9gms Panax ginseng
Baked Licorice (Zhi Gan Cao)	9gms Glycyrrhiza uralensis
Jujube Dates (Da Zao)	12pcs Zizyphus jujuba

Properties and Actions:

a) Reverses the flow of rebellious Stomach Qi

b) Relieves both Hot and Cold Stagnation in the gastrointestinal tract

Indications: For disharmony between the Stomach and Intestines with Stagnation of either or both Cold and Heat. The symptoms may include abdominal fullness, retching and vomiting, borborygmus, loose stool and/or diarrhea. It can be used for acute gastroenteritis.

Tongue: thin yellow and greasy coat

Pulse: wiry or tight and rapid

Variations:
1. With Heat and Dampness eliminate Dry Ginger (Gan Jiang) and substitute Fresh Ginger (Sheng Jiang). This is called Pinellia and Ginger Combination (Sheng jiang xie xin tang).
2. For Deficient Stomach Qi increase the amount of Baked Licorice (Zhi Gan Cao) to 12-15 grams. This is called Pinellia and Licorice Combination (Gan Cao Xie Xin Tang).

Polyporus Combination (Zhu ling tang)

Polyporus (Zhu Ling)	3gms Polyporus umbellata
Poria (Fu Ling)	3gms Poria cocos
Water Plantain (Ze Xie)	3gms Alisma plantago-aquatica
Talcum (Hua Shi)	3gms Hydrous magnesium silicate
Donkey-Hide Gelatin (E Jiao)	3gms Equus asinus

Properties and Actions:
a) Diuretic
b) Clears Damp-Heat
c) Nourishes Yin

Indications: It is indicated for urinary tract infections with accompanying Yin Deficiency. Can be used for cystitis, acute and chronic nephritis.

Tongue: white and moist

Pulse: floating, slippery

Poria, Cinnamon, Atractylodes and Licorice Combination
(Ling gui zhu gan tang)*

Poria (Fu Ling)	9-12gms Poria cocos
Cinnamon twig (Gui Zhi)	6-9gms Cinnamomum cassia
White Atractylodes (Bai Zhu)	6-9gms Atractylodes alba
Baked Licorice (Zhi Gan Cao)	3-6gms Glycyrrhiza uralensis

Properties and Actions:
a) Diuretic, dispels Spleen Dampness
b) Warms the Spleen and resolves Phlegm

Indications: For Cold, stagnant mucus caused by Cold and Damp Spleen and lack of Heat in the Stomach. There will be symptoms of Phlegm blocking the passages of the Lungs, with shortness of breath, sinusitis, rhinitis, asthma, emphysema, cardiac asthma. There may also be various cardiovascular and renal (urinary) conditions such as valvular disease, heart palpitations, chronic nephritis, renal atrophy, hypertension caused by fluid retention.

Tongue: pale with a moist white coat

Pulse: wiry, deep and tight

Variations:

1. For vomiting with water and Phlegm add Pinellia (Ban Xia) and Citrus peel (Chen Pi). This also increases its drying properties.

2. For Spleen Qi Deficiency with tiredness add Ginseng (Ren Shen) or Codonopsis (Dang Shen).

Poria Five Herbs Formula (Wu ling san)*

Poria (Fu Ling)	6-9gms Poria cocos
Water Plantain (Ze Xie)	9-12gms Alisma plantago-aquatica
Polyporus (Zhu Ling)	6-9gms Polyporus umbellatus
Cinnamon twig (Gui Zhi)	6-9gms Cinnamomum cassia
White Atractylodes (Bai Zhu)	6-9gms Atractylodes alba

Properties and Actions:

a) Diuretic, clears edema

b) Diaphoretic

c) Digestive, strengthens the Spleen

Indications: This is the primary diuretic formula. It is used for Spleen Dampness conditions, edema, thirst, headache, nausea and vomiting after drinking water, urinary retention, ascites, cardiac edema, digestive problems including acute gastritis, gastrectasis, ascites caused by liver cirrhosis, acute enteritis with diarrhea as well as swollen testicles.

Tongue: white and moist

Pulse: floating, slippery

Variations:

1. For jaundice and/or blood in the urine, hepatitis, add Capillaris (Yin Chen Hao).

2. Modified Poria Five Herbs formula (Wu ling san) with Curculiginis (Xian Mao) 15 gms, Epimedium (Yin Yang Huo) 15 gms, Astragalus root (Huang Qi) 15 gms, Cuscuta seed (Tu Si Zi) 15 gms and Ginseng (Ren Shen) 9 gms.

For Deficient Spleen and Kidney Yang type Lupus with symptoms of a pale complexion, edema of the face and limbs, distended and full abdomen, cold extremities, shortness of breath, loose stool, frequent urination, pale, possibly swollen and scalloped tongue with moist fur, deep and thready or thready and weak pulse.

Pueraria Combination (Ge gen tang) *

Pueraria (Ge Gen)	6-9gms Pueraria lobata
Ephedra (Ma Huang)	6-9gms Ephedra sinica
Cinnamon twig (Gui Zhi)	6-9gms Cinnamomum cassia

White Peony (Bai Shao)	3gms Paeoniae alba
Baked Ginger (Zhi Gan Jiang)	3gms Zingiberis officinalis
Licorice (Gan Cao)	3gms Glycyrrhiza uralensis
Jujube Dates (Da Zao)	3-5pcs Zizyphus jujuba

Properties and Action:
a) Diaphoretic, treats External Wind-Cold-Damp
b) Antispasmodic, relieves stiffness and pain of the shoulders and neck

Indications: Used for Greater Yang (Tai Yang) conditions including colds, coughs, acute bronchitis, influenza, emphysema, asthma, upper respiratory allergies, stiffness of the neck and shoulders, intolerance of wind and cold, lack of perspiration. It is also effective for individuals who upon deep palpation have tenderness around the navel with associated sweet cravings. This formula is for individuals with acute upper respiratory ailments, including fevers, whose constitution is neither too strong nor too weak and for whom Ephedra Combination (Ma huang tang) may be too strong and Cinnamon Combination (Gui zhi tang) too weak. The indications of neck and shoulder pain and stiffness particularly indicates its usage. It has been used by chiropractors and Chinese herbalists simply for this indication alone.

It is also very valuable for the Stomach and Intestines because it is a complex carbohydrate that breaks down into simpler sugars more slowly and therefore helps to overcome all conditions that have occurred as a result of any Internal or External sympathetic nervous stimulation (Yang). One such stimulation is a by-product of overconsumption of simple sugars from refined sugar and fruit. Pueraria (Ge Gen), or in Japanese, Kuzu, has become the botanical scourge of the Southeastern states. Having been transplanted in that area for erosion control, over the last several decades it has become highly invasive and very difficult to control or eradicate. It helps to overcome sweet cravings and the negative effects of sweets.

Tongue: pink with a white coat

Pulse: floating and tight

Rehmannia and Gypsum Combination (Yu nu jian)

Gypsum (Shi Gao)	10-15gms Calcium sulfate
Prepared Rehmannia (Shu Di Huang)	10-15gms Rehmannia glutinosa
Ophiopogon (Mai Men Dong)	3-6gms Ophiopogon japonicus
Anemarrhena (Zhi Mu)	3-6gms Anemarrhena asphodeloides
Achyranthes (Niu Xi)	3-6gms Achyranthis bidentata

Properties and Actions:
a) Clears Heat and Fire from the Stomach

b) Nourishes Yin Essence

Indications: Inflammation of the oral cavity, toothache, gingivitis, periodontitis, glottitis, diabetes mellitus.

Tongue: red, dry with a yellow, dry coat

Pulse: large, slippery, floating

Contraindication: Not for conditions of loose stool or diarrhea.

Variations:

1. For dehydration and thirst add Schisandra (Wu Wei Zi).

2. For greater Deficiency of Yin Essence add Dendrobium (Shi Hu) and Glehnia root (Sha Shen).

3. For extreme Heat and Fire add Gardenia (Zhi Zi) and Lycium bark (Di Gu Pi).

Rehmannia Eight Combination

(Jin gui shen qi wan or Ba wei di huang wan)*

Prepared Aconite (Fu Zi)	10-15 gms Aconitum praeparata
Cinnamon twigs (Gui Zhi)	6-9 gms Cinnamomum cassia
Prepared Rehmannia (Shu Di Huang)	20-30 gms Rehmannia glutinosa
Cornus (Shan Zhu Yu)	10-15gms Cornus officinalis
Dioscorea (Shan Yao)	10-15gms Dioscorea opposita
Water Plantain (Ze Xie)	9-12gms Alisma plantago-aquatica
Moutan Peony (Mu Dan Pi)	6-9gms Paeonia suffruticosa
Poria (Fu Ling)	9-12gms Poria cocos

Properties and Actions:

a) Tonifies Yang

b) Warms the Kidneys and lower extremities

Indications: For symptoms of Kidney Yang Deficiency with lower back ache, coldness in the lower extremities, impotence, spermatorrhea, prostatic hypertrophy, frequent urination, nocturia, cough, asthma, persistent diarrhea, dysuria, spasms of the lower abdomen. It can be considered for diabetes mellitus and insipidus, hyperaldosteronism, Addison's disease, hypothyroidism, arteriosclerosis, hypertension, edema, cystitis, chronic nephritis, kidney stones, albuminuria, chronic bronchitis, edema, chronic diarrhea, rectal prolapse, chronic gonorrhea, arthritis, menopausal problems, eczema, senile pruritis, vaginal itching, urticaria, neurasthenia, cataracts, glaucoma, keratitis.

Tongue: pale

Pulse: sunken, slow and weak

Contraindications: Not for individuals with symptoms of Excess Heat or Yin Deficiency. Avoid using for individuals with gastrointestinal weakness.

Variations:

If Coldness is greater substitute Cinnamon twig with Cinnamon bark (Rou Gui).

For impotence add Morinda (Bai Ji Tian), Cistanches (Rou Cong Rong), Cynomorii (Suo Yang), Epimedium (Yin Yang Huo), Circuliginis (Xian Mao), Alli fistulosi (Cong Bai), Alli tuberosi (Jiu Zi), Actinolitum (Yang Qi Shi), and Lycii berries (Gou Qi Zi).

For low back pain add Dipsacus (Xu Duan) and Eucommia (Du Zhong).

For hypertension add Dragon bone (Long Gu) and Oyster shell (Mu Li).

For poor memory and/or hair loss add Polygonum multiflorum (He Shou Wu).

Rehmannia Six Combination (Liu wei di huang wan)*

Prepared Rehmannia (Shu Di Huang)	20-30gms Rehmannia glutinosa
Cornus (Shan Zhu Yu)	10-15gms Cornus officinalis
Dioscorea (Shan Yao)	10-15gms Dioscorea opposita
Water Plantain (Ze Xie)	9-12gms Alisma plantago-aquatica
Moutan Peony (Mu Dan Pi)	6-9gms Paeonia suffruticosa
Poria (Fu Ling)	9-12gms Poria cocos

Properties and Actions:

a. Nutritive tonic for the Liver and Kidney Yin Essence (nourishes the parasympathetic nervous system)

Indications: Formula for Kidney Yin, Essence Deficiency. This formula and its companion Rehmannia Eight (which, with the mere addition of Prepared Aconite (Fu zi) and Cinnamon bark (Rou Gui) is a Kidney Yang tonic) are good for retarded growth or mal-development in children and all chronic degenerative diseases.

Symptoms of Yin Deficiency may include dizziness, tinnitus, chronic sore throat, afternoon tidal fevers, night sweats and spontaneous emissions, thirst and dryness, burning sensation in the palms, soles and chest and toothache. It is useful for a variety of Deficiency conditions including lower back pain, pulmonary tuberculosis, various eye disorders, chronic urinary infections, hypertension, Addison's disease, diabetes, hyperthyroidism, retarded growth and difficulty in maintaining health, tinnitus and deafness.

Tongue: reddish and with a shiny appearance

Pulse: thin and rapid

Contraindication: Not for a person with weak digestion or a lack of Yang

Variations:
1. For Yin Deficiency with Fire and severe inflammation add Anemarrhena (Zhi Mu) and Phellodendron (Huang Bai) and substitute Unprepared Rehmannia for Prepared Rehmannia. This formula, called Anemarrhena, Phellodendron with Rehmannia Six (Zhi bai di huang wan), is for inflammation and Heat conditions associated with constitutional Yin Deficiency.
2. For visual weakness add Lycii berries (Gou Qi Zi) and Chrysanthemum flowers (Ju Hua). This is Lycium, Chrysanthemum and Rehmannia Six Combination (Qi ju di huang wan).
3. For consumptive Lung disorders with cough add Ophiopogon (Mai Men Dong) and Schisandra berries (Wu Wei Zi).
4. For Yang Deficiency add Cinnamon bark (Rou Gui) and Prepared Aconite (Fu Zi). This becomes Rehmannia Eight Combination (Ba wei di huang wan or what is also known as Jin gui shen qi wan), one of the classic Kidney Yang tonic formulas.

Remove Blood Stagnation Below the Diaphragm Decoction (Ge xia zhu yu tang)

Angelica (Dan Gui)	6-9gms Angelica sinensis
Ligusticum (Chuan Xiong)	6-9gms Ligusticum wallichii
Persica seed (Tao Ren)	6-9gms Prunus persica
Carthamus (Hong Hua)	6-9gms Carthamus tinctorius
Pteropus Feces (Wu Ling Zhi)	6-9 Pteropus feces
Lindera (Wu Yao)	6-9gms Lindera strychnifolia
Corydalis (Yan Hu Suo)	3-6gms Corydalis yanhusuo
Cyperus (Xiang Fu)	3-6gms Cyperus rotundus
Red Peony (Chi Shao)	6-9gms Paeonia lactiflora
Moutan Peony (Mu Dan Pi)	6-9gms Paeonia suffruticosa
Bitter Orange (Zhi Ke)	3-6gms Citrus aurantium
Licorice (Gan Cao)	1-3gms Glycyrrhiza uralensis

Properties and Actions:
a) Relieves abdominal pains
b) Circulates Qi and Liver Blood

Indications: Stagnant Qi and Blood conditions with symptoms of fixed abdominal pains and hard spots, sharp chest pains, irritability, indigestion, constipation. It can be considered for hypochondriac pain, painful menstruation, stopped menstruation, irregular menstruation, breast distention and abdominal tumors.

Tongue: purple with spots (maculae) on the sides

Pulse: tight and hesitating

Modified Remove Blood Stagnation Below the Diaphragm Decoction (Ge xia zhu yu tang) with Bupleurum (Chai Hu) 10 gms, Angelica sinensis (Dang Gui) 10 gms, White Paeonia (Bai Shao Yao) 10 gms, Polygonium cuspidatum (Hu Xiang) 10 gms, Fructus Meliae toosendan (Chuan Lian zi) 10 gms, Curcuma root (Jiang Huang) 12 gms and Cirsium thistle(Da ji) 10 gms. For Lupus from Blood and Liver Qi Stagnation with symptoms of jaundice, hypochondriac distention, abdominal fullness, anorexia, spitting blood, nosebleed and an enlarged liver, the strategy is to relieve Liver Heat, soothe the Liver, regulate circulation of Qi and Blood and remove Stagnation.

Remove Blood Stagnation in the Chest Decoction (Xue fu zhu yu tang)*

Persica seed (Tao Ren)	9-12gms Prunus persica
Safflower (Hong Hua)	6-9gms Carthamus tinctorius
Angelica (Dang Gui)	6-9gms Angelica sinensis
Ligusticum (Chuan Xiong)	6-9gms Ligusticum wallichii
Red Peony (Chi Shao Yao)	6-9gms Paeonia lactiflora
Achryanthes (Chuan Niu Xi)	6-9gms Achyranthis bidentata
Bupleurum (Chai Hu)	3-6gms Bupleurum falcatum
Platycodon (Jie Geng)	3-6gms Platycodon grandiflorum
Bitter Orange (Zhi Ke)	6-9gms Citrus aurantium
Unprepared Rehmannia (Sheng Di Huang)	6-9gms Rehmannia glutinosa
Licorice (Gan Cao)	3-6gms Glycyrrhiza uralensis

Properties and Actions:
a) Promotes blood circulation
b) Relieves pain

Indications: For pains in the head and chest caused by poor circulation. Symptoms include chronic head and chest pains which are fixed and sharp (indicating Blood Stagnation), chronic hiccup, anxiety, irritability and insomnia. It can be considered for many painful conditions caused by Blood Stagnation including coronary heart disease, angina pectoris, rheumatic heart disease, chest injury, concussion.

Tongue: dark red with purplish spots

Pulse: wiry, tight and difficult

Variations:
1. For angina add Salvia root (Dan Shen) and eliminate Platycodon (Jie Geng).
2. For stopped or painful menstruation add Cyperus (Xiang Fu) and Motherwort (Yi Mu Cao) and eliminate Platycodon (Jie Geng).
3. For Blood clots and bleeding add Salvia root (Dan Shen) and Tian Qi Ginseng (San Qi) and eliminate Platycodon (Jie Geng).

Replenishing the Yang (You gui wan)

Prepared Rehmannia (Shu Di Huang)	20-30gms Rehmannia glutinosa
Prepared Aconite (Fu Zi)	6-9gms Aconitum carmichaeli
Cinnamon bark (Rou Gui)	6-9gms Cinnamomum cassia
Dogwood berries (Shan Zhu Yu)	10-15gms Cornus officinalis
Lycii Berries (Gou Qi Zi)	10-15gms Lycium chinensis
Dioscorea root (Shan Yao)	15-20gms Dioscorea batata
Eucommia bark (Du Zhong)	10-15gms Eucommia ulmoides
Angelica (Dang Gui)	10-15gms Angelica sinensis
Dodder seed (Tu Si Zi)	10-15gms Cuscuta chinensis
Colloid of Deer antler (Lu Jiao Jiao)	15-20gms Cervus nippon

Properties and Actions:

a) Replenishes the Yang function of the Kidney-adrenals

Indications: For individuals with cold intolerance, pale complexion and cold extremities, involuntary perspiration, premature ejaculation, impotence, spermatorrhea, weakness and soreness of the lower back and knees, dizziness, frequent and nighttime urination. It may be considered for chronic nephritis, impotence, spermatorrhea and diabetes.

Tongue: pale

Pulse: slow and weak

Rhinoceros and Rehmannia Combination (Xi jiao di huang tang)*

Rhinoceros horn (Xi Jiao)	3-6gms Rhinoceros unicornis
Unprepared Rehmannia (Sheng Di Huang)	8gms Rehmannia glutinosa
Red Peony (Chi Shao Yao)	3gms Paeonia lactiflora
Moutan Peony (Mu Dan Pi)	2gms Paeonia suffruticosa

Properties and Actions:

a) Treats severe fevers and Heat in the Blood system

b) Removes Blood Stagnation

Indications: For severe high febrile diseases, delirium, spitting of blood, epistaxis, hematuria, dark black stools (blood in the feces). It can be used for high fevers with bleeding, acute leukemia, uremia, hepatic coma, septicemia, boils and severe local inflammations.

Tongue: dark red Tongue with prickly coating

Pulse: thin and rapid

Note: For ecological reasons, today Water Buffalo or Cow's horn is used in triple the amount in substitution for Rhinoceros horn.

Variations:

1. For spitting of blood and nosebleeds add Imperata (Bai Mao Gen) and Biota tops (Ce Bai Ye).

2. For blood in the feces add Sophora flower (Huai Hua) and Lithospermum (Zi Cao).

3. For delirium and mania add Scutellaria (Huang Qin) and Rhubarb (Da Huang).

Modified Rhinoceros and Rehmannia Combination (Xi jiao di huang tang) with Gypsum (Shi Gao) 30 gms, Anemarrhena (Zhi Mu) 10 gms, Scrophularia (Xuan Shen) 15 gms, Lonicera flower (Jin Yin Hua) 30 gms, Forsythia (Lian Cao) 15 gms, Lithospermum root (Zi Cao) 12 gms, Ophiopogon root (Mai Men Dong) 12 gms and Imperatae (Bai Mao Gen) 15 gms (substitute 3 times the amount of Water buffalo horn for Rhinoceros horn). Use for Excess Heat type Lupus with symptoms of sudden onset, high fever, flushed face, red skin rash, blotches dotted over the skin, irritability, thirst, possible coma, delirium in severe cases, arthritic symptoms, constipation, scanty and dark urine, deep crimson Tongue with a yellow greasy fur and a full, rapid or tight and rapid Pulse.

Rhinoceros and Antelope Horn Formula (Zi xue dan)

Rhinoceros horn (Xi Jiao)	1gm Rhinoceros unicornis
Musk (She Xiang)	0.5gm Moschus
Antelope horn (Ling Yang Jiao)	1gm Antelopis cornu
Aristolochia root (Qing Mu Xiang)	9gms Aristolochia debilis
Aquilaria (Chen Xiang)	3gms Aquilariae lignum
Clove (Ding Xiang)	3gms Syzygium aromaticum
Gypsum (Shi Gao)	5gms Gypsum fibrosum
Calcitum (Han shui shi)	5gms Calcitum
Gold (Huang Jin)	10-15gms Gold
Lodestone (Ci Shi)	9gms Magnetitum
Talc (Hua Shi)	9gms Talcum
Mirabilitum (Mang Xiao)	6gms Natrum sulfuricum
Niter (Xiao Shi)	6gms Nitrum
Scrophularia (Xuan Shen)	9gms Scrophulariae ningpoensis
Black Cohosh (Sheng Ma)	6gms Cimicifuga foetida
Licorice (Gan Cao)	3gms Glycyrrhizae uralensis
Cinnabar (Zhu Sha)	0.5gms Cinnabaris

Preparation: Grind to a powder and take 3-6gms two or three times a day

Properties and Actions:

a) Febrifuge, clears severe high fever

b) Anticonvulsive

Indications: Used to treat severe high fever with irritability, delirium, convulsions, extreme thirst, dry lips, red urine, constipation.

Tongue: red

Pulse: rapid Pulse

Note: For ecological reasons, today Water Buffalo or Cow's horn is used in triple the amount in substitution for Rhinoceros horn. Gold is often omitted from the formula.

Rhubarb and Mirabilitum Combination (Tiao wei cheng qi tang)

Rhubarb (Da Huang)	10-20gms Rheum palmatum
Mirabilitum (Mang Xiao)	10-20gms Natrum sulphate
Baked Licorice (Zhi Gan Cao)	3-6gms Glycyrrhiza uralensis

Properties and Actions: For Heat and Dryness in the lower bowel. It is a similar purgative to the previously mentioned Rhubarb formulas and can be used for constipation.

Tongue: yellow coat

Pulse: deep and strong

Rhubarb and Moutan Combination (Da huang mu dan pi tang)

Rhubarb (Da Huang)	6gms Rheum palmatum
Mirabilitum (Mang Xiao)	12gms Mirabilitum
Moutan Peony (Mu Dan Pi)	12gms Paeonia suffruticosa
Benincasa (Dong Gua Ren)	18gms Benincasa hispida
Persica seed (Tao Ren)	1.2gms Prunus persica

Properties and Actions:

a) Laxative, clears Stagnant Heat in the intestines

b) Reduces swelling and disperses lumps

Indications: For Excess conformation with constipation and Blood Stagnation. It can be used for acute appendicitis, intestinal abscess, pelvic inflammation, Blood Stagnation in the pelvic cavity with cysts and uterine inflammation. It is especially effective for the right lower abdomen.

Tongue: pale with a yellow greasy coat

Pulse: rapid and tight

Contraindications: Use with caution for the weak, pregnant or elderly individuals with constipation.

Schizonepeta and Forsythia Combination (Jing jie lian qiao tang)

Angelica (Dang Gui)	3gms Angelica sinensis

Paeonia (Bai Shao Yao)	3gms Paeonia lactiflora
Ligusticum (Chuang Xiong)	3gms Ligusticum wallichii
Scutellaria (Huang Qin)	3gms Scutellaria baicalensis
Gardenia (Zhi Zi)	3 gms Gardenia jasminoides
Forsythia (Lian Qiao)	3gms Forsythia suspensa
Schizonepeta (Jing Jie)	3gms Schizonepeta tenuifolia
Bitter Orange (Zhi Ke)	3gms Citrus aurantium
Ledebouriella(Fang Feng)	3gms Ledebouriella seseloides
Platycodon (Jie Geng)	6gms Platycodon grandiflorum
Angelica (Bai Zhi)	6gms Angelica dahurica
Bupleurum (Chai Hu)	6gms Bupleurum falcatum
Licorice (Gan Cao)	3gms Glycyrrhiza uralensis
Phellodendron (Huang Bai)	3gms Phellodendron amurense
Prepared licorice (Zhi Gan Cao)	3gms Glycyrrhiza uralensis
Coptis (Huang Lian)	3gms Coptis chinensis
Field Mint (Bo He)	3gms Mentha haplocalyx
Raw Rehmannia (Sheng Di Huang)	3gms Rehmannia glutinosa

Properties and Actions:
a) Detoxifies
b) Clears Heat
c) Nourishes the Blood

Indications: It can be used for a variety of Upper Warmer inflammations including middle ear infection, rhinitis, nasal suppuration, tonsillitis, epistaxis, acne, tuberculosis and alopecia.

Schizonepeta and Ledebouriella Combination (Jing fang bai du san)

Schizonepeta (Jing Jie)	6-9gms Schizonepeta tenuifolia
Ledebouriella (Fang Feng)	6-9gms Ledebouriella seseloides
Notopterygium (Qiang Huo)	6-9gms Notopterygium incisium
Angelica (Du Huo)	6-9gms Angelica pubescens
Ligusticum (Chuan Xiong)	6-9gms Ligusticum wallichii
Bupleurum (Chai Hu)	6-9gms Bupleurum falcatum
Peucedanum (Qian Hu)	6-9gms Peucedanum praeruptorum
Platycodon (Jie Geng)	6-9gms Platycodon grandiflorum
Bitter Orange (Zhi Ke)	6-9gms Citrus aurantium
Poria (Fu Ling)	6-9gms Poria cocos
Mentha (Bo He)	3-6gms Mentha haplocalyx

Licorice (Gan Cao) — 3-6gms Glycyrrhiza uralensis
Forsythia (Lian Qiao) — 3-6gms Forsythia suspensa
Lonicera (Jin Yin Hua) — 3-6gms Lonicera japonica
Fresh Ginger (Sheng Jiang) — 3gms Zingiberis officinalis

Properties and Actions:
a) Warming diaphoretic, clears Wind-Heat
b) Antipyretic, anti-inflammatory, lowers fevers and clears Heat
c) Diuretic, clears Dampness

Indications: Fever, lack of perspiration, chills, head and body aches, nasal congestion, conjunctivitis.

Tongue: thin white coat

Pulse: floating and rapid

Scrophularia and Ophiopogon Combination (Zeng ye tang)
(Increase the Fluids Decoction)

Unprepared Rehmannia (Sheng Di Huang) — 3gms Rehmannia glutinosa
Scrophularia (Xuan Shen) — 3gms Scrophularia ningpoensis
Ophiopogon (Mai Men Dong) — 3gms Ophiopogon japonicus

Properties and Actions:
a) Nourishes Yin and Essence
b) Lubricates Dryness

Indications: For Yin deficiency, injured Fluids from a febrile disease. Loss of Fluids can cause or be associated with constipation, thirst, irritable bowel syndrome, aphthous ulcers (mouth sores), hyperthyroid, chronic pancreatitis.

Tongue: dry red Tongue

Pulse: thready, slightly rapid and weak pulse

Seaweed Decoction (Hai zao yu hu tang)

Sargassum (Hai Zao) — 6-9gms Sargassum fusiforme
Ecklonia (Kun Bu) — 6-9gms Ecklonia kurome
Kelp (Hai Dai) — 6-9gms Laminaria japonica
Fritillaria (Zhe Bei Mu) — 6-9gms Fritillaria thunbergii
Pinellia (Ban Xia) — 6-9gms Pinellia ternata
Citrus peel (Chen Pi) — 3-6gms Citrus reticulata
Green Tangerine peel (Qing Pi) — 3-6gms Citrus tangerina
Forsythia (Lian Qiao) — 6-9gms Forsythia suspensa
Angelica (Dang Gui) — 6-9gms Angelica sinensis

Ligusticum (Chuan Xiong)   3-6gms Ligusticum wallichii
Angelica (Du Huo)   6-9gms Angelica pubescens
Licorice (Gan Cao)   3-6gms Glycyrrhiza uralensis

Properties and Actions:
a) Soften hardenings and eliminates Phlegm

Indications: Primarily used for hyperthyroid conditions with goiter, caused by deficiency of iodine. It also promotes blood circulation and regulates Liver Qi, relieving symptoms of chest fullness. It may also be considered for treating swollen, hardened lymph nodes, for which Persica seed (Tao Ren) and Safflower (Hong Hua) can be added to break Blood Stagnation.

Tongue: thin greasy coat
Pulse: slippery and wiry

Six Major Herbs (Liu jun zi tang)
Ginseng (Ren Shen)   6-9gms Panax ginseng
White Atractylodes (Bai Zhu)   6-9gms Atractylodes alba
Poria (Fu Ling)   6-9gms Poria cocos
Citrus peel (Chen Pi)   3-6gms Citrus reticulata
Pinellia (Ban Xia)   6-9gms Pinellia ternata
Licorice (Gan Cao)   3-6gms Glycyrrhiza uralensis

Properties and Actions:
a) Tonifies Qi
b) Tonifies the Spleen and Stomach
c) Clears Phlegm and mucus
d) Promotes appetite

Indications: For individuals with low energy and lack of appetite, loose stool, nausea and vomiting, acid regurgitation, abdominal and chest fullness. It may be considered for anorexia, gastric and duodenal ulcers, chronic gastritis, acid regurgitation, and bloated abdomen and chest fullness.

Tongue: pale with white greasy coat
Pulse: weak and soft

Variations:
1. With increased chest fullness, add: Saussurea (Mu Xiang), Cardamon (Sha Ren), Fresh Ginger (Sheng Jiang). This is Saussurea and Cardamon Combination (Xiang sha liu jun zi tang).

Six to One Powder (Liu yi san)*
Talcum (Hua Shi)   6 parts Talcum
Licorice (Gan Cao)   1 part Glycyrrhiza uralensis

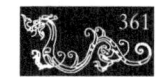

Properties and Actions:
a) Clears Summer Heat
b) Drains Dampness
c) Supplements Qi

Indications: Summer Heat conditions associated with high fever, Dampness, thirst, difficult urination, irritability. It can also be used for urinary tract infections.

Tongue: greasy coat

Pulse: slippery

Contraindications: Not for the elderly or those with Yin Deficiency. It is also not for those without signs of Dampness.

Small Thistle Decoction (Xiao ji yin zi)

Unprepared Rehmannia (Sheng Di Huang)	12-25gms Rehmannia glutinosa
Small Thistle (Xiao Ji)	9-15gms Cephalanoplos aegetum
Cattail Pollen (Pu Huang)	6-9gms Typha angustata
Lotus Node (Ou Jie)	6-9gms Nelumbo nucifera
Talcum (Hua Shi)	9-15gms Talcum
Akebia (Mu Tong)	3-6gms Akebia trifoliata
Black Bamboo leaves (Dan Zhu Ye)	6-9gms Lophatherum gracile
Gardenia fruit (Zhi Zi)	6-9gms Gardenia jasminoides
Angelica (Dang Gui)	6-9gms Angelica sinensis
Baked Licorice (Zhi Gan Cao)	3-6gms Glycyrrhiza uralensis

Properties and Actions:
a) Anti-inflammatory, stops bleeding
b) Clears Damp-Heat

Indications: It is specifically used for hematuria. Symptoms include signs of blood in the urine and burning pain with Heat.

Tongue: red with a yellow coat

Pulse: rapid and strong

Sophora Flower Powder (Huai hua san)

Sophora flower (Huai Hua)	9-15gms Sophora japonica
Biota tops (Ce Bai Ye)	6-9gms Biota orientalis
Schizonepeta (Jing Jie Sui)	6-9gms Schizonepeta tenuifoliae
Bitter Orange (Zhi Ke)	6-9gms Citrus aurantium

Properties and Actions:
a) Hemostatic, stops bleeding

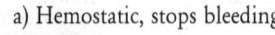

b) Cools the intestines

c) Disperses Wind and promotes Qi circulation

Indications: For bleeding from the rectum during defecation, blood in the stools, hemorrhoids.

Tongue: red

Pulse: rapid and tight

Variations:

1. For severe Heat in the Intestines add Coptis (Huang Lian) and Phellodendron (Huang Bai).
2. For hemorrhoids add Sanguisorba (Di Yu) and Cuttlefish bone (Hai Piao Xiao).
3. For amebic dysentery take with Anemone Decoction (Bai tou weng tang).
4. For Blood Deficiency add Dang Gui.
5. For ulcerative colitis omit Bitter Orange (Zhi Ke) and add White Peony (Bai Shao), Sanguisorbae (Di Yu), Bletilla (Bai Ji), Cuttlefish bone (Hai Piao Xiao) and Scutellariae (Huang Qin).

Spermatorrhea Pills (Jin suo gu jing wan)

Rose Hips (Jin Ying Zi)	12gms Rosa laevigata
Cynomorium (Suo Yang)	12gms Cynomorium songaricum
Astragalus seed (Sha Yuan Zi)	25gms Astragalus complanatus
Euryale (Qian Shi)	10gms Euryale ferox
Lotus stamen (Lian Xu)	10gms Nelumbo ferox
Lotus seed (Lian Rou Zi)	10gms Nelumbo nucifera
Dragon Bone (Long Gu)	10gms Stegedon orientalis
Oyster shell (Mu Li)	10gms Ostrea spp.

Properties and Actions:

a) Consolidates and astringes the Kidney Essence

b) Astringent

Indications: It is used for spermatorrhea, wet dreams, enuresis or frequent urination, insomnia, leukorrhea.

Tongue: pale with white coat

Pulse: deep and weak

Contraindications: It is not good for conditions of inflammation and Heat or if the discharge is yellow (Damp-Heat).

Variations:

1. For impotence add: Epimedium (Yin Yang Huo).

2. For lower back pain add: Eucommia bark (Du Zhong) and Dipsacus root (Xu Duan).

3. For loose stool and diarrhea add: Psoralea (Bu Gu Zhi) and Schisandra (Wu Wei Zi).

Spleen Warming Decoction (Wen pi tang)

Rhubarb (Da Huang)	6-9gms Rheum officinale
Prepared Aconite (Fu Zi)	6gms Aconitum carmichaeli
Ginseng (Ren Shen)	6gms Panax ginseng
Dry Ginger (Gan Jiang)	6gms Zingiberis officinale
Licorice (Gan Cao)	3gms Glycyrrhiza uralensis

Properties and Actions:

a) Laxative

b) Tonifies Spleen Yang, clears Cold accumulation

Indications: For chronic constipation or diarrhea caused by Spleen Yang Deficiency. Symptoms include constipation, dysentery with pus or blood, abdominal pains, cold extremities.

Tongue: pale, white coat

Pulse: deep, wiry and tight

Variations:

1. With acute abdominal pain add: Cinnamon bark (Rou Gui), Saussurea (Mu Xiang).

2. With nausea and vomiting add: Pinellia (Ban Xia) and Cardamon (Sha Ren).

Stagnation Relieving Pills (Yue qu wan)

Cyperus (Xiang Fu)	9-12gms Cyperus rotundus
Black Atractylodes (Cang Zhu)	9-12gms Atractylodes lancea
Ligusticum (Chuan Xiong)	9-12gms Ligusticum wallichii
Medicated Leaven (Shen Qu)	9-12gms Massa fermentata medicinalis
Gardenia fruit (Zhi Zi)	9-12gms Gardenia jasminoides

Preparation: Grind into a powder, mix with water into pills the size of an azuki bean or take 6-9gms with warm water.

Properties and Actions:

a) Carminative, regulates and circulates Qi

b) Removes all kinds of Stagnation, including Stagnation of Food, Blood, Phlegm, Dampness and Fire.

Indications: Used to treat all five kinds of Stagnation. Symptoms include a feeling of Stagnation in the chest and abdomen, possible hypochondriac pain, bloating, belching, acid belching, nausea, vomiting, mild coughing, indigestion with a lack of appetite. It may be considered for nervous stomach, gastro-intestinal ulcers, pain in the chest, hepatitis, cholecystitis, gallstones.

Tongue: pale with a thin or greasy coat

Pulse: rapid, tight and/or slippery

Contraindications: Not for an individual whose Stagnation is caused by Deficiency and weakness.

Variation:

1. For Cold with Stagnant Qi add Galangal (Gao Liang Jiang).

Stephania and Astragalus Combination (Fang ji huang qi tang)

Stephania (Fang Ji)	6gms Stephania tetrandra
Astragalus (Huang Qi)	9gms Astragalus membranaceus
White Atractylodes (Bai Zhu)	6gms Atractylodes alba
Fresh Ginger (Sheng Jiang)	6gms Zingiberis officinalis
Jujube Dates (Da Zao)	3-5pcs Zizyphus jujuba
Licorice (Gan Cao)	1.5gms Glycyrrhiza uralensis

Properties and Actions:

a) Diuretic, clears Excess fluid and removes edema

b) Tonifies the Spleen Qi

c) Calms External Wind

Indications: For swollen abdomen, ascites, edema with a Deficient Exterior. Other symptoms include spontaneous perspiration, pale and puffy skin, obesity (especially useful with Ledebouriella and Platycodon Combination), arthritis and rheumatic problems. It can be considered for congestive heart conditions and nephritic edema.

Tongue: pale with a white coat

Pulse: floating, weak, soft or thready

Contraindications: Not used if there are no signs of fluid retention.

Variations:

1. With low energy add either Ginseng (Ren Shen) or Codonopsis (Dang Shen).

2. If there is severe abdominal distention add Citrus peel (Chen Pi) and Bitter Orange (Zhi Ke).

3. For extreme Dampness and heaviness add Poria (Fu Ling) and Coix (Yi Yi Ren).

Sweet Wormwood and Tortoise Shell Formula (Qing hao bie jia tang)*

Sweet Wormwood (Qing Hao)	6-9gms Artemisia annua
Tortoise shell (Bie Jia)	10-15gms Amyda sinensis
Unprepared Rehmannia (Sheng Di Huang)	6-9gms Rehmannia glutinosa
Anemarrhena (Zhi Mu)	6-9gms Anemarrhena Asphodeloides
Moutan Peony (Mu Dan Pi)	6-9gms Paeonia suffruticosa

Properties and Actions:
a) Nourishes the Yin Essence
b) Clears Heat

Indications: For symptoms of Yin Deficiency with afternoon tidal fever, weakness and emaciation and lack of appetite. It can be used for summer fevers in children, chronic pyelonephritis and kidney tuberculosis.

Tongue: red, with no coat

Pulse: rapid

Variations:
1. For pulmonary tuberculosis add Glehnia (Bei Sha Shen), Eclipta (Han Lian Cao) and American Ginseng (Xi Yang Shen).
2. For pyelonephritis and kidney tuberculosis add Imperata (Bai Mao Gen).
3. For fever of unknown origin add Swallow Wort (Bai Wei), Dendrobium (Shi Hu) and Lycium bark (Di Gu Pi).

Modified Sweet Wormwood and Tortoise Shell Formula (Qing hao bie jia tang) with the addition of Lycii bark (Di Gu Pi) 15 gms, Picrorhiza bark (Hu Huang Lian) 10 gms, Stellaria root (Yin Chai Hu) 10 gms, Anemarrhenae (Zhi Mu) 12 gms, Phellodendron cortex (Huang Bai) 10 gms, Arisaema (Tian Nan Xing) 12 gms, Ophiopogon (Mai Men Dong) 12 gms and Honey prepared Licorice (Zhi Gan Cao) 6 gms. If there is both Liver and Kidney Yin Deficiency with symptoms of blurred vision, tinnitus, vertigo, dry mouth and throat, add Ligustrum fruit (Nu Zhen Zi) 12 gms and Eclipta herb (Han Lian Cao) 12 gms. For Yin Deficient Lupus with symptoms of low grade fever with tidal afternoon fever, heat sensation in the palms and soles of the feet, deep red colored eruption, night sweats, fatigue, irritabililty, insomnia, aching pain and soreness of the joints and waist, hair loss, mirror-like red Tongue with a thin yellowish fur, thin and rapid pulse.

Threatened Abortion Powder (Tai shan pan shi san)

Ginseng (Ren Shen)	6-9gms Panax ginseng
Astragalus (Huang Qi)	6-9gms Astragalus membranaceus
Angelica (Dang Gui)	6-9gms Angelica sinensis
Dipsacus (Xu Duan)	6-9gms Dipsacus aspire

Scutellaria (Huang Qin)	3-6gms Scutellaria baicalensis
Ligusticum (Chuan Xiong)	6-9gms Ligusticum wallichii
White Peony (Bai Shao Yao)	6-9gms Paeonia alba
Prepared Rehmannia (Shu Di Huang)	9-12gms Rehmannia glutinosa
White Atractylodes (Bai Zhu)	6-9gms Atractylodes alba
Cardamon (Sha Ren)	3-6gms Amomum villosum
Baked Licorice (Zhi Gan Cao)	3-6gms Glycyrrhiza uralensis
Glutinous Rice (Nuo Mi)	20-30gms Oryza sativa

Properties and Actions:
a) Tonifies Qi and Blood
b) Prevents miscarriage

Indications: For a woman who is disposed to miscarriage with Qi and Blood Deficiency. There may be accompanying symptoms of light red blood, pale complexion, palpitations, insomnia, lack of appetite, low energy.

Tongue: pale with a thin coat

Pulse: slippery and weak

Variations:
1. If there is excessive bleeding add Donkey-Hide Gelatin (E Jiao).
2. With low back pain add Eucommia bark (Du Zhong).

Two Effective Ingredients (Er miao san) *

Phellodendron (Huang Bai)	6-9gms Phellodendron amurense
Black Atractylodes (Cang Zhu)	9-12gms Atractylodes lancea

Properties and Actions: Clears Damp-Heat.

Indications: Lower back pain caused by Damp-Heat with symptoms of pain in the knees, eczema, leukorrhea, dark colored and scanty urine, tinea pedis (athlete's feet), eczema, gonorrhea.

Tongue: yellow and greasy coat

Pulse: soft and rapid

Variations:
1. To strengthen the Liver and Kidney add Achyranthes (Niu Xi).
2. To clear Dampness add Coix (Yi Yi Ren).

Vitality Combination (Zhen wu tang - also called Black Warrior Decoction)

Prepared Aconite (Fu Zi)	9-12gms Aconitum carmichaeli
White Atractylodes (Bai Zhu)	10-15gms Atractylodes alba
Poria (Fu Ling)	10-15gms Poria cocos

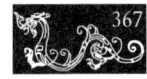

White Peony (Bai Shao)	6-9gms Paeonia alba
Fresh Ginger (Sheng Jiang)	6-9gms Zingiberis officinalis

Properties and Actions:
a) Warm and tonify the Yang and Qi of the Spleen and Kidney
b) Diuretic, eliminate Dampness

Indications: For symptoms of low metabolism, including hypo or asthenic conditions such as hypothyroidism, hypoadrenalism as well as edema, ascites, hyperaldosteronism, cardiac failure, coldness and tiredness, chronic nephritis, chronic enteritis, leukorrhea, rheumatoid arthritis, intestinal tuberculosis, diarrhea and loose stool.

Tongue: white coat

Pulse: deep and thin

Variations:
1. For Deficient Yin add Prepared Rehmannia (Shu Di Huang)
2. For Blood Deficiency add Angelica sinensis (Dang Gui)
3. For Qi Deficiency add Ginseng (Ren Shen) or Codonopsis (Dang Shen).
4. For arthritis add Cinnamon twigs (Gui Zhi).
5. For increased edema add Coix (Yi Yi Ren) and Water Plantain (Ze Xie).

Warm and Activate the Circulation of the Heart Pills (Guan xin su he wan)

Musk (She Xiang)	0.03-0.01gms Moschus moschiferus
Liquidamber (Su He Xiang)	1-3gms Styrax liquidamber
Alpinia (Cao Dou Kou)	9-15gms Alpinia katsumadai
Cinnamon bark (Rou Gui)	9-21gms Cinnamomum cassia
Prepared Aconite (Fu Zi)	9-30gms Aconitum carmichaeli
Wild Ginger (Xi Xin)	15-30gms Asarum heterophylii

Preparation: Powder and mix with honey. Dose is 1/4 to 1/2 teaspoon at a time.

Properties and Actions: Restores and activates Yang, warmth and circulation to the Heart and Kidney.

Indications: Coma, loss of consciousness, stroke, angina, heart disease

Tongue: pale

Pulse: deep, slow, forceful, wiry, tight

Contraindications: Not to be used during pregnancy

White Tiger Decoction (Bai hu tang)*

Gypsum (Shi Gao)	20-30gms Calcium sulfate
Anemarrhena (Zhi Mu)	9-12gms Anemarrhena asphodeloides

Rice (Jing Mi)	15-30gms Oryza sativa
Baked Licorice (Gan Cao)	3-6gms Glycyrrhiza uralensis

Properties and Actions:

a) To eliminate Heat in the Qi (secondary defense) system and the Yang Ming channel

b) To promote the secretion of body fluids

Indications: For high fever, children's fever, meningitis, diabetes, gingivitis, encephalitis B.

Tongue: yellow and dry coat

Pulse: large and forceful or slippery and rapid

Variations:

1. For accompanying Deficient Qi add Ginseng (Ren Shen). This formula is called White Tiger Plus Ginseng (Bai hu ren shen tang). It may be considered for diabetes, encephalitis B, epidemic meningitis.

2. For arthritic pain add Cinnamon twig (Gui Zhi).

3. For encephalitis and meningitis add Forsythia (Lian Qiao) and Honeysuckle (Jin Yin Hua).

4. If there are convulsions with fever add Antelope horn (Ling Yang Jiao) and Uncaria (Gou Teng).

Xanthium Powder (Cang er san)

Xanthium fruit (Cang Er Zi)	6-9gms Xanthium sibiricum
Magnolia flower (Xin Yi Hua)	3-6gms Magnolia officinalis
Angelica (Bai Zhi)	3-6gms Angelica dahurica
Mint (Bo He)	3-6gms Mentha haplocalyx

Properties and Actions:

a) Disperses Wind

b) Opens the nasal passages

Indications: Relieves allergy symptoms and opens the sinuses. It is useful for nasal sinusitis, chronic rhinitis, allergic rhinitis, relieves temporal and frontal headaches.

Tongue: white coat

Pulse: floating

Note: The Magnolia flowers (Xin Yi Hua) and Mint (Bo He) should not be boiled, rather they should be added in at the end of the preparation.

Variations:

1. For increased Lung inflammation add Lycium bark (Di Gu Pi) and Mulberry bark (Sang Bai Pi).

2. For excessive nasal discharge add Honeysuckle (Jin Yin Hua), Centipeda (E Bu Shi Cao) and Licorice (Gan Cao).

Zizyphus Combination (Suan zao ren tang)*

Zizyphus (Suan Zao Ren)	10-15gms Zizyphus spinosa
Poria (Fu Ling)	9-12gms Poria cocos
Ligusticum (Chuan Xiong)	6-9gms Ligusticum wallichii
Anemarrhena (Zhi Mu) asphodeloides	6-9gms Anemarrhena
Licorice (Gan Cao)	3-6gms Glycyrrhiza uralensis

Properties and Actions:
a) Sedative for insomnia and nervousness
b) Nourishes Liver Blood
c) Clears Liver Heat

Indications: For Deficient Liver Blood with symptoms of restlessness, insomnia, nervous anxiety, excessive dreams, palpitations, dizziness, dryness of the mouth and throat.

Tongue: red

Pulse: thready, rapid and bowstring

Variations:

1. For night sweats add Biota seeds (Bai Zi Ren), Schisandra (Wu Wei Zi).

2. For insomnia and nervous restlessness add Eclipta (Han Lian Cao) and Ligustrum (Nu Zhen Zi).

3. For Heart and Spleen Deficiency add Codonopsis (Dang Shen) and Dragon's Teeth (Long Chi).

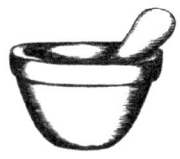

THREE
TREATMENT OF SPECIFIC DISEASE

THE DIGESTIVE SYSTEM

Most traditional herbal systems regard the digestive system and the process of digestion as pivotal to health. Traditional Chinese herbalism considers the Stomach as the more superficial Yang aspect where food is broken down, while its Yin counterpart, represented by the Chinese concept of the Spleen, is the deeper aspect where food and fluids are transformed.

The Spleen is the source of "Acquired Qi" that occurs from the gastrointestinal tract down to the level of cellular mitochondria (see chapter footnote). Coldness, adversely affecting the TCM Stomach and Spleen, is equivalent to low metabolism and is usually accompanied with low energy and low immunity along with poor digestion and assimilation.

Dampness is a Pernicious Evil that can injure Spleen Qi, causing edema, feelings of heaviness, bloating and loose stools or diarrhea. Dampness refers not only to external climatic conditions such as high humid environments, but also foods and herbs that are oily and mucilaginous such as fatty, oily foods and mucilaginous herbs like Rehmannia root (Di Huang). The combination of Coldness (or lack of Spleen Yang), Dampness and Deficient Qi encompasses most metabolic gastrointestinal imbalances. When there are Heat signs associated with the GI tract, it is usually described as Damp Heat of the Liver or Stomach Heat, since one understanding is that the Spleen's assimilative capacity can never be too Yang. Other theories state that the Spleen can have Damp Heat, which becomes a moot point since the same formulas that treat Damp Heat in the Liver also treat Damp Heat of the Spleen.

To treat the Spleen, spicy-warm carminatives are employed such as citrus peel (Chen Pi) and Saussurea (Mu Xiang). These are both Drying and help to stimulate Spleen Yang (functional activity). In addition, diuretics are used to resolve Dampness, such as Poria cocos (Fu ling),

and Qi tonics such as Ginseng (Ren Shen) and Atractylodes (Bai Zhu) are used to tonify Spleen Qi.

The Stomach secretes hydrochloric acid and other secretions that initially serve to dissolve and break down food. To counteract a prolonged acidic tendency, however, the actual lining of the stomach must be alkaline. If the degree of alkalinity is less than the degree of acidity, acid stomach, indigestion and eventual ulcers result. Thus, TCM says that the Stomach must be cool (alkaline) while the Spleen should be warm.

The oral cavity, being a continuation of the gastrointestinal tissues, is a direct manifestation of the health of the Stomach. Excess Stomach Heat causing digestive upset and gastrointestinal ulcers may also manifest as mouth sores, gingivitis, periodontal disease and toothaches. Formulas that contain cooling, anti-inflammatory herbs such as Coptis (Huang Lian), and demulcent Yin tonics such as Ophiopogon (Mai Men Dong) are used to clear Excess Stomach Heat and nourish Stomach Yin.

Finally, emotional upset and stress can adversely affect digestion by overly stimulating the secretion of adrenaline and other stress hormones. When the sympathetic nervous system is overly active, digestion is adversely affected. Formulas that affect the mind and nervous system, containing Pacify Spirit herbs that are high in calcium such as Oyster shell (Mu Li) and Dragon Bone (Long Gu), are used together with herbs such as Bupleurum (Chai Hu) that harmonize and regulate the Liver-Spleen relationship and help to neutralize the toxic effects on the body.

INDIGESTION
1. Excess Type
    a. Food Stagnation: use Citrus and Crataegus Formula (Bao he wan) for symptoms associated with abdominal bloating, acid regurgitation, loss of appetite and either constipation or diarrhea.
    b. Qi Stagnation: Stagnation Relieving Pills (Yue qu wan) for symptoms of abdominal distention and bloating and acid regurgitation.
    c. Liver Qi Stagnation: Disperse Vital Energy in the Liver Powder (Chai hu su gan san) for symptoms of mental depression and chest fullness.
2. Spleen Deficiency type: with accompanying symptoms of weakness, fatigue, loss of appetite, vomiting, diarrhea, anemia, edema Ñ Ginseng, Poria and Atractylodes Powder (Sheng ling bai zhu san) and/or Six Gentlemen Decoction (Liu jun zi tang), which is the model formula for Spleen Deficiency causing Dampness; or Four

Gentlemen (Si jun zi tang), a somewhat milder formula that tonifies Qi more than correcting functional weaknesses and Dampness.

3. Spleen Yang Deficient type: This encompasses similar symptoms to Spleen Qi Deficiency except it also has accompanying Coldness. It usually represents a further complication of the Spleen Deficient type when it has not been properly treated. The main formula is Ginseng and Ginger Combination or Regulate the Middle Pill (Li zhong wan).
4. Spleen and Kidney Yang Deficient Type: This is similar to Spleen Yang Deficiency except it also has symptoms of early morning diarrhea (around 5 AM). Use Aconite, Ginger and Ginseng Combination (Fu zi li zhong wan).

A well known Chinese patent remedy, called Curing Pills, is specific for indigestion, Food Stagnation, alcoholic hangover and conditions caused by sudden change of diet and other conditions that may occur when traveling.

STOMACH ACHE

This is related to the relationship of the Stomach and Liver. There are three types:

1. Food Stagnation: use Citrus and Crataegus Formula (Bao he wan).
2. Disharmony between Stomach and Liver: the most common cause. Use Bupleurum and Chih Shih Formula (Si ni san or Frigid Extremities Powder). Two other formulas to consider are Disperse Vital Energy in the Liver Powder (Chai hu su gan san) and Stagnation Relieving Pills (Yue qu wan). Finally, Bupleurum and Peony Combination (Xiao yao wan) can also be considered for stomach pains caused by disharmony between Stomach and Liver.
3. Damp Heat: consider using Bamboo and Poria Combination (Wen dan tang).

FLATULENCE

There are many causes for this condition, including a too rapid change of diet, lack of liver enzymes, overeating and nervousness while eating, but undoubtedly the most common is bad food combining. The combination of lighter foods such as juices, fruits and raw vegetables with heavier complex carbohydrates, such as whole grains and beans, is the major cause of flatulence in most instances. Many find that when they first change to a vegetarian diet, they tend to experience more gas. Because Indian cuisine was originally predominantly lacto-vegetarian, traditional Indian and Asian cuisine is served with the addition of various

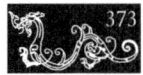

spices such as Ginger, Garlic, Asafoetida and several curry combinations to make them more Yang and warming.

Vegetable charcoal tablets can be purchased in many natural food stores and will absorb a considerable amount of digestive gases. The use of Ginger tea and Asafoetida powder is also very effective for preventing and removing gas.

Formulas: see the formulas for stomach ache.

ANOREXIA, NAUSEA, VOMITING

Most common causes are:
1. Deficient Spleen Qi: Use Six Gentlemen Decoction (Liu jun zi tang) or Saussurea and Cardamon Combination (Xiang sha liu jun zi tang).
2. Liver Qi Attacking the Spleen and the Stomach: use Bupleurum and Peony Combination (Xiao yao wan).
3. If nausea is more pronounced consider Agastache Formula (Huo xiang zheng qi san).
4. If vomiting is severe: consider Inula Flower and Hematite Combination (Xuan fu dai zhe tang). When Stomach Qi ascends with Dampness and vomiting, Inula flowers are excellent to use.

PEPTIC ULCER AND GASTRITIS

Peptic ulcer is a disease characterized by circular erosions or ulcers in the lining of the stomach or duodenum. Gastritis is a more diffuse mucosal inflammation and irritation of the stomach lining that is the cause of many symptoms similar to peptic ulcers. Both conditions can cause bleeding, but this is usually more associated with peptic ulcer disease. Overall, peptic ulcer and gastritis are chronic diseases that can relapse depending upon various External and Internal dietary stress factors. In both cases the bacteria helicobacter pylori has been found to be part of the etiology.

Common symptoms of simple peptic ulcer or gastritis include a "burning" sensation in the upper-central abdomen (immediately below the rib cage). There is also a "full" sensation after every meal and an experience of weight loss. The pain is commonly worse on an empty stomach, at night or between meals and may radiate to the back.

Complications associated with these conditions are:
1. Hemorrhage: usually a slow bleeding that can discolor the stool black, or a more rapid bleeding associated with vomiting blood.
2. Obstruction: a blockage that impedes the passage of the contents of the stomach into the intestines. The obstruction is the result of

a scar formed from a previous ulcer. Symptoms include abdominal pain that gradually increases in severity, vomiting and bloating.
3. Perforation: this occurs when the peptic ulcer completely penetrates through the stomach into the abdominal cavity. Symptoms include a sudden and rigid stiffening of the abdomen. This condition should be considered a medical emergency, possibly requiring surgical intervention.

Patients with these conditions should stop smoking, decrease stress and avoid aspirin, anti-inflammatory drugs, alcohol and caffeine.

1. Stagnant Liver Qi: Disperse Vital Energy in the Liver (Chai hu su gan tang).
2. Heat Stagnation in the gastrointestinal tract: Bupleurum and Peony Formula (Xiao yao san).
3. Blood Stagnation with accompanying symptoms of Food Stagnation: with fixed abdominal pain, indigestion and constipation. Remove Blood Stagnation Below the Diaphragm Decoction (Ge xia zhu yu tang)
4. Yin Deficiency: Liver Strengthening Decoction (Yi guan yuan) with accompanying symptoms of dryness caused by diminishing of vital Essence of the Liver and Kidney.
5. Spleen Qi Deficiency: Ginseng and Ginger Combination (Li zhong wan) when there is accompanying weakness with symptoms of tiredness and indigestion.

HICCUPS

The Chinese mainly consider this a condition of Rebellious Qi with Liver and Stomach Qi having a strong upward movement. Inula Flower and Hematite Combination (Xuan fu dai zhe tang) is specifically effective for this condition. Another specific treatment utilizes the calyx of the Persimmon in a formula called Clove and Persimmon Calyx Combination (Shi di tang). Use Evodia Combination (Wu zhu yu tang) when there is accompanying gas and Internal Coldness and laxity of the G.I. tract. If hiccups are caused by Heat, then Minor Rhubarb (Xiao cheng qi tang) can be used.

CONSTIPATION

Rhubarb is the major herb for constipation. It is routinely added to any formula when constipation is an associated symptom. The most commonly used formula for constipation is Major Rhubarb Combination (Da cheng qi tang). Otherwise, the following may be considered:

1. Excess type: Major Rhubarb Combination (Da cheng qi tang)
2. Deficient type (elderly and weak): Cannabis Seed Pills (Ma zi ren wan).
3. Yang and Blood Deficient type: Blood Replenishing Decoction (Ji chuan jian).
4. Yin Deficient type: Increase Body Fluids Decoction (Zhen yi tang).

DIARRHEA

Excessive Type

a) Damp Heat type: associated with bacterial and amebic dysentery. Consider Coptis, Scute and Pueraria Combination (Ge gen huang qin huang lian tang) or Anemone Combination (Bai tou weng tang) for this type of diarrhea.

b) Damp Cold type: use Agastache Formula (Huo xiang zheng qi san) for Cold Damp turbidity of the Spleen and Stomach.

Deficiency Type

a) Spleen Qi and Yang type: Use Saussurea and Cardamon Combination (Xiang sha liu jun zi tang) or Vitality Combination (Zhen wu tang).

b) Spleen and Kidney Yang type: use Aconite, Ginger and Ginseng Combination (Fu zi li zhong wan).

c) Spleen Qi Deficiency with symptoms of prolapse: use Ginseng and Astragalus Combination (Bu zhong yi qi tang).

d) Symptoms of either Cold or Heat: Pinellia Combination (Ban xia xie xin tang) is used to restore the normal flow of energy in the G.I. tract.

HEMORRHOIDS (PILES)

Any fleshy masses that are found at the internal or external areas of the anus are called hemorrhoids. Piles refers to a hemorrhoidal lump.

EXTERNAL HEMORRHOIDS

There are generally four types of external hemorrhoids:

1) Varicose: This is usually associated with bowel movements or when the patient assumes a squatting position, although a small local mass can sometimes be found at other times as well.

2) Connective tissue external hemorrhoid: This is a prolapse of the skin caused by perianal hyperplasia. It can be of different sizes and there may be local itching, especially after defecation (because there is a problem cleaning the area); it is usually not inflamed.

3) Thrombotic external hemorrhoid: This will present with Stagnated Blood caused by a rupture of vessels around the anal area. The resulting lump may be purplish-blue colored. When palpated, there is a small hard ball of Stagnated Blood at the center of the lump.

4) Inflammatory external hemorrhoid: Here there is an acute inflammatory swelling around the anus with severe pain. When palpated, there is no ball of Stagnated Blood at the center.

INTERNAL HEMORRHOID

The hemorrhoid begins inside the rim of the anus with the swelling of a blood vessel. This can gradually enlarge until it protrudes externally. As the disease progresses, it can become significantly enlarged with prolapse and bleeding. There are three stages:

1) Bleeding with a small hemorrhoid.

2) Bleeding with more severe prolapse, but the hemorrhoid can be either pushed back into the anus or will automatically retract after defecation.

3) Bleeding is more severe and the hemorrhoid is not able to be slipped back into the anus.

Treatment should be both internal and external. In all cases a salve of Oak bark (Quercus sp.), Agrimony herb (Agrimonia pilosula), Bayberry bark (Myrica cerifera), Yarrow herb (Achilea millifolia), Echinacea root (Echinacea species), Comfrey root (Symphytum officinalis) and Calendula flower (Calendula officinalis) can be topically applied and/or inserted into the rectum.

Internal treatment: use Sophora Flower Powder (Huai hua san) or a highly effective Chinese patent formula called Fargelin Pills.

ULCERATIVE COLITIS

Symptoms are inflammation of the large intestine with symptoms of abdominal pain, the passage of stools with mucus and pus, a tendency to recurrent bouts of diarrhea, and occasional intermittent fever. In more advanced cases, rectal bleeding may also occur with diarrhea (more than 6 bowel movements a day), fever and nausea. This in turn can cause weight loss and a low blood count (anemia).

Any of the following formulas can be used, especially with the addition of Moutan Peony, Red Peony and Persica seed.

a) General colitis: Bupleurum and Cinnamon Combination (Chai hu gui zhi tang).

b) Acute colitis: Pueraria, Coptis and Scutellaria Combination (Ge gen huang qin huang lian tang).

c) Chronic colitis caused by Spleen Yang Deficiency with Coldness: Aconite, Ginger and Ginseng Combination (Fu zi li zhong wan).

SPASTIC OR IRRITABLE COLON

Symptoms include a tendency to colonic hyperperistalsis, sometimes with colicky pains and diarrhea and possibly alternating with constipation. This is caused by either Liver Qi Stagnation or disharmony between the Liver, Colon and Stomach.

a) Liver Qi Stagnation and disharmony of Liver and Spleen with accompanying depression and loss of appetite and tiredness: Bupleurum and Dang Gui Formula (Xiao yao san or Rambling Powder).
b) Liver Qi and Blood Stagnation with pain and symptoms of abdominal fullness, indigestion, hypochondriac pain and mental depression: Use Disperse Vital Energy in the Liver Powder (Chai hu su gan san) with Corydalis (Yan Hu Suo) and Melia toosendan (Chuan Lian Zi).
c) Cold Spleen when the condition is caused by pain that is not relieved after diarrhea, accompanied by a thin white tongue coat and a slow bowstring pulse: White Atractylodes and White Peony Powder (Tong xie yao fang). For diarrhea add Cyperus (Xiang Fu), Areca seed (Bing Lang) and Saussurea (Mu Xiang).

ESOPHAGEAL SPASM

A spasm of the esophagus results in a sensation of tightness, cramping, pain or a foreign body deep in the throat or chest. This sensation may come and go irregularly. Pinellia and Magnolia Combination (Ban xia hou pou tang) is specifically indicated for this condition. Inula Flower and Hematite Combination (Xuan fu dai zhe tang) is also very effective for this condition. Inula flower is a primary herb for the treatment of esophageal spasm.

METABOLIC DISEASES

GALLBLADDER DISEASE

This includes cholelithiasis (gallstones), cholecystitis (inflammation of the gallbladder secondary to gallstones) and choledocholithiasis (a stuck gallstone in the common bile duct where bile normally drains from the gallbladder to the small intestine).

The gallbladder is a digestive organ that stores bile produced by the liver. Bile is important in the digestion of fats within the intestines. Approximately 30% of the population over 40 develops gallstones, females being at greater risk than males.

Each year, about 5000 to 8000 deaths are attributed to the sudden blockage of the gallbladder. Common symptoms include sharp "knifelike" pains in the upper right abdomen along the margin of the ribcage. Nausea and vomiting are also present. Fever is a complication in more serious cases. The sudden onset of pain is often felt after eating a fatty meal.

It is important for patients with gallbladder disease to reduce their weight and lower their cholesterol.
1. Acute: When Excess symptoms predominate, use Major Rhubarb Combination (Da cheng qi tang) or Major Bupleurum Combination (Da chai hu tang).
2. Chronic: Minor Bupleurum Combination (Xiao chai hu tang).
3. If neither of these formulas are effective: consider Decoction of Three Golds (San jin tang), Biliary Lithagogue Decoction (Dan dao pai shi tang) or Capillaris Combination (Yin chen hao tang).

The major herbs for gallstones are Bupleurum (Chai Hu), Capillaris (Yin Chen Hao), Turmeric (Jiang Huang), Scutellaria (Huang Qin), Chicken Gizzard (Ji Nei Jin), Desmodium (Jin Qian Cao), Corydalis (Yan Hu Suo: high doses relaxes the sphincter of the gallbladder and relieves pain), White Peony (Bai Shao Yao), Cyperus (Xiang Fu) and Rhubarb (Da Huang).

HEPATITIS

Hepatitis is inflammation of the liver. This can occur as a result of an externally contacted virus, usually from fecal matter, a secondary symptom of alcohol abuse, drug side effect, acetaminophen overdose, fungal infection (cryptococcal infection) or viral infection. Cytomegalovirus hepatitis is a relatively rare form of hepatitis. There are 5 major types of hepatitis, of which three are most commonly seen.
1. Hepatitis A, or Infectious Hepatitis.
2. Hepatitis B, or Serum Hepatitis.
3. Hepatitis C, (transfusion hepatitis) also known as non-A non-B hepatitis.
4. Hepatitis D, a rarer form of transfusion hepatitis that can also be transmitted sexually.
5. Hepatitis E, which is a generic name for all types of hepatitis that test negative for the other forms.

Hepatitis A (infectious hepatitis) is spread through personal contact with infected oral secretions or stools. The common route of transmission is from insects such as flies that land on stools and later contaminate food. Symptoms include nausea, vomiting, indigestion, right upper quadrant abdominal pain, weakness, tiredness, yellowing of the eyes and skin, irritability, dark urine and pale or chalky colored stool.

In Traditional Chinese Medicine it is commonly caused by Damp Heat in the Liver or Gallbladder. It can also be caused by Spleen Qi weakness with accumulated Dampness and an aggressive Liver.

1. Damp Heat of the Liver: The specific formula for this, Capillaris Combination (Yin chen hao tang), is also good for gallstones and cholecystitis.

2. Liver Qi Stagnation: Bupleurum Powder to Disperse Stagnant Liver Qi (Chai hu su gan san).

3. Liver Yin Deficiency: Liver Strengthening Decoction (Yi guan jian).

Some herbs particularly useful to treat hepatitis may be added to the above: Isatis leaf or root (strong antiviral against hepatitis B) and Schisandra are very good herbs for hepatitis. Chinese research has shown that Schisandra is very effective in reducing abnormal liver enzymes.

CIRRHOSIS

Cirrhosis represents irreversible damage to the liver, usually as a secondary toxic effect of alcohol. There are many symptoms attendant to cirrhosis, including gastrointestinal bleeding, congestive heart failure, peptic ulcer disease, malnutrition, and other complications accompanying inadequate liver function. This also represents the direct toxic effects of the buildup of the ethanol molecule on the bodily tissues.

This is a very serious condition that combines both Excess and Deficiency together. Deficiency refers to Spleen, Kidney and Liver while Excess refers to Cold Dampness, Heat Dampness, Blood and Qi Stagnation.

1. Stagnant Liver Qi: Bupleurum Powder to Disperse Stagnant Liver Qi (Chai hu su gan san).
2. Stagnant Liver Heat and toxicity: Capillaris Combination (Yin chen hao tang).
3. Damp Stagnation: Magnolia and Hoelen Combination (Wei ling tang).
4. Liver Yin Deficiency: Liver Strengthening Decoction (Yi guan jian) together with Polyporus Combination (Zhu ling tang) or Rehmannia Six Combination (Liu wei di huang wan).

5. Severe ascites and swelling: Boat and Carriage Pills (Zhou che wan).
6. Blood Stagnation: Remove Blood Stagnation Below the Diaphragm Decoction (Ge xia zhu yu tang) when there is pain in the liver.
7. Other: Vitality Combination (Zhen wu tang) with Poria, Akebia, Areca peel, Alisma, and Polyporus is also clinically effective.

HYPOGLYCEMIA (LOW BLOOD SUGAR)

Symptoms may include sudden sweating, nausea, faintness or fainting, weakness, flushed complexion and rapid heart rate. Low blood sugar at night can cause nightmares or interrupted sleep.

There are seven causes and types:
1. Drug side effect
2. Adrenal insufficiency (considered a rare form).
3. Post-prandial hypoglycemia (low blood sugar after a meal).
4. Exertional (low blood sugar after exercise).
5. Fasting
6. Alcohol (Alcohol can inhibit the liver's ability to convert stored glycogen into glucose).
7. Insulin (this may not be directly caused by an overdose but by a skipped meal). A simple fingerstick blood sugar test is available in pharmacies. A small drop of blood is placed on a color coded chemical strip. The resultant color will correlate with the current blood sugar level.
1. Spleen and Heart Deficiency with associated emotional and neurological symptoms: Ginseng and Longan (Gui pi tang).
2. Spleen Qi Deficiency with associated appetite disorders: Six Gentlemen Combination (Liu jun zi tang).
3. Spleen Qi and Yang Deficiency with apparent malnourishment: Minor Cinnamon and Paeonia Combination (Xiao jian zhong tang).

DIABETES MELLITUS

Diabetes is divided between childhood type, which is definitely inherited, and adult onset type, which may or may not be inherited. The major difference is that childhood diabetes may not be cured but only managed, while in many cases adult onset type may be cured with the limitation of simple sugars and the use of herbs.

The disease is characterized by carbohydrate intolerance because of insufficient insulin. Symptoms include polyuria, thirst, itching, hunger, weakness and weight loss. Because of the large amount of urine that is passed daily, skin dryness may also result. Definitive diagnosis is through routine urine and blood examination.

In Chinese medicine, diabetes is a condition of Inner Wasting and Thirst. It is divided between Upper Wasting, Middle Wasting and Lower Wasting. The cause is irregular diet, unstable emotions and a Yin Deficient body type. Kidney Yin Deficiency is the basic cause of diabetes.

Upper Wasting diabetes manifests as Heat and Yin Deficiency of the Lung with thirst, excessive urination, red tipped tongue with a thin and yellow tongue coat and a forceful pulse.

Middle Wasting diabetes has similar symptoms except there is greater appetite and hunger.

Lower Wasting, or Kidney Yin Deficiency, manifests with symptoms of tinnitus, nocturnal emission, night perspiration, heat in the palms, soles, chest ("five burning spaces"), dry mouth, red tongue and a deep, thready and rapid pulse.

1. Upper Wasting: White Tiger Plus Ginseng (Bai hu ren shen tang).
2. Middle Wasting: Rehmannia and Gypsum Combination (Yu nu jian) or Ophiopogon and Trichosanthes Combination (Mai men dong yin si).
3. Lower Wasting:
   a. Depletion of Kidney Yin
   Rehmannia Six Combination (Liu wei di huang wan) or
   Anemarrhena, Phellodendron with Rehmannia Six (Zhi bai di huang wan).
   b. Depletion of both Kidney Yin and Yang: Rehmannia Eight Combination (Ba wei di huang wan).

HYPERTHYROIDISM

Hyperthyroidism is an abnormal increase of thyroid gland activity. It is commonly associated with enlargement of the thyroid gland (goiter) as a result of low levels of iodine (commonly found in sea vegetables). Another cause of goiter and hyperthyroidism is known as Graves' disease and is believed to be the result of an autoimmune imbalance.

Common symptoms of hyperthyroidism include heart palpitations, weight loss, heat intolerance, bulging eyes, high blood pressure and anxiety.

1. Obstruction of Phlegm and Qi: Goiter Pills (Xiao lei wan) or Seaweed Decoction (Hai zao yu wu tang).
2. Excessive Liver Fire: Gentiana Combination (Long dan xie gan tang).
3. Deficient Heart and Liver Yin: Ginseng and Zizyphus Combination (Tian wang bu xin tang: Emperor of Heaven's Tonic

Pill for the Mind) or Scrophularia and Ophiopogon Combination (Zeng ye tang).

HYPOTHYROIDISM

Hypothyroidism refers to the low production of thyroid hormone by the thyroid gland. Enlargement of the thyroid gland resulting from inadequate intake of iodine can cause the formation of a thyroid goiter (this is rare in developed countries). The thyroid regulates metabolism and growth in the body and in turn is regulated by another gland, known as the pituitary gland, located at the base of the brain.

There are two forms of hypothyroidism:
1. Primary hypothyroidism: occurs as a result of Hashimoto's thyroiditis which leads to autoimmune destruction of the thyroid and the eventual lack of thyroid hormone.
2. Secondary hypothyroidism: caused by the under-production of thyroid hormone from lack of stimulation from the pituitary gland.

Symptoms of hypothyroidism include cold intolerance, thin, dry, brittle hair, fatigue, weakness, muscle weakness, hyporeflexia, low body temperature (less than 98 degrees F.), unexplained weight gain and dry skin.

In general, traditional Chinese herbalism recommends the use of a variety of seaweeds as part of the diet and treatment program. In addition, herbs and formulas that stimulate Kidney and Spleen Yang are used such as: Rehmannia Eight Combination (Ba wei di huang wan) and Vitality Combination (Zhen wu tang, also called Black Warrior Decoction).

LUPUS ERYTHEMATOSUS (SLE)

Lupus, or SLE, is considered an autoimmune disease and may have a strong genetic factor. It can involve many organs and connective tissues of the body accompanied by blood and immunological changes.

Early diagnosis is difficult because the symptoms are atypical and include fatigue, anorexia, emaciation, arthralgia, low fever, photosensitization and skin rash (with a characteristic mask-like rash on the center of the face). Subsequent functional damage of multiple internal organs occurs as the disease progresses, with damage to the liver, kidneys and cardiovascular, digestive and nervous systems. Cardiovascular and renal damage are most prominent, with kidney failure being the primary cause of death.

An anemic condition with decreased white blood cells and platelets is also characteristic. Serum albumin is reduced with elevated globulin.

IgG (Immune globulin G) is markedly elevated. In some patients there will also be elevation of A2 globulin with noticeable renal lesions. Some patients will also test positive for rheumatoid factor (RF).

In TCM, there are three main system complexes involved:

1. Excess Heat: The primary symptoms and signs for Excess Heat type Lupus are sudden onset, high fever, flushed face, red skin rash, blotches dotted over the skin, irritability, thirst, possible coma, delirium in severe cases, arthritic symptoms, constipation, scanty and dark urine, deep crimson tongue with a yellow greasy fur and a full, rapid or tight and rapid pulse.
Formula: Modified Rhinoceros and Rehmannia Combination (Xi jiao di huang tang).

2. Internal Heat caused by Yin Deficiency: The symptoms and signs for Yin Deficient Lupus are low grade fever with tidal afternoon fever, heat sensation in the palms and soles of the feet, deep red colored eruption, night sweats, fatigue, irritability, insomnia, aching pain and soreness of the joints and waist, hair loss, mirror-like red tongue with a thin yellowish fur, thin and rapid pulse.
Formula: Modified Sweet Wormwood and Tortoise Shell Formula (Qing hao bie jia tang).

3. Deficient Spleen and Kidney Yang: Symptoms include a pale complexion, edema of the face and limbs, distended and full abdomen, cold extremities, shortness of breath, loose stool, frequent urination, pale, possibly swollen and scalloped tongue with moist fur, deep and thready or thready and weak pulse.
Formula: Modified Poria Five Herbs Formula (Wu ling san).

THROMBOCYTOPENIC PURPURA

This is an autoimmune disease involving a hyperactive spleen, destruction of platelets, threatened hemorrhage and easy bruising with subsequent infections. It most commonly affects children and young adults, with its incidence being higher in females than males.

Acute type: This is found more commonly in adolescents. There is usually a previous history of viral infection. It begins suddenly with chills, fever, bruises and hemorrhaging of the skin and mucosa. The chronic type is usually found in females with periods of remission and recurrence of symptoms.

Chronic type: Other than the characteristic easy bruising, there may be no other obvious symptoms, except in the chronic type there is

usually an enlargement of the spleen. Blood tests show a marked reduction in platelet count with the life of platelets being shorter than usual.

There are three general types of TCM treatment approaches for thrombocytopenic purpura:
1. Bleeding caused by Blood-Heat: sudden onset with fever, many deep purplish bruises, hematuria, flushed face, a crimson tongue with dry and yellowish fur and a slippery and rapid pulse: Use Modified Rhinoceros and Rehmannia Combination (Xi jiao di huang tang).

2. Hyperactivity of Fire caused by Yin Deficiency: This type displays more purpuras with purple and red color especially in the lower extremities, dizziness, tinnitus, heat in the palms and soles of the feet, night sweats, bleeding gums, epistaxis, excessive menstruation, red, dry tongue, thready and rapid pulse. Formula: Achyranthes and Rehmannia Combination (Zuo gui wan - Restore the Left Pill).

3. Deficient Spleen Qi: Lighter or more pinkish purpuras that appear and disappear intermittently, fatigue, dizziness, palpitations, lack of appetite, pale tongue with little fur, weak pulse: Use Modified Ginseng and Longan Combination (Gui pi tang).

CANCER AND MALIGNANCY

Today in China, cancer is seldom treated solely with herbs. Whenever possible, the cancer is first removed surgically or some other medical intervention is undergone, with herbs being used in adjunct to counteract the side effects of drugs and other cancer therapies. The herbs are also extremely useful to restore health and prevent the reoccurrence of the cancer.

There are several strategies that are generally used in the treatment of cancer. Some of these are as follows:
1) Moving Qi and Blood: This approach is used to relieve pain and disperse congestion of Qi and Blood and aid in the process of breaking up the tumorous growth.

   a) Regulate Qi: Citrus peel (Chen Pi), Green Citrus (Qing Pi), Sandalwood (Tan Xiang), Saussurea root (Mu Xiang), Fennel seed (Xiao Hui Xiang), Aquilaria (Chen Xiang), Cyperus (Xiang Fu), Lindera (Wu Yao) and Magnolia (Hou Po) to name a few.

   b) Regulate Blood: Angelica sinensis (Dang Gui), Ligusticum (Chuan Xiong), Red Peony (Chi Shao), Peach kernel (Tao Ren), Carthami flower (Hong Hua), Red Salvia (Dan Shen), Trogopterori (Wu Ling Zhi), Corydalis (Yan Hu Suo), Olibanum (Ru Xiang) and Myrrh (Mo Yao).

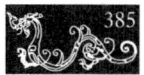

2) Soften Hardness and Disperse Nodules: Sargassum seaweed (Hai Zao), Laminariae seu Eckloniae (Kombu), Sparganim (San Leng), Prunella spike (Xia Ku Cao), Fritillary (Chuan Bei Mu) and Trichosanthes fruit (Gua Lou).

3) Transforming Phlegm and Clearing Dampness: Pinellia (Ban Xia), Poria (Fu Ling), Polyporus (Zhu Ling), Ganoderma (Ling Zhi), Alisma (Ze Xie), Plantain seed (Che Qian Zi), Lobelia (Ban Bian Lian), Apricot seed (Xing Ren), Fritillary bulb (Chuan Bei Mu), Trichosanthes fruit (Gua Lou) and Coix (Yi Yi Ren).

4. Anti Cancer and Toxin Expelling Herbs: Prunella spike (Xia Ku Cao), Coptis (Huang Lian), Scutellaria (Huang Qin), Dandelion (Pu Gong Ying), Houttuynia herb (Yu Xing Cao), Sophora (Ku Shen), Oldenlandia herb (Bai Hua She She Cao), Lobelia (Ban Bian Lian), Poria (Fu Ling), Polyporus (Zhu Ling), Ganoderma (Ling Zhi), Fritillary (Chuan Bei Mu), Trichosanthes fruit (Gua Lou), Arisaematis (Tian Nan Xing), Solani nigri (Long Gui) and Solanum lyratum (Bai Ying).

5. Supporting the Righteous Qi:

a) Tonifying Qi and Blood: Astragalus (Huang Qi), Angelica (Dang Gui), Ginseng (Ren Shen), Codonopsis (Dang Shen), Pseudostellaria (Tai Zi Shen), Ganoderma (Ling Zhi), Prepared and Unprepared Rehmannia (Di Huang), Donkey-hide gelatin (E Jiao) and Human Placenta (Zi He Che).

b) Nourishing Yin and Generating Fluid: Rehmannia (Di Huang), Scrophularia (Xuan Shen), Ophiopogonis (Mai Men Dong), Asparagi cochinchinensis (Tian Men Dong), Adenophora (Nan Sha Shen), Plastrum testudinis (Gui Ban), Carapax amydae (Bie Jia), Dendrobium (Shi hu), Polygonatum (Yu Zhu) and Trichosanthes root (Gua Lou).

An effective general formula to treat most cancers is Coptis and Scutellaria Combination (Huang lian jie du tang).

To support the immune system and help counteract the effects of radiation and chemotherapy use a combination of Ganoderma lucidum (Ling Zhi), Astragalus (Huang Qi) and Ligustrum (Nu Zhen Zi).

THE RESPIRATORY SYSTEM

In general, for upper respiratory problems caused by Wind Cold with symptoms of coldness, chills, body aches, cough with thin, watery sputum, lack of sweating and a floating, tight pulse, use Ephedra Decoction (Ma huang tang). For Wind Heat with symptoms of fever, aversion to heat, sore throat, slight chills, perspiration, cough with thicker yellow mucus, a floating and rapid pulse and a reddish tongue with a white or yellow coat, use Lonicera and Forsythia Combination (Yin

qiao san). Western medicine differentiates the first Wind Cold condition as the common cold type condition while the second is associated with influenza.

COMMON COLD, COUGHS AND BRONCHITIS

1. Chills and lack of sweating: Use Ephedra Decoction (Ma huang tang), especially for those with a stronger constitution.
2. Wind-Cold symptoms associated with stiff neck and shoulders: Use Pueraria Combination (Ge gen tang), especially for those with an average constitution.
3. Wind-Cold symptoms of sweating caused by weakness: Use Cinnamon Combination (Gui zhi tang), especially for those with a weaker, more delicate constitution.

With symptoms of cough:

4. Coughs caused by Cold Dampness in the Lungs: Ephedra Combination (Ma huang tang)
5. Coughs caused by Heat and Dampness: Use Ephedra, Apricot, Gypsum and Licorice decoction (Ma xing shi gan tang).
6. Other formulas that may be considered for colds and coughs are: Wind Cold and Wind Heat: Use Bupleurum and Cinnamon Combination (Chai hu gui zhi tang). This is one of the most commonly effective formulas for most colds.
7. Severe symptoms of chills, sore throat and cough: Use Ma Huang, Aconite and Asarum Combination (Ma huang fu zi xi xin tang).
8. Colds and coughs that tend to linger and recur: Use either Minor Bupleurum Combination (Xiao chai hu tang) or Jade Screen Powder (Yu ping feng san).
9. Colds, coughs and allergies with symptoms of clear watery phlegm: Use Minor Blue Dragon (Xiao qing long tang).
10. For Internal Coldness, and to prevent recurring colds and flu: Use Jade Screen Formula (Yu ping feng san).

BRONCHIAL ASTHMA AND EMPHYSEMA

Asthma is described as a reversible narrowing (bronchospasm) of the smaller airways (bronchioles) in the lungs. It can be caused by allergic reactions, changes in weather, stress, colds, emotions, exercise or unknown factors. Common symptoms include: rapid onset of wheezing (difficulty breathing out), chest tightness, dry or productive cough and a prior history of similar attacks.

Emphysema, or chronic obstructive pulmonary disease, is similar to asthma but without a sense of lung constriction and the symptoms

of wheezing, shortness of breath and coughing tend to develop more slowly. Smoking is a common cause of emphysema. Other causes include cystic fibrosis, alpha-antitrypsinase enzyme deficiency (an inherited condition) and chronic exposure to certain chemicals and irritants such as asbestos, silica and coal dust.

1. Lack of sweating: Use Ephedra Combination (Ma huang tang) for bronchial asthma and emphysema, especially combined with Aster (Zi Wan), Apricot seed (Xing Ren), Farfarae (Kuan Dong Hua), Trichosanthes fruit (Gua Lou) and Stemona (Bai Bu).
2. For External Wind Cold with Internal Phlegm: Use Minor Blue Dragon (Xiao qing long tang).
3. For chronic asthma: Use Minor Bupleurum Combination (Xiao chai hu tang), which should also be used intercurrently between the use of any of the previous Ephedra formulas.
4. Heat: Use Ma Huang and Ginkgo Combination or Decoction for Asthma (Ding chuan tang) for asthma with associated symptoms of Heat including thick, yellow phlegm, increased thirst, red complexion.

INFLUENZA AND PNEUMONIA

Influenza is a common viral upper respiratory infection that affects a large percentage of adults, especially during the winter months. It is transmitted through inhalation of particle droplets containing the virus, such as a sneeze from an infected individual. Other common methods of transmission are through the eyes and mouth. The risk of exposure is lessened by maintaining proper protective measures such as washing the hands and not touching one's face after direct contact with an infected person.

The incubation period may be anywhere from 1 to 6 days before the onset of symptoms. Common symptoms include: fever (differentiating influenza from the common cold), chills, runny nose, sore throat, swollen glands, frontal headache, muscle and body aches, joint pains, dry cough, chest pains, coughing and weakness. Children and infants can have wheezing or asthma-like symptoms.

Influenza viruses are generally self-limiting. However, Chinese formulas such as Lonicera and Forsythia Combination (Yin qiao san) can be taken to both prevent and shorten the duration. Influenza can lead to pulmonary complications such as pneumonia, which can be caused by either bacterial or viral infection of the lungs. The most common forms of bacterial pneumonia are caused by Pneumococcus

and Mycoplasma. Viral pneumonia is more severe and can lead to complete respiratory failure.

1. Wind-Heat symptoms with associated chills, high fever and sore throat: Lonicera and Forsythia Combination (Yin qiao san).

    2. Wind-Heat symptoms with coughing and bronchitis: Use Morus and Chrysanthemum Combination (Sang ju yin).

    3. Wind Cold conditions: Use Nine Herbs with Notopterygii Decoction (Jiu wei qiang huo tang).

Other formulas to consider are:

    a. With symptoms of high fever: Use White Tiger Decoction (Bai hu tang).

    b. For symptoms of lingering pneumonia: Use Minor Bupleurum Formula (Xiao chai hu tang).

Chinese herbs that are highly effective against viruses can be taken alone or added to any of the above formulas. These are Isatis tinctoria leaf (Da Qing Ye) and root (Ban Lan Gen), Polygala (Yuan Zhi) and Houttuyniae (Yu Xing Cao).

TUBERCULOSIS

Tuberculosis is a bacterial disease that infected nearly 80% of the population in the early 1900's. Since 1950 there was a slow and steady decline of TB. However, in recent years, with the increase of AIDS and poverty conditions, the disease has been on the rise since the 1980's. In 1993, 25,313 TB cases were reported, down 5% from 1992, but 14% higher than where it was in 1985.

Approximately 2-5% of children in the U.S. are infected, most of these in lower social and economic levels, with African Americans, Hispanics and Native Americans having a significant number. The bacillus is spread through coughing and presents a variety of wasting symptoms based on its location in the body. While it is most commonly associated as a lung condition, it can also be the cause of meningitis, kidney infections and blood borne infections.

One of the most problematic aspects of its current manifestation is the increasing number of TB cases that have been resistant to current tuberculosis medications. Most of these are to be found in AIDS patients.

TB presents typical Yin Deficient symptoms such as dry chronic cough, sometimes with blood, weight loss, five burning spaces Heat, night sweats, fevers and chills. TCM describes it as a condition of Lung Yin Deficiency and treatment is considered only mildly effective.

Anyone suspected of or possibly exposed to TB should undergo a medical skin test. Once an individual has TB, their skin test will remain

positive for life. Ultimately the most successful treatment of this disease is through prevention by identifying those who carry TB.

Chinese herbal treatment for tuberculosis is not very effective, but the primary herbal formula to consider is Lily Bulb Decoction to Consolidate the Lung (Bai he gu jin tang).

Other formulas that can be considered are:
1. Minor Bupleurum Combination (Xiao chai hu tang) is a primary formula because it both clears Heat and inflammation and tonifies Deficiency and wasting. It can be used simultaneously with any other formula.
2. Ophiopogon Combination (Mai men dong tang) is indicated for Lung and Stomach Yin Deficiency with symptoms of dry mouth and throat.

PLEURISY OR PLEURITIS

Pleurisy is described as a painful condition of the lungs which can be associated with a variety of both serious and non-serious diseases. The immediate cause is an inflammation of the pleura, or lining, of the lungs. The sensation is described as sharp or stabbing and is most severe with the inhaled breath. It can be either one or two-sided and is aggravated with movement of the thorax. If pleurisy is associated with shortness of breath, it is usually considered a more serious disease.

Some of the causes of pleurisy can be: pneumonia (either viral or bacterial), pulmonary embolism, pneumothorax (punctured lung), lung cancer, rheumatic diseases such as rheumatoid arthritis or lupus, and tuberculosis. Chinese herbalism regards pleurisy in the category of chest pain caused by Stagnation and congestion.

The major formula used for this condition is Trichosanthes, Bakeri and White Wine (Gua lou xie bai bai jiu tang). The combination of Trichosanthes and Bakeri (Macrostem onion) are the two most important ingredients and can be combined with Pinellia (Ban Xia) to help clear Dampness and Phlegm, Salvia (Dan Shen) to remove Stagnation of Blood, Poria (Fu Ling) to help clear Dampness, Corydalis (Yan Hu Suo) to stop pain, and/or Magnolia bark (Hou Pou) to regulate the Qi of the Lungs.

UPPER RESPIRATORY ALLERGIES

Allergic rhinitis results from the inflammation and irritation of the lining of the nose in response to a variety of stimuli such as pollen, house dust, animal dander, fungus, molds, foods, grasses and so forth. It can either be seasonal (when the particular stimulus is around), or throughout the year, possibly with multiple environmental allergies.

Chronic allergic rhinitis can lead to the growth of nasal polyps in the nose and paranasal sinuses. These in turn can impair normal breathing. Common symptoms include clear, watery discharge, itchy nose, sneezing, watery and itchy eyes.

1. For upper respiratory allergies, nasal sinusitis, frontal and temporal headache: Use Xanthium Powder (Cang er san).
2. When there is clear nasal discharge: Use Minor Blue Dragon (Xiao qing long tang).

Trikatu is an East Indian Ayurvedic combination of three spicy Hot herbs: Black Pepper, Pippali pepper and Ginger. These warm digestion (tonify Spleen Yang) and dry Dampness. As a result, the combination is very useful for overcoming Cold mucus conditions both by preventing and treating respiratory allergies. One can also combine the powders of Echinacea, Golden Seal, Garlic and Goldenrod. Take 2 capsules three or four times daily. To clear the sinuses more quickly, chew one teaspoon of Horseradish root with a teaspoon of apple cider vinegar and a teaspoon of honey until all or most of the flavor is gone.

SORE THROAT AND LARYNGITIS

1. Sore throat with dry, burning sensation, and hoarse voice: Ophiopogon Combination (Mai men dong tang).
2. Sore throat and laryngitis caused by excessive singing and talking: Use Gasping Formula (Xiang sheng po tai luen).
3. Laryngitis: Chew a piece of Sweet Flag root (Calamus), which in India is called the singer's herb, because it clears the throat and strengthens the voice. Also, Licorice tea with honey is very effective.

THE CIRCULATORY SYSTEM

Heart disease is the major cause of death in Western industrialized nations, accounting for half of all deaths that occur in the United States alone. The prevalence of these conditions, however, is mostly the direct result of lifestyle and diet.

Heart attack, or what is called myocardial infarction, is usually an end result of a variety of circulatory problems including hypertension, strokes, arteriosclerosis (hardening and obstruction of the arteries), and angina pectoris, with possible symptoms of peripheral coldness, palpitations, tachycardia, anemia and varicose veins.

Research supports the presence of a number of predictable factors, namely: (1) heredity, (2) emotional stress, (3) obesity, (4) lack of physical activity, (5) hypertension, (6) high cholesterol and blood lipids, (7) diabetes mellitus and (8) smoking. The obvious fact of all this is that, to a major

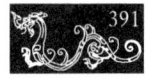

extent, heart disease, with all its precipitating conditions, is largely preventable.

Many of the formulas used for the treatment of circulatory and heart diseases include Salvia miltiorrhiza (Dan Shen), Polygonum multiflorum (He shou wu), Angelica sinensis (Dang Gui), Ganoderma lucidum (reishi mushroom or Ling zhi), Tienchi Ginseng (Panax notoginseng) and Ginseng (Panax ginseng). These can be used both to prevent and treat circulatory heart diseases.

HEART DISEASE (GENERAL)

The Heart governs Blood and Blood circulation. Heart disease, therefore, is caused by Stagnation of Blood and Qi and Deficiency of Qi and Yang (which strengthens the Qi).

If there are symptoms of heart pain (angina) it is most often caused by Stagnation of Heart Blood. It can also be caused by weakness of heart muscles attendant to Heart Qi Deficiency, or edema caused by Deficiency of Heart Yang.

Herbs have food-like general effects on the whole body and tend to be weaker in specific properties than drugs. Because of this, many of the same formulas can be considered for a variety of heart diseases such as valvular disease, tachycardia, palpitations, cardioneurosis, angina pectoris and myocardial infarction. Besides herbal treatments, the successful treatment of circulatory heart disease must be supported by appropriate dietary and lifestyle changes.

Deficiency of Qi and Yin with general weakness, shortness of breath, palpitation, fatigue, insomnia: Baked Licorice Combination (Zhi gan cao tang) and its variations are specific for all heart disease, especially when there are associated palpitations.

Hawthorn berries and flowers, Linden flowers, Cactus grandiflorus, Lily of the valley (regarded by some to have toxic properties), Garlic, and Cayenne Pepper are also used singly or in special formulations for the treatment of heart problems.

HYPERTENSION (HIGH BLOOD PRESSURE)

Hypertension is measured by a standard blood pressure instrument that registers two numbers, an upper (systolic) number and a lower (diastolic) number. The systolic, or first number, represents the strength of the heart beat as it contracts to push the blood through the arteries. The lower, or diastolic, number is the period of relaxation between contractions that represents the peristaltic action of the arterial wall

that is activated by the nerves. A reading that is greater than 140 over 90 is considered high.

Hypertension, in itself, is not considered a disease in Traditional Chinese Medicine but one of a complex of conditions representing a general imbalance. As with most circulatory heart disorders, appropriate lifestyle and dietary factors are primary for reducing hypertension.

Traditional Chinese Medicine recognizes four basic causes:
1. Hypertension Caused by Hyperactive Liver Yang:
a) Obese and strong with a large, swollen abdomen: Ledebouriella and Platycodon Combination (Fang feng tong sheng san).
b) Excess types but with a more pronounced tendency towards lung congestion and constipation: Major Bupleurum (Da chai hu tang).
c) Excess Damp Heat: With toxicity but with less tendency towards abdominal fullness or lung congestion: Gentiana Combination (Long dan xie gan tang) or Coptis and Scutellaria Combination (Huang lian jie du tang).
d) Stuffiness and fullness in the chest with nervousness, insomnia and emotional volatility: Bupleurum and Dragon Bone Combination (Chai hu jia long gu mu li tang).

In addition herbs such as Abalone shell (Shi Jue Ming), Prunella (Xia Ku Cao) and Gentiana (Long Dan Cao) can be added as needed. Cassia tora seeds (Jue Ming Zi) can be lightly toasted in an open skillet, crushed and brewed as a substitute for coffee. Where coffee is Heating and aggravates hyperactive Liver Yang, Cassia tora seeds are cooling and detoxifying.

2. Hypertension Caused by Deficiency:
a) Weakness of the urinary organs and Coldness: Rehmannia Eight Formula (Ba wei di huang wan) is especially indicated when there is hypertension in the elderly.
b) Yin Deficiency: Use Rehmannia Six Formula (Liu wei di huang wan).

These constitute a root symptom treatment to which one would add accordingly:
For Wind: Add Uncaria (Gou Teng) and Gastrodia (Tian Ma).
For Heat: Add Prunella (Xia Ku Cao) and Gentiana (Long Dan Cao).
For Dampness: Add Plantago (Che Qian Zi) and Gentiana (Long Dan Cao).

For Yang Deficiency: Add Eucommia (Du Zhong), Loranthes (Sang Ji Sheng) and Cuscuta (Tu Si Zi).

Both Triphala and Guggul are also indicated as well as Garlic and Hawthorn, the latter being two herbs that are most commonly used for hypertension by Western herbalists.

HYPOTENSION (LOW BLOOD PRESSURE)

Individuals whose systolic blood pressure reads 90 or less have low blood pressure. Again, this is considered more a potential symptom of imbalance rather than a disease in itself. Frequently low blood pressure is associated with low thyroid function, anemia, dizziness, anorexia and fatigue.

When Qi is chronically Deficient, it can result in low blood pressure. Tonics are prescribed.

1. Qi Deficiency: use Ginseng and Astragalus (Bu zhong yi qi tang) and Ginseng and Ginger Combination (Li Zhong wan).

2. Deficiency of Spleen Yang: Use Vitality Combination (Zhen wu tang) when there is weak digestion and fatigue.

Herbs that can be added to formulas for hypotension when there is Qi Deficiency are: Astragalus (Huang Qi), Ginseng (Ren Shen) and Codonopsis (Dang Shen).

Chinese research supports the benefits of taking high doses of Cinnamon twig (Gui Zhi) to increase blood pressure. This is especially true with doses of Astragalus (Huang Qi). Further, Garlic and/or Cayenne Pepper are commonly used by Western herbalists.

ARTERIOSCLEROSIS AND ATHEROSCLEROSIS

Arteriosclerosis is hardening of the arteries, while atherosclerosis is the accumulation of lipids and other substances that impair the arterial passages.

1. Excess Conditions:

    Treatment is similar to hypertension. Ledebouriella and Platycodon Combination (Fang feng tong sheng san) or Coptis and Scutellaria Combination (Huang lian jie du tang) can be used with the addition of Rhubarb root (Da Huang) if there is a tendency towards constipation.

2. Yang or Qi Deficiency, Deficient Conditions: Rehmannia Eight Combination (Ba wei di huang wan) or Ginseng and Dang Gui Ten Combination (Shi chuan da bu tang).

Two specific Chinese herbs that reduce cholesterol are Polygonum multiflorum (He Shou Wu) and Salvia miltiorrhiza (Dan Shen).

In Ayurvedic medicine, Triphala and Guggul are specifically used to help reduce high blood lipids and cholesterol. Western herbalism uses Hawthorn berries and flowers (Crataegus oxycanthus), Linden flowers (Tilia europa), and Garlic (Allium sativa), as well as herbs for the liver such as Oregon Grape or Barberry root (Berberis species) and Artichoke leaves which increase the liver's ability to regulate lipid metabolism.

ANGINA PECTORIS (HEART PAINS)
Symptoms of angina are severe chest pains, difficult breathing and a feeling of chest constriction that is not the result of overeating or strenuous exercise.
The major cause is Blood Stagnation.
1. Trichosanthes, Bakeri and White Wine (Gua lou xie bai bai jiu tang) is the primary formula used for this condition, but one must add other herbs that move Blood to increase its effectiveness. Select four from the following: Salvia (Dan Shen), Carthamus (Hong Hua), Panax notoginseng (Tienchi Ginseng), Red Peony (Chi Shao), Ligusticum (Chuan Xiong), Corydalis (Yan Hu Suo) and Cinnamon twigs (Gui Zhi).
2. Bupleurum and Dragon Bone Combination (Chai hu long gu mu li tang) is generally effective for most types.
3. Salvia Pills is a patent Chinese formula that combines Salvia miltiorrhiza with Borneolum (Bing Pian). It relieves angina by dispersing Stagnant Qi and Blood. Salvia miltiorrhiza root (Dan Shen) is very effective as a single herb or can be taken together with Motherwort herb (Leonurus cardiaca).

Other herbs include Hawthorn berries (Crataegus oxycantha), Linden flower (Tilia europea), Motherwort (Leonurus cardiaca), Cayenne (Capsicum frutescens) and Garlic (Allium sativa), which can be used singly or in various combinations appropriate to the individual.

VARICOSE VEINS
In TCM this is considered a symptom of Blood Stagnation rather than a primary disease. The primary strategy is moving Blood. The major formula: Removing Blood Stasis in the Lateral Abdomen (Xue fu zhu yu tang).

For Blood Stagnation with Blood Deficiency or anemia: Dang Gui Four (Si wu tang) with Carthamus (Hong Hua), Persica seed (Tao Ren) and Salvia (Dan Shen).
Other: Carthamus and Persica Seed Decoction (Hong hua tao ren jian).

Another remedy is to make a strong tea of Witch Hazel bark (Haemamelis), White Oak bark (Quercus alba) and/or Horse Chestnut (Aesculus hippocastanum) and a dash of Cayenne Pepper (Capsicum). Soak a flannel cloth in the tea and apply over the affected areas as hot as possible for 20 to 30 minutes twice daily.

LYMPHADENITIS (SWOLLEN LYMPH GLANDS)
Caused by Stagnation of Heat and Phlegm:
The representative formula for this condition is Seaweed Decoction (Hai zao yu wu tang).

Other formulas to consider are:
1. Goiter caused by Congestion of Heat and Phlegm and for swollen thyroid and for swollen lymph glands characterized by hard lumps or swellings in front of and behind the ears: Pills for Goiter (Xiao lei wan).
2. Wind-Cold or Wind-Heat: Bupleurum and Schizonepeta Formula (Japanese: Shih wei pai tu tang).

Prunella (Xia Ku Cao), Oyster shell (Mu Li), Sargassum (Hai Zao) and Kelp (Kun Bu) used alone or in combination are the major herbs used for goiter and swollen lymph glands.

THE URINARY SYSTEM

URINARY TRACT INFECTION:
Symptoms include painful or burning urine and difficult and frequent urination. Cystitis is the more chronic form while nephritis is often accompanied with lower back pain.

In TCM the urinary system generally relates to the Kidney system and Urinary Bladder (UB) system. The Kidney is the primary Organ relating to the opening and closing of the Urinary Bladder system. In TCM, urinary tract infections are usually caused by Damp Heat in the Urinary Bladder area.

TCM distinguishes between two types of urinary infections as follows:
1. Acute: This is an Excess condition and the representative formula is Dianthus Formula (Ba zheng san).

2. Chronic: This is caused by Kidney Yin Deficiency and it can be treated with Anemarrhena and Phellodendron Combination (Zhi bai di huang wan).

Other possible formulas to consider are:

Polyporus Combination (Zhu ling tang) is for acute and chronic cystitis, strangury, tendency to dribble after urination and occasional discharge of blood.

Gentiana Combination (Long dan xie gan tang) is for urinary tract inflammation with severe painful urination.

Gardenia and Poria Combination (Wei wu lin san) is for more chronic cystitis with Internal Heat in the Bladder, painful urination, fatigue, urinary calculus and hematuria.

EXCESSIVE URINATION OR POLYURIA

There are several causes, with the most common of those being:

Excess caused by Heat and Dampness in the Bladder: For this type one can use Dianthus Formula (Ba zheng san) or Gentiana Combination (Long dan xie gan tang) to release the Damp Heat.

Deficiency: Use Rehmannia Eight Combination (Ba wei di huang wan) for associated Kidney Yang Deficiency or Rehmannia Six Formula (Liu wei di huang wan) for Yin Deficiency.

Other possible causes for excess urination are nephritis and prostatic enlargement. Because there can be many causes for this condition, there are many possible formulas.

HEMATURIA OR BLEEDING IN THE URINARY TRACT

This has symptoms of burning pain upon urination and inflammation: Use Polyporus Combination (Zhu ling tang) or Small Thistle Decoction (Xiao ji yin zi).

DYSURIA (SCALDING OR BURNING URINE)

This is commonly caused by Damp Heat, and Gentiana Combination (Long dan xie gan tang) is most commonly indicated.

NEPHRITIS

Nephritis is regarded as a type of auto-immune disease in Western scientific medicine. In TCM there are different types of nephritis which are broadly categorized as Excess or Deficient.

1. Excess: Use Decoction of Three Golds (San jin tang) when the condition is caused by Excess Damp Heat in the urinary tract, sometimes associated with urinary stones.

2. Deficiency: TCM commonly views nephritis under the category of Kidney Deficiency. Recent TCM understanding also indicates the possibility of some Blood Stagnation as a contributory factor in the disease complex, so that the addition of Blood moving herbs are added, such as Salvia (Dan Shen), Cirsium (Da Ji), Moutan (Mu Dan Pi), and Leonorus (Yi Mu Cao) to address the problem of protein in the urine (which in TCM might be considered as a kind of Blood Stagnation). One possibility is to combine a variety of these Blood moving herbs with Rehmannia Six (Liu wei di huang wan) for Kidney Yin Deficiency or Rehmannia Eight Combination (Ba wei di huang wan) when there is Kidney Yang Deficiency.

KIDNEY STONES

If the stone is very small, it can usually be flushed out. Interestingly, one can use the same herbs for urinary stones as one would use for gallstones. Capillaris (Yin Chen Hao), Akebia (Mu Tong), Rhubarb (Da Huang) and Turmeric (Jiang Huang) are effective for dissolving and expelling urinary stones.

Other formulas that are indicated include:
Polyporus Combination (Zhu ling tang) and Dianthus Formula (Ba zheng san).

EDEMA

As with many disease conditions in TCM, there are at least two types. These are:
1. Excess: Caused by Excess fluid retention; use Poria Five Herbs formula (Wu ling san). This is a good general formula for edema caused by a Damp Spleen.
2. Deficient: This type of edema is associated with general Spleen Deficiency and the most representative formula is Stephania and Astragalus Combination (Fang qi huang qi tang). This formula is also very effective for lymphedema.

THE FEMALE REPRODUCTIVE SYSTEM

LEUKORRHEA (VAGINAL DISCHARGE)
1. Damp Heat type: Gentiana Combination (Long dan xie gan tang) is used when there are symptoms of thick yellow discharge.
2. Liver Qi Stagnation : Bupleurum and Peony Combination (Xiao yao san) is used when there is PMS with depression and mood swings.

3. Coldness from Deficiency of the Spleen and Kidney: Aconite Combination (Si ni tang) is used with the addition of Codonopsis (Dang Shen), Poria (Fu Ling) and Alisma (Ze Xie) if leukorrhea is associated with digestive weakness, lower back and joint pains and general fatigue.
4. Tendency towards anemia: Dang Gui and Peony Formula (Dang gui shao yao san) is used if the discharge is clear or whitish and there is anemia.
5. Stagnation of Coldness and Deficiency: Dang Gui and Evodia Combination (Wen jing tang) is used when the discharge is clear or whitish with pronounced symptoms of Coldness.
5. Qi and Blood Deficiency: Ginseng and Dang Gui Ten Combination (Shi chuan da bu tang).
6. Stagnation of Blood and/or Fluid: Cinnamon and Poria Combination (Gui zhi fu ling wan) for any condition where there is both Blood and Fluid Stagnation, especially with pelvic pains.

AMENORRHEA (STOPPED MENSTRUATION)

Dang Gui Four (Si wu tang) is the base gynecological formula for Blood Deficiency.
1. Deficient Blood, with Spleen (digestive) and Kidney (endocrine) Deficiency: Use Dang Gui and Peony Combination (Dang gui shao yao san).
2. Stagnation of Coldness and Deficiency with irregular menstruation: Dang Gui and Evodia Combination (Wen jing tang).

DYSMENORRHEA (PAINFUL MENSTRUATION)

Blood Deficient types: Dang Gui Four (Si wu tang). Cyperus (Xiang Fu), Corydalis (Yan Hu Suo) and Leonurus (Yi Mu Cao) added to Dang Gui Four will enhance the effectiveness of this most representative gynecology formula.
1. Frail and sensitive types: Dang Gui and Peony Combination (Dang gui shao yao tang).
2. Blood Stagnation: Cinnamon and Poria Combination (Gui zhi fu ling tang) or Persica and Rhubarb Combination (Tao he cheng qi tang).
Caution: Be careful to avoid Dang Gui when there is excessive menstrual bleeding, because it has a very strong dispersing effect and causes more bleeding.

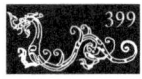

MENORRHAGIA, METRORRHAGIA OR FLOODING

Qi Deficiency: Ginseng and Longan Combination (Gui pi tang) with the addition of Donkey-hide Gelatin (Equus asinus, called E jiao) is used when there is both Qi and Blood Deficiency, with paleness, poor memory, insomnia and a tendency towards low blood sugar.

Dang Gui and Gelatin Combination (Jiao ai tang) is especially used to stop menstrual bleeding and to prevent miscarriage (This is available as a patent formula from Chinese pharmacies in a modified form as Tang Kwei Gin)

Blood Heat: use a combination of Agrimony (Xian He Cao) and Tienchi Ginseng. This simple two-herb combination is also effective for excessive bleeding caused by Qi Deficiency.

Functional uterine bleeding associated with menopause: use either Dang Gui Four Combination (Si wu tang) or Agrimony (Xian He Cao) and Tienchi Ginseng along with herbs for the Kidney such as Dipsacus (Xu Duan), Cuscuta (Tu Si Zi), Lycii berries (Gou Qi Zi) and both Prepared Rehmannia (Shu Di Huang) and Unprepared Rehmannia (Sheng Di Huang).

INFERTILITY

1. Deficient Liver and Kidney Type: use the Five Seeds of Creation Formula (Wu zi wan).
2. Blood Stagnation associated with endometriosis: use Dang Gui Four (Si wu tang) with Blood and Qi moving herbs such as Cyperus (Xiang Fu), Corydalis (Yan Hu Suo) and Leonurus (Yi Mu Cao).
3. Stagnation of Blood, ovaritis, endometritis or malposition of the uterus: Cinnamon and Poria Combination (Gui zhi fu ling wan).
3. Excessive Dampness and Heat: For infertility associated with obesity in women use: Gentiana Combination (Long dan xie gan tang) or Citrus and Pinellia Combination (Er chen tang) together with Dang Gui Four (Si wu tang) if there is Blood Deficiency.
4. Yin Deficiency: Rehmannia Six Combination (Liu wei di huang wan) or Achyranthes and Rehmannia Combination (Restore the Left Pill: Zuo gui wan) are used with accompanying symptoms of night sweats, insomnia, thirst and dryness with either uterine bleeding or amenorrhea. One should be careful to not give these formulas if there is associated Dampness.
5. Yang Deficiency: Eucommia and Rehmannia Combination (Restore the Right: You gui wan) is used when there are accompanying symptoms of coldness, weakness and spontaneous perspiration.

6. Cold Stagnation in the meridians: Dang Gui and Evodia Combination (Wen jing tang) is used when there are symptoms of irregular menstruation caused by Coldness and Deficiency.
7. Deficient Blood: Use Dang Gui and Peony Combination (Dang gui shao yao tang) if infertility is caused by anemia and/or defective uterine development.

MISCARRIAGE

1. Deficient Kidney Yang: Associated with weakness of the Belt (Dai Mo) or Chong (Chong Mo) extra meridians. Use Rehmannia Eight Combination (Ba wei di huang wan) for Deficient Kidney Yang with the addition of Cuscuta (Tu Si Zi), Dipsacus (Xu Duan), Eucommia (Du Zhong), Lycii berries (Gou Qi Zi), Ligustrum (Nu Zhen Zi) and sometimes Prepared Aconite (Fu Zi).
2. Deficient Yin: Rehmannia Six Combination (Liu wei di huang wan).
3. Cold Deficiency: Dang Gui and Evodia Combination (Wen jing tang).
4. Qi and Blood Deficiency: Threatened Abortion Powder (Tai shan pan shi san) or Dang Gui and Peony Combination (Dang gui shao yao san) can be taken throughout pregnancy if in previous pregnancies there has been a tendency to miscarriage.

ABNORMAL LABOR

1. To hasten delivery: Ephedra Combination (Ma huang tang) with 1 gram of Aconite is taken.
2. Weakness from prolonged labor: Ginseng tea is given if a woman has lost her amniotic fluid and is nearing delivery.
3. To Strengthen Contractions: Use Dang Gui and Peony Combination (Dang gui shao yao san). This formula can be taken daily throughout pregnancy if needed.

MASTITIS

1. Fire in the Liver Meridian: Considered the primary cause of mastitis, and the most representative formula for this condition is Antiseptic Decoction with Five Ingredients (Wu wei xiao du yin) with Trichosanthes peel (Gua Lou Pi), Fritillary bulb (Bei Mu) and Moutan Peony (Mu Dan Pi).
2. Acute mastitis during the early stage: Pueraria Combination (Ge gen tang) with Gypsum (Shi Gao) can be taken.

3. Anti-inflammatory for the mammary glands: Coptis, Scute and Pueraria Combination (Ge gen huang lian huang qin tang) with Dandelion root is effective.

INSUFFICIENT LACTATION
Pueraria Combination (Ge gen tang) is given.

Fennel seed, Dandelion root and Borage, either singly or together in formula, will increase lactation. To make the milk richer, use Marshmallow root.

MORNING SICKNESS
1. Dampness and Phlegm: Minor Pinellia and Poria Combination (Xiao ban xia jia fu ling taxng) is commonly used to relieve nausea, vomiting and stomach upset. This is effective both alone or with fresh Ginger tea.
2. Spleen Qi weakness: Six Major Herbs with Saussurea and Cardamon (Xiang sha liu jun zi tang) (see Liu Jun zi tang) is used when there is associated abdominal pains, nausea, diarrhea, loss of appetite, thin body, pale tongue with a white coat, and a thready and weak pulse. If there is associated Coldness add Dry Ginger (Gan Jiang). If there is a tendency towards Heat add Black Bamboo shavings (Zhu Ru).

Apply a Mustard seed poultice to the abdomen during the early stages of pregnancy to stop nausea and vomiting. Take a mixture of one part powdered Coriander seeds (Dhanya) and four parts of sugar with rice water.

CHANGE OF LIFE (CLIMACTERIC)
Menopausal symptoms such as hot flashes, nervousness, palpitations, moodiness and insomnia are primarily caused by Deficient Kidney Yin and/or Liver Qi Stagnation.

Formulas to consider are:
1. Kidney Yin Deficiency: Rehmannia Six (Liu wei di huang wan) can be effective either alone or together with Lycii bark (Di Gu Pi), Cynanchum (Bai Wei), Ligustrum fruit (Nu Zhen Zi), Unprepared Rehmannia (Sheng Di Huang) and Angelica sinensis (Dang Gui).
2. Liver Qi Stagnation: Bupleurum and Peony Combination (Xiao yao wan) is used.

UTERINE PROLAPSE

This is usually caused by Qi Deficiency and the representative formula to consider is Ginseng and Astragalus Combination (Bu zhong yi qi tang) with high doses of Astragalus root (up to 30 grams daily) and 35 gms of Bitter Orange (Zhi Ke).

Much contemporary Chinese research has substantiated Bitter Orange (Zhi Ke: Citrus aurantium) as being highly effective for prolapsed uterus, rectum or stomach.

FIBROIDS AND CYSTS

1. Blood and Fluid Stagnation: Cinnamon and Poria Combination (Gui zhi fu ling wan) is used for lumps in the lower pelvic cavity. However, this formula is stronger when Squama Manitis (Anteater scales: Chuan Shan Jia), Zedoaria (E Zhu) and Vaccaria seed (Wang Bu Liu Xing) are added to remove Blood Stagnation, and Liquidambar (Su He Xiang), Trichosanthes fruit (Gua Lou) and Fritillary (Chuan Bei Mu) are included to remove Phlegm Stagnation.

Vitex agnus castus is considered essential in Western herbalism for the treatment of fibroids and cysts. It can be accompanied with 20 minute topical applications daily of warm castor oil compresses and a heating pad.

THE MALE REPRODUCTIVE SYSTEM

IMPOTENCE

Impotence is usually caused by Kidney Yang Deficiency. If impotence follows an operation on the prostate or colon it can be caused by Blood stagnation.

1. Blood Deficiency and Stagnation: Use Blood moving formulas such as Dang Gui Four Combination (Si wu tang) with Zedoaria (E Zhu), Carthamus (Hong Hua), Vaccaria seeds (Wang Bu Liu Xing) and Achyranthes (Niu Xi).
2. Yang Deficiency: Use Rehmannia Eight Combination (Ba wei di huang wan) when there is Yang Deficiency or Eucommia and Rehmannia Combination (Restore the Right: You gui wan) when there is Yang Deficiency with accompanying symptoms of Coldness, weakness and spontaneous perspiration.
3. Yin Deficiency: Rehmannia Six (Liu wei di huang wan) or Achyranthes and Rehmannia Combination (Restore the Left Pill: Zuo gui wan) are used when impotence and/or infertility is

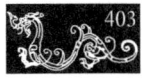

associated with Yin Deficient symptoms such as night sweats, insomnia, thirst, and dryness.

The East Indian herb, Ashwagandha (Withania somnifera), is effective and can be taken for impotence in doses of one teaspoon mixed with honey 3 times daily.

PREMATURE EJACULATION

Pills for Spermatorrhea (Jin suo gu jing wan: Lotus Stamen Formula) is used for spermatorrhea and premature ejaculation. It is available as a patent formula in pill form.

1. Yang Deficiency: Use Eucommia and Rehmannia Combination (Restore the Right: You gui wan) if there is accompanying Coldness and weakness. Use Rehmannia Eight (Ba wei di huang wan) when there are symptoms of Kidney Yang Deficiency with possible lower back aching and joint pains.

Again, the East Indian herb, Ashwagandha (Withania somnifera) is effective and can be taken in doses of one teaspoon mixed with honey 3 times daily.

ORCHITIS (INFLAMMATION OF THE TESTICLES)

Coptis and Scutellaria Combination (Huang lian jie du tang) is taken for all infections and inflammations and is effective for this condition.

One can also take a mixture of Echinacea, Goldenseal and Garlic, taken as a powder or alcoholic extract every two or three hours and diminishing the dosage as symptoms subside.

In India, Gotu Kola (Hydrocotyle asiatica) oil is applied directly to the scrotum. This is easily made by lightly heating an ounce of the leaves with sesame oil over a low flame for a few minutes. Allow it to stand and cool. Then strain for use. At the same time, mix a teaspoon of powdered Gotu Kola with honey and take internally three times daily.

SPERMATORRHEA (GLEET OR PENILE DISCHARGE)

1. Kidney Yang Deficiency: Pills for Spermatorrhea (Jin suo gu jing wan: Lotus Stamen Formula) is a patent formula for spermatorrhea and premature ejaculation. Eucommia and Rehmannia Combination (Restore the Right: You gui wan) is also used for spermatorrhea caused by Kidney Yang Deficiency.
2. Yin Deficiency: Achyranthes and Rehmannia Combination (Restore the Left Pill: Zuo gui wan) is used when there is acute inflammation and possible symptoms of night sweats, insomnia, thirst and dryness.

Anemarrhena and Phellodendron Combination (Zhi bai di huang wan) can also be considered for Kidney Yin Deficiency with Fire (inflammation).
3. Damp Heat: Gentiana Combination (Long dan xie gan tang) is indicated when there is a yellowish discharge.

Echinacea, Golden Seal, Chaparral and Garlic tincture is taken three or four times daily or a powder of the dried herbs is taken in a dose of two 'OO' sized capsules three or four times daily with a tea of Yellow Dock and Dandelion root. This is especially indicated if the discharge is yellowish.

In India, a tea comprised of one teaspoon each of Ginger, Turmeric and unrefined sugar is taken three times daily. Saffron cooked ghee (clarified butter) can be taken three times a day for three days. The mucilage of the seeds of Sacred Basil (Tulasi) can be taken in teaspoonful doses three times a day.

PROSTATE PROBLEMS

Many men nearing the age of 50 experience a tendency towards prostate enlargement. This is usually caused by Kidney Deficiency, for which one might choose either Rehmannia Six Combination (Liu wei di huang wan) if there is Kidney Yin Deficiency, or Rehmannia Eight Combination (Ba wei di huang wan) if there is Kidney Yang Deficiency. In addition one would consider adding Blood moving herbs such as Salvia (Dan Shen), Ligusticum (Chuan Xiong), Red Peony (Chi Shao Yao), Zedoaria (E Zhu), Carthamus (Hong Hua), Vaccaria seeds (Wang Bu Liu Xing) and Achyranthes (Niu Xi). If urine is slow or incomplete, add diuretics such as Alisma (Ze Xie) or Poria (Fu Ling). To soften and reduce swellings, add Sargassum (Hai Zao) and Kelp (Kun Bu).

Another cause is inflammation and Dampness in the Liver and Urinary Bladder meridians, for which Gentiana Combination (Long dan xie gan tang) can be used. Additionally, another combination of herbs that is effective consists of Phellodendron, Scutellaria, Dandelion, Talcum, Akebia and Capillaris.

The Chinese patent pills, called "Kit Kat Pills", are effective for many men suffering from enlarged prostate with a tendency towards frequent urination. A benign enlarged prostate is treated with Saw Palmetto berries (Serenoa), two '00' capsules of the powdered berries three times daily.

NEUROLOGICAL, MENTAL AND EMOTIONAL PROBLEMS

HEADACHES, INCLUDING MIGRAINE HEADACHES

Headaches are usually a primary indicator of an imbalanced diet, lifestyle, weather and other External Influences as well as various Internal causes such as an imbalance of the emotions. Chronically recurring headaches such as migraines, while directly affected by stress and dietary factors, are more immediately the result of Internal circulatory, metabolic and neurological imbalances. The characteristic sensation of flashes of light, distorted vision and other symptoms associated with migraine headaches are caused by the constriction of blood vessels in the cerebrum. Migraines tend to run in the family, especially with women between the ages of ten and thirty. These headaches tend to recede after the age of fifty in most individuals.

TCM designates four different types of headaches.
1. Forehead or frontal headache is described as a Yang Ming headache and involves the Stomach and Intestines.
2. Vertex headache is caused by the Liver.
3. A headache at the temples is caused by the Gallbladder.
4. Occipital headache at the back of the head and neck involves the Urinary Bladder meridian.

Some of the most important single herbs for headaches that may be added to the following formulas are Ligusticum wallichii (Chuan Xiong), Angelica dahurica (Bai Zhi), and Ligusticum sinense (Gao Ben).

1. External or acute headaches:

    a. Cnidium and Green Tea Combination (Chuan xiong cha tiao san) is the indicated formula for headaches (bilateral, frontal, occipital, vertical and migraine) caused by Wind (tension and spasms), with possible symptoms of vertigo, chills, fever and nasal congestion.

    b. Evodia Combination (Wu zhu yu tang) is used for headaches caused by Wind, Cold and Damp but with more Liver and Stomach involvement than the previous.

    c. Chianghuo and Turmeric Combination (Chuan bi tang) is used to treat headaches caused by Wind, Cold and Dampness and is antirheumatic, suggesting that it is more involved with blocked meridians.

2. Headaches caused by Internal, chronic conditions:
   d. Gastrodia and Uncaria Combination (Tian ma gou teng yin) is used for headaches caused by Internal Liver Wind (hypertension).
   e. Replenishing the Yang (You gui wan) is used for headaches caused by Deficient Kidneys (low adrenals).
   f. Eight Precious Herbs (Ba zhen tang) is indicated for headaches caused by Deficient Qi and Blood.

STRESS, ANXIETY, HYSTERIA AND INSOMNIA

Most emotional conditions are regarded as Heart and Liver system disorders. The Heart is considered the home of the spirit. Various Heart imbalances such as Heart Fire, Heart Yin Deficiency and Heart Blood Deficiency can cause panic attacks, hysteria, restlessness, impatience and insomnia.

Liver Qi Stagnation is another major cause of emotional feelings such as frustration, stressful feelings and depression. Liver Qi Stagnation can affect the Heart and Stomach and further give rise to GI tract disturbances with anxiety type problems.

Tranquilizing sedative: Licorice, Sprouted Wheat and Jujube Date Decoction (Gan mai da zao tang) has antispasmodic and Spleen tonifying properties. It can be used by itself or added to any formula when there are symptoms of stress, anxiety, mania, insomnia and convulsions. To increase its sedative action, add Jujube seeds (Suan Zao Ren), Biota seeds (Bai Zi Ren), Poria (especially the part that attaches to the tree and is called "Fu Shen") and Albizzia flower (He Huan Hua).

Liver Blood Deficiency with Liver Heat: Zizyphus Combination (Suan zao ren tang) is indicated for insomnia, especially when one awakens soon after going to sleep, and nervousness. It is particularly useful for symptoms of frustration, anxiety and nervousness. The addition of Dragon's Teeth (Stegodon orientalis, called "Long Chi"), which are the ossified teeth of prehistoric mammals, and Oyster shell (Mu Li), increases the effectiveness of these and any other formulas for treating palpitations and insomnia.

Liver Fire uprising: Gentiana Combination (Long dan xie gan tang) is for insomnia with symptoms of hypertension, headache, anger, restless nervousness, feeling of fullness or pain in the chest.

Heat and mucus: Bamboo and Poria Combination (Wen dan tang) is for insomnia with symptoms of restlessness, palpitations, dizziness, nausea, profuse white sputum and timidity.

Heart and Kidney Yin Deficiency: Ginseng and Zizyphus Combination (Tian wang bu xin tang) is indicated for insomnia caused by over-work and excess study. Symptoms include forgetfulness, restlessness, fatigue, nocturnal emission and dry stool. Because this formula contains Cinnabar, it should only be taken for 2 weeks at a time followed by a 2 week break before resuming.

Neurosis, hysteria, mania, fearfulness, melancholy: Bupleurum and Dragon Bone Combination (Chai hu jia long gu mu li tang) is indicated for insomnia, palpitations, neurotic impotence, hypertension, angina pectoris, epilepsy, convulsions and alopecia (caused by worry and stress).

Fire of the Heart: Cinnabar Sedative Pills (Zhu sha an shen wan) is an available patent formula used to relieve many problems associated with mental derangement, including nervousness, insomnia, forgetfulness, palpitations, shortness of breath, anxiety and hysteria. Since Cinnabar is mildly toxic, this preparation should only be taken for short periods of one or two weeks at a time.

Deficiency of Qi and Blood of the Spleen and Heart: Ginseng and Longan Berries Combination (Gui pi tang) is indicated for nervousness, insomnia, forgetfulness, nightmares, palpitations and fatigue, especially mental fatigue resulting from low blood sugar.

A wide variety of mental and neurological symptoms: Bupleurum and Cinnamon Combination (Chai hu gui zhi tang), is the most versatile of all Chinese formulas, here useful for neurosis, nervous exhaustion, irritability, insomnia, premenstrual syndrome, hysteria, epilepsy and heart problems.

The primary herbs that are currently available and used by Western herbalists for stress-related mental problems are: Skullcap (Scutellaria lateriflora), particularly for alcohol and drug withdrawal, because it also has detoxifying properties and is more useful for Liver Heat; Valerian officinalis as a mild hypnotic and sedative for insomnia and nervousness. It is more indicated for Cold conditions. Others are Passion Flower (Passiflora incarnata) primarily used for insomnia; Hops (Humulus lupulus) for insomnia especially, when it is caused by digestive disturbance and as a digestive bitter; Chamomile (Matricaria chamomila) has a calming effect because it seems to powerfully nourish the myelin sheath of the nerves much like calcium and magnesium. It can be used when one has a tendency towards tearfulness; and Poppy (different varieties) has a mild analgesic property and is also useful for insomnia. Usually various combinations of any of the above herbs can have greater effectiveness than the use of a single herb. The addition of American Ginseng is also calming and strengthening to the nervous system.

Ayurvedic herbs useful for stress, anxiety, hysteria and insomnia include: Nardostachys jatamamsi (Jatamamsi), an Indian species of Valerian. It has a mildly sedative effect but does not have such a strong drug-like effect as Western Valerian (Valeriana officinalis); Calamus root (Acorus calamus), also called Sweet Flag (Sanskrit: "vacha"), has the properties of increasing one's focus and concentration. It can be taken internally as a powder, about 1 quarter to a half teaspoon mixed with honey. It is also good to accompany it with an exclusive diet of rice and warm milk for a period of 10 days. This will enhance its centering effects by promoting detoxification. This herb is regularly taken in India to help overcome the effects of marijuana. In fact, many who use marijuana (Cannabis sativa) combine calamus with it. Asafoetida (Sanskrit: Hing or Chinese: E wei) is a common Ayurvedic resin that was also used for hysteria both in India and in the West. One preparation is to combine it with the gel of Aloe barbadensis (Kumari), taking a teaspoon of the preparation three times daily. Asafoetida is also efficacious when it is made into an emulsion of 30 grains of the gum in 4 oz of water and injected as a rectal enema.

In India Brahmi is a specific remedy for all mental conditions, including its use as an aid to increase memory. There are actually two species that are called Brahmi. The more common one is Gotu Kola (Centella asiatica or Hydrocotyle asiatica) while the other is Bacopa monierri, a semi-aquatic plant which is generally regarded as the more efficacious of the two Brahmis for mental conditions.

Either herb can be used internally, approximately one teaspoon of the powdered herb mixed with honey taken three times daily. A formula with broader action is the combination of Brahmi (either variety), Calamus root (Acorus calamus), Indian Valerian (Nardostachys jatamamsi) and Ashwagandha (Withania somnifera). A teaspoon of a combination of the powdered herbs is similarly taken three times daily mixed with honey and ghee.

A very effective therapy used in Ayurvedic medicine to treat all nervous conditions is called Shira Basti. This is a technique of applying warm Brahmi oil directly to the head. Various methods can be used, ranging from simply massaging the oil into the scalp a half hour or so before showering, to slowly dripping the oil directly onto the forehead for 1/2 to 1 hour. This latter method must be applied by a provider who is trained in the technique of Ayurvedic Panchakarma. The combination of Gotu Kola and sesame oil is specifically beneficial for all mental, emotional and stress related problems, including neurosis, schizophrenia, anxiety, insomnia and so forth. The method of making a quart of Brahmi oil is to simmer 4 ounces of dried Brahmi in a quart of sesame oil and a half quart of water. Allow it to continue simmering until only the sesame oil remains. Strain and bottle for use.

MEMORY WEAKNESS, INCLUDING SENILE AND PRE-SENILE DEMENTIA

Caused by Kidney Deficiency: Rehmannia Eight Combination (Ba wei di huang wan) is commonly indicated since the condition is usually caused by a degeneration of Kidney and Liver function. Herbs that are useful to add for the mind include Polygala (Yuan Zhi) for poor memory, He Shou Wou (Polygonum multiflorum) which is anti-aging in general and useful for strengthening the brain and memory, Lycii fruit (Gou Qi Zi) and Deer Antler (Lu Rong), both of which are beneficial for the brain.

Other formulas to consider are: Heart Yin and Blood Deficiency: Cinnabar Sedative Combination (Zhu sha an shen wan) tranquilizes the mind, calms the emotions and clears Heat from the Heart.

Heart Blood and Yin Deficiency: Ginseng and Zizyphus Combination (Tian wang bu xin tang) is especially useful for brain fatigue.

Western herbalism routinely uses Ginkgo biloba, especially in a 24:1 extract, to improve vascular circulation to the brain. The Indian combination of equal parts Brahmi (especially Bacopa monnieri), Calamus root (Acorus calamus), Indian Valerian (Nardostachys) and Ashwagandha (Withania somnifera) is effective for improving all mental functions. Grind the herbs to a fine powder and mix with ghee. Take one teaspoon three times daily.

DEPRESSION, MANIA AND SCHIZOPHRENIA

1. Excess type:

    A. Internal Heat: Coptis and Scutellaria Combination (Huang lian jie du tang) is for manic conditions.

    B. Obese and somewhat constipated conditions: Major Rhubarb Combination (Da cheng qi tang) is for depressed, manic individuals.

    C. Stagnant Liver Qi and premenstrual and change of life cycles in women: Bupleurum and Dang Gui Formula (Xiao yao san or Rambling Powder).

    D. Stagnant Qi and Phlegm: Pinellia and Magnolia Combination (Ban xia hou po tang) or Bamboo and Poria Combination (Wen dan tang) are indicated.

2. Deficient Type:

A. Deficient Qi and Blood: Ginseng and Longan Combination (Gui pi tang) is for individuals with hypoglycemia with weak digestion.

B. Spleen Deficiency: Licorice, Sprouted Wheat and Jujube Date Decoction (Gan mai da zao tang) is for mania and depression associated with forgetfulness and hysteria.

C. Caused by restless spirit with Stomach Heat: Dragon Bone and Oyster Shell Combination (Long gu mu li tang) is a tonic sedative and tranquilizer, and relieves acid stomach.

For conditions associated with Heat (the more usual type), use equal parts powdered Gotu Kola (Hydrocotyle asiatica), Calamus (Acorus calamus), Asafoetida (E wei) and Nardostachys jatamamsi mixed into a pill mass with a combination of 2 parts ghee and 1 part honey. This should be taken 3 times daily.

JOINT AND NERVE DISORDERS

BACK PAIN AND SCIATICA

1. Wind Cold Damp Stagnation: Du Huo and Loranthes Combination (Du huo ji sheng tang) for back pain with symptoms of Coldness in the lower back, pain radiating down the spine and legs, a general aversion to coldness, pale tongue with a thin coat and a floating and tight pulse.
2. Kidney Deficiency: Symptoms include lower back ache, pain that is relieved with pressure massage, weakness extending to the lower legs, worse after exertion, better with rest, chronic and recurring. Differentiate between Kidney Yin and Kidney Yang related back pain.

    a. Kidney Yin Deficiency: This complex displays Yin Deficient signs of restlessness, anxiety, insomnia, thirst, dry throat, flushed complexion, feeling of heat on the palms and soles of the feet, night sweats, afternoon fever, shiny red tongue and a rapid and thin pulse. Use Rehmannia Six Combination (Liu wei di huang wan), Anemarrhena, Phellodendron and Rehmannia Combination (Zhi bai di huang wan) or Achyranthes and Rehmannia Combination (Restore the Left Pill: Zuo gui wan).

    b. Kidney Yang Deficiency: Symptoms include general Kidney Deficiency with pale complexion, cold extremities and low libido, pale tongue and a thin and deep pulse. Rehmannia Eight Combination (Ba wei di huang wan), Eucommia and Rehmannia Combination (Restore the Right: You gui wan), or Blue Fairy Pills for Lower Back Pain (Qing e wan) can be considered.

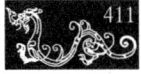

3. Blood and Kidney Deficiency: Use Blood Replenishing Decoction (Ji chuan jian).
4. Damp Spleen back pain: For symptoms of Dampness with a feeling of drawing in the lower back, pale complexion, lack of appetite, loose stool, greasy white coated tongue and a slippery and soft pulse, use Magnolia and Ginger Formula (Ping wei san) or Stephania and Astragalus Combination (Fang qi huang qi tang).
5. Liver Qi Stagnation back pain: With symptoms of lumbar pain radiating from the back to the hypochondriac and abdominal area, difficulty standing for a long period, a red tongue and wiry and thin pulse, use Lindera Formula for Regulating Qi (Wu yao shun qi wan).
6. Damp Heat back pain: With accompanying symptoms of knee and lower back pain, dark colored urine, a greasy tongue with a yellow coat and a soft and rapid pulse, use Two Effective Ingredients (Er Miao San).

NECK PAIN AND NEURALGIA
1. Caused by External Cold factors: Use Pueraria Combination (Ge gen tang) or Cinnamon Combination (Gui zhi tang) with Pueraria.
2. Caused by inflammation: Use Coptis, Scute and Pueraria Combination (Ge gen huang qin huang lian tang).

OSTEOARTHRITIS AND RHEUMATIC ARTHRITIS
1. Caused by Coldness: Aconite Combination (Si ni tang) with Cinnamon twigs and Peony root.
2. Fixed pains: Chianghuo and Turmeric Combination (Chuan bi tang).
3. Migratory pains: Cinnamon Twig, Paeonia and Anemarrhena Decoction (Gui zhi shao yao zhi mu tang).
4. Caused by Heat: Two Effective Ingredients (Er miao san).
5. Chronic and rheumatoid arthritis: Du huo and Loranthes Combination (Du huo ji sheng tang).
6. Caused by Dampness: Ma Huang and Coix Combination (Ma xing yi gan tang) or Coix combination (Yi yi ren tang).

MUSCULAR ATROPHY
Muscular atrophy, or "wei syndrome", displays symptoms of muscular weakness and motor impairment and, in advanced stages, paralysis. These include various pathogenic conditions such as multiple

sclerosis, muscular dystrophy, myotonic syndromes, myasthenia gravis, endocrine myopathies, periodic paralysis and hysterical paralysis.
1. Caused by weakness of Spleen and Stomach Qi: Use Ginseng and Dang Gui Ten combination (Shi quan da bu tang) or Ginseng and Longan Combination (Gui pi tang).
2. Caused by Internal Wind: Big Pearl for Internal Wind (Da ding feng zhu).
3. Caused by Liver and Kidney Deficiency: Rehmannia Six Combination (Liu wei di huang wan) for Kidney and Liver Yin Deficiency or Rehmannia Eight Combination (Ba wei di huang wan) for Kidney Yang Deficiency.
4. Caused by Heat and Dampness: Coix Combination (Yi yi ren tang).

EPILEPSY

Epilepsy is a nervous system disease where the patient is periodically seized by a sudden loss of consciousness or acute spasms. It is potentially dangerous because the patient may experience a sudden fall with frothing at the mouth, eyes turned upward, spasms and convulsions of the limbs and epileptic screams. It is a recurring symptom, with the patient feeling afterwards as if they had awakened exhausted from sleep. The attacks can last anywhere from a few seconds to a few minutes. Western medicine classifies primary epilepsy as being of hereditary origin while secondary epilepsy is the result of cerebral trauma.

TCM considers epilepsy a condition of Internal Liver Wind and Dampness. It can be triggered by stress, dietary or hereditary factors, or by an obstruction of turbid Phlegm. Epilepsy involves the Liver, Spleen and Kidney systems which ultimately affect the Heart, resulting in seizures.

Under emotional stress, the Liver and Kidneys can be acutely depleted, resulting in Yin Deficiency. Yin is therefore unable to control Yang with the result of Stagnation of Heat with Internal Wind. This in turn congeals Bodily Fluids to a further degree of Wind and Phlegm, causing an obstruction of the nervous system.

Epilepsy can also be triggered by imbalanced dietary influences that injure the Spleen and Stomach and result in turbid Phlegm and Wind. When Phlegm Stagnates in the Internal Organs, an internal tension or spasms occur, called Internal Wind which rises and obstructs the Heart. The result is the sudden loss of consciousness characterized by the disease.

The treatment approach involves tonifying the Liver, Kidneys and Spleen and clearing Stagnant Liver Qi, Internal Wind and Phlegm.

Use Bupleurum and Peony Combination (Xiao yao wan) or the appropriate formula listed below with the addition of Pinellia (Ban Xia), Arisaema (Tian Nan Xing), Polygala (Yuan Zhi), Bamboo skin (Zhu Ru), Oyster shell (Mu Li), Smilax (Tu Fu Ling) and Acorus (Chang Pu) as indicated by the symptoms.
1. Deficient Liver and Kidney Yin: Achyranthes and Rehmannia Combination (Restore the Left Pill: Zuo gui wan).
2. Deficient Spleen and Stomach: Six Major Herbs (Liu jun zi tang).
3. Liver Fire with Damp Heat: Gentiana Combination (Long dan xie gan tang), with the addition of 3 gms of Polygala (Yuan Zhi) and 6 gms of Acorus (Chang Pu).

INJURIES

TRAUMATIC INJURY INCLUDING WOUNDS, BURNS AND CUTS

External Application: Bruise Relieving Powder (Qi li san).
Internal use: Remove Blood Stagnation in the Chest Decoction (Xue fu zhu yu tang).

In general, medicated oils are used for bruises that break the skin while alcoholic liniments are applied on those that do not. Liniments and medicated oils are superior to the application of cold packs to injuries and bruises because they are anti-inflammatory and disperse Blood without impairing the body's healing capacity. They should be rubbed on liberally. Another method is to use a soft cloth saturated with the oil or liniment, and apply it topically over the affected area for a period of an hour or two.

To make a medicated oil, simmer a combination of Calamus root (Shi Chang Pu), Tienchi Ginseng (Tian Qi), Gardenia fruit (Zhi Zi), Rhubarb root (Da Huang), Ligusticum root (Chuan Xiong) and Safflower (Hong Hua) in water until most of the water is evaporated, strain and add sesame oil. Continue simmering until all the water is evaporated.

To make an alcoholic liniment, use either alcohol or pure grain turpentine. Macerate a combination of the same herbs with Myrrh (Mo Yao), Calamus (Shi Chang Pu), Tienchi Ginseng (Tian Qi), Ligusticum (Chuan Xiong), Rhubarb root (Da Huang), and Safflower (Hong Hua) in the alcohol or turpentine. Cover the herbs completely with approximately one or two inches of the liquid above the top of the herbs. This can stand for anywhere from 2 weeks to 6 months before straining through a cloth. To make the alcohol or turpentine liniment

more cooling, add Menthol, Wintergreen, and Camphor oils. To make it more heating, add Cinnamon oil.

Two simple oils can be made by using either or both grated Garlic and Ginger in sesame or olive oil. Further, the same two substances can be added to either rubbing alcohol or apple cider vinegar to make a liniment.

THE SKIN

ECZEMA, DERMATITIS, PRURITIS, ACNE, ERYSIPELAS AND PSORIASIS

Dermatitis includes a wide range of skin conditions with symptoms of reddening, oozing and dry scaling skin. Eczema is a chronic form of this disease. It may involve problems of Qi, Blood, Lungs, Large Intestines, Spleen, Stomach, Kidneys and Heart. In later stages there is usually Blood Stagnation, which makes the condition more difficult to cure.

External causes of skin disease are Wind, Cold, Dampness or Heat that cause a disharmony of Lung and Wei (immune) Qi.

Stagnated Stomach and Intestinal Heat is the result of overindulgence in fatty and heating foods such as fatty meat, oily foods, sugar, alcohol and spices. Shellfish, which has a Cold, Damp energy, can also stagnate the GI tract and eventually generates Heat Stagnation. Dampness is always a result of impaired digestion and injury of the Spleen and Stomach function that in turn injures the Lungs, which govern the skin.

Blood Heat is the result of excess stress that overtaxes Kidney Qi and ultimately causes Deficiency. As a result, the Heart (emotions and vessels) are adversely affected. The Evil Qi floats to the surface, affecting the skin.

Deficiency of Qi and Blood results in poor nourishment and assimilation that affects the skin.

1. Caused by External Wind:

   a. Wind-Cold: With symptoms of pale, whitish skin eruptions, adversely effected by Wind and Coldness, thin, white tongue coat, floating and slow or tight pulse. Schizonepeta and Ledebouriella Combination (Jing fang bai du san) or Cinnamon Combination (Gui zhi tang).

   b. Wind- Heat: With symptoms of eruptions all over the body, including the face and hands, with feelings of heat, itching, edema, suppurating, swelling, worse at night, thin, greasy tongue coat and either a floating or a floating slow pulse (especially occurring with

young children). Use Bupleurum and Schizonepeta Formula (Shih wei pai tu tang) or Ledebouriella and Platycodon Formula (Fang feng tung sheng).
2. Caused by Damp Heat: Two Effective Ingredients (Er miao san).
3. Liver Fire: Gentiana Combination (Long dan xie gan tang).
4. Stagnant Heat of the Heart and Lungs: Ginseng and Zizyphus Combination (Tian wang bu xin tang: Emperor of Heaven's Tonic Pill for the Mind).
5. Deficient Qi and Blood: Eight Precious Herbs (Ba zhen tang) or Ginseng and Dang Gui Ten Combination (Shi quan da bu tang).

FROSTBITE

Use Cinnamon Combination (Gui zhi tang) for frostbite or cold extremities. Use Dang Gui and Jujube Combination (Dang gui si ni tang) when there is Blood Deficiency and impaired circulation to the extremities.

HERPES SIMPLEX AND HERPES ZOSTER (SHINGLES)

Herpes simplex is a recurrent viral infection that appears as small fever blisters, cold sores or multiple inflamed vesicles on the mucus membranes of the lips, mouth or genital area. There are two types: 1) Heat in the Blood and 2) Damp Heat in the Liver meridian.

Anti-viral herbs, such as Isatis root and leaf (Ban Lan Gen and Da Qing Ye), Polygala (Yuan Zhi) and Dandelion (Pu Gong Ying) can be used. To reduce Heat in the Blood, use Moutan (Mu Dan Pi), Scrophularia (Xuan Shen) and Unprepared Rehmannia (Sheng Di Huang).
Formulas:
Gentiana Combination (Long dan xie gan tang), Bupleurum and Schizonepeta Formula (Shih wei pai tu tang), Lonicera and Forsythia Combination (Yin qiao san) and Morus and Chrysanthemum Combination (Sang ju yin).

TINEA PEDIS (ATHLETE'S FOOT) AND FUNGUS INFECTIONS

This is a Damp-Heat condition: Use Two Effective Ingredients (Er Miao San) or Gentiana Combination (Long dan xie gan tang). Topically, apply Garlic and olive oil, Tea Tree oil or Bloodroot tincture (Sanguinaria canadensis).

ALOPECIA (BALDNESS)

TCM generally considers alopecia a condition of Blood Stagnation. Often it can begin with nervousness that Stagnates the Qi and later evolves into Blood Stagnation and hair loss.

Blood and Qi Stagnation: Salvia Root Decoction (Dan shen yin). Blood Deficiency: add Dang Gui (Angelica sinensis) and Prepared Rehmannia (Shu Di Huang) to the above formula.
Other formulas to consider are:
Rehmannia Six Combination (Liu wei di huang wan), Achyranthes and Rehmannia Combination (Restore the Left Pill or Zuo gui wan) and Dang Gui Four (Si wu tang). These are all useful because the first two serve as Yin tonics while the latter is a Blood tonic.

FURUNCLE AND CARBUNCLE

A furuncle is a pyogenic (pus) infection that forms around a hair follicle and its sebaceous gland and spreads to the subcutaneous tissue. A carbuncle is a more serious purulent infection that is deeper and larger than a furuncle. Both are conditions associated with toxic Damp Heat and can be treated with either of the following: Bupleurum and Schizonepeta Formula (Shi wei bai du tang) or Coptis and Scutellaria Combination (Huang lian jie du tang).

ORAL CAVITY

Usually conditions affecting the gums and mouth are caused by Stomach Heat. Therefore the approach is to clear Internal Stomach Heat for the following:

TOOTHACHE
Coptis and Scutellaria Combination (Huang lian jie du tang).

GINGIVITIS

White Tiger Decoction (Bai hu tang) for short term relief of acute symptoms, or use a Western herbal combination of the powders of Oak bark (Quercus), Rhatany bark (Krameria triandra), Bayberry bark (Myrica cerifera), Echinacea (Echinacea species), Myrrh (Comiphora myrrha) and Hydrastis (H. canadensis). Macerate 4 ounces in a pint of water for two weeks. Strain through a cloth, add a few drops of mint oil to taste and bottle for use. Put a teaspoon of this extract in a commercial waterpick and rinse the mouth and gums twice daily.

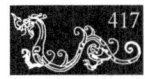

In India, individuals with spongy, ulcerated gums brush their teeth two or three times daily with a fine powder of Chebulic myrobalan (Harada). This herb is used as an astringent in TCM where it is known as "He Zi". It is available from either Chinese herb pharmacies or Indian import stores and is one of the three ingredients of Triphala. Additionally, Triphala should be taken internally, three times daily.

THE EYES

The eyes are generally governed by the Liver while the power to see relates to the Kidneys. Because of this, herbal formulas that clear Liver Heat and Kidney and Liver Yin Deficiency are used together with Heat clearing herbs.

CONJUNCTIVITIS
a. Caused by Wind-Heat: Morus and Chrysanthemum Combination (Sang ju yin).
b. Caused by Liver Fire: Gentiana Combination (Long dan xie gan tang).

CATARACTS
Caused by Deficient Kidney Essence and Heart Fire: With accompanying symptoms of nervousness, anxiety, palpitations, insomnia and blurred vision. Use Magnetite and Cinnabar Sedative (Ci zhu wan) or Lycium, Chrysanthemum and Rehmannia Combination (Qi ju di huang wan).

IMPROVING VISION
Use Improve the Vision with Rehmannia (Ming mu di huang wan). This is similar to Lycium, Chrysanthemum and Rehmannia Combination (Qi ju di huang wan) but has more Blood nourishing properties, making it more useful for strengthening eyesight.

EARS AND HEARING

Earache (Otitis Media): Earaches are usually a problem classified as Damp Heat, for which Gentiana Combination (Long dan xie gan tang) or Pueraria Combination (Ge gen tang) is used. Also, Echinacea, Golden Seal and Garlic tincture can be taken internally three or four times daily. Macerate Mullein flowers and/or Rue herb (Ruta graveolens) in olive oil and apply one or more drops in each ear to help relieve discomfort and speed recovery. Further, Garlic juice mixed with equal parts olive oil can be used as ear drops.

DEAFNESS AND TINNITIS

These are difficult diseases to cure, especially if the problem has occurred for more than a year.

1. Caused by Kidney Deficiency: With symptoms of lumbar and joint aches, dizziness, blurred vision, impotence, nocturnal emission, pale tongue with a thin coat, a deep, wiry and thready pulse. Use Magnetite and Cinnabar Sedative (Ci zhu wan) with Lycii berries (Gou Qi Zi), Ligustrum fruit (Nu Zhen Zi), Cuscuta (Tu Si Zi) and Prepared Rehmannia (Shu Di Huang) or Rehmannia Eight Combination (Ba wei di huang wan).

   2. Caused by Liver Fire: Gentiana Combination (Long dan xie gan tang).
   3. Acute syndrome caused by External Wind-Heat: With symptoms of partial hearing loss, headache, fever, aversion to cold and wind, aching joints, itching ears, thin, white tongue coat and floating pulse. Use Ledbouriella and Platycodon Formula (Fang feng tung sheng) for Excess conditions with Wind-Heat and Internal Lung Heat; Schizonepeta and Ledebouriella Combination (Jing fang bai du san) for Wind attacking the Lungs.
   4. Caused by Phlegm with symptoms of Heat and turbid Phlegm: Use Bamboo and Poria Combination (Wen dan tang) to clear Liver Fire and Phlegm, or Citrus and Pinellia Combination (Er chen tang) for Damp-Phlegm conditions.
   5. Caused by Qi Deficiency: With symptoms of fatigue, weak digestion, pale complexion, loose stool, pale tongue and thready and weak pulse. Use Ginseng and Astragalus Combination (Bu zhong yi qi tang) or Ginseng and Ginger Combination or Regulate the Middle Pill (Li zhong wan).
   6. Caused by Blood and Yin Deficiency: With symptoms of pale complexion, pale finger nails, dry tongue and thready and weak pulse. Use Eight Precious Herbs (Ba zhen tang).

PARASITES

WORMS
Coldness with Deficient Spleen Qi: Use Mume formula (Wu mei wan).

BACTERIAL AND AMEBIC DYSENTERY
Anemone Combination (Bai tou weng tang) or Coptis, Scute and Pueraria Combination (Ge gen huang qin huang lian tang).

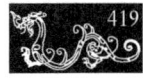

BIBLIOGRAPHY

Traditional Chinese Medicine Theory
Chen and Chen. *A Comprehensive Guide to Chinese Herbal Medicine.* Long Beach: Oriental Healing Arts (Ohai), 1992.

Chen and Chen. *Tongue Diagnosis.* Long Beach: Ohai, 1989. (One of the best books on tongue diagnosis with color plates and scientific references).

Cheung, C.S. *Treatment of Traditional Chinese Medicine.* San Francisco: Traditional Chinese Medicine Publisher, 1980.

Connelly, Diane. *Traditional Acupuncture: The Law of the Five Elements.* Maryland Center for Traditional Acupuncture, 1979.

Diagnostics of Traditional Chinese Medicine. Shandong Science and Technology Press, 1990.(an excellent reference to diagnostic principles).

Flaws, Bob. *How To Write A TCM Herbal Formula.* Boulder: Blue Poppy Press, 1993.

Flaws, Bob. *The Secret of Chinese Pulse Diagnosis.* Boulder: Blue Poppy Press, 1995.

Maciocia, Giovanni. *The Foundations of Chinese Medicine.* Edinburgh: Churchill Livingston, 1989. (the best book on Chinese medical theory).

Maciocia, Giovanni. The *Practice of Chinese Medicine.* Edinburgh: Churchill Livingston, 1994.

Kaptchuk, Ted. *The Web That Has No Weaver.* New York: Congdon and Weed, 1983. (along with *Between Heaven and Earth*, a very good introduction to the principles of Traditional Chinese medicine).

Korngold, Efrem and Harriet. *Between Heaven and Earth.* Pub. NY: Ballantine, 1991. (A highly fascinating and outstanding introduction to Traditional Chinese Medicine).

Ross, Jeremy, Zang Fu. *The Organ Systems of Traditional Chinese Medicine*, Second Edition. Edinburgh London, Melbourne and New York: Churchill Livingstone, 1985.

Ross, Jeremy. *The Organ Systems of Traditional Chinese Medicine.* Second Edition. Edinburgh: Churchill Livingstone, 1985.

Teegarden, Iona Marsaa. *The Joy of Feeling.* NY: Japan Publications, Inc., 1984.

Wicke, Roger Wm. *Traditional Chinese Herbal Science*, Vol. 1 and 2. Hot Springs, Montana: Rocky Mountain Herbal institute, 1994. (PO Box 579, Hot Springs, Montana 59845, USA).

Zhen, Li Shi. *Pulse Diagnosis*. Brookline, MA: Paradigm Publications, 1981.

Zhang Enqin, Shi Lanhua and Wang Min, *Basic Theory of Traditional Chinese Medicine Vol. 1 and 2*. Shanghai: TCM Pub. House Books, 1988.

Kanpo (Japanese Chinese Medicine)
Bulletins of the Oriental Healing Arts Institute of U.S.A. and The International Journal of Oriental Medicine. Long Beach: Oriental Healing Arts Institute, 1945. (Palo Verde Ave. Suite 208, Long Beach, California 90815. An excellent quarterly journal on Chinese Herbalism).

Hong-Yen Hsu & Preacher, William. *Chinese Herb Medicine and Therapy*. Long Beach, California: Oriental Healing Arts Institute, 1976.

Hong-Yen Hsu. *How To Treat Yourself with Chinese Herbs*, New Canaan, CT: Keats Publishing Inc, and Oriental Healing Arts Institute, Long Beach, CA, 1993.

Hyatt, Richard. *Chinese Herbal Medicine*. New York: Schocken Books, 1978. (also includes Kanpo Chinese Theory)

Food Therapy and Chinese and Macrobiotic Nutrition
Ballentine, Rudolph, MD. *Diet and Nutrition*. Honesdale, PA: Himalayan International Institute, 1978. (Includes Ayurvedic nutrition. One of the best books on holistic nutrition).

Colbin, Annemarie. *Food and Healing*. New York: Ballentine Books, 1980.

Flaws, Bob and Honore Wolfe. , *Prince Wen HuiÕs Cook: Chinese Dietary Therapy*. Brookline, MA: Paradigm Publications, 1983.

Kushi, Michio. *Book of Macrobiotics*. New York: Japan Publications, 1977.

Kushi, Michio. *Macrobiotic Diet*. New York: Japan Publications, 1985.

Kushi, Michio. *Macrobiotic Home Remedies*. New York: Japan Publications, 1985.

Kushi, Michio. *Macrobiotic-Way*. Wayne, NJ: Avery Publications, 1985.

Lu, Henry C. *Chinese System of Food Cures*. New York: Sterling Publishing Co., 1986.

Muramoto, Naboro. *Healing Ourselves*. New York: Avon Press, 1973.

Ni, Maoshing. *The Tao of Nutrition*. LA, CA: Union of Tao and Man, 1987. (117 Stonehaven Way, LA, CA 90049 USA,. An excellent book on food energetics and Chinese food therapy).

History of Chinese Medicine

Hoizey, Dominique and Marie-Joseph. *A History of Chinese Medicine*. Vancouver, BC: UBC Press, 1993.

Unschuld, Paul U. *Medicine in China: A History of Ideas*. Berkeley: University of California Press, 1985.

Unschuld, Paul U. *Medicine in China: A History of Pharmaceutics*. Berkeley: University of California Press, 1985.

Herbals and Philosophy, Ayurvedic

Lad, Dr. Vasant. *Ayurveda, the Science of Self-Healing*. Twin Lakes: Lotus Press, 1984.

Lad, Dr. Vasant & David Frawley. *The Yoga of Herbs*. Twin Lakes: Lotus Press, 1986.

NOTES

Introduction
   [1] Flaws, Bob, *Something Old, Something New,* Blue Poppy Press, Boulder, CO. 1991

Chapter 2
   [1] In Japan, there is a Buddhist monastery where the monks chant the entire Shang Han Lun formulary each morning.

GLOSSARY

TERMS OF TRADITIONAL CHINESE MEDICINE

Aromatic Stomachic: herbs which are aromatic and assist digestion by moving Dampness.

Blood: though broader in definition, it encompasses the physical blood in the body which moistens the tissues, muscles, skin and hair and nourishes cells and organs.

Blood Deficiency: a lack of blood with signs of anemia, dizziness, scanty menses or amenorrhea, thin emaciated body, spots in the visual field, impaired vision, numb arms or legs, dry skin, hair or eyes, lusterless, pale face and lips, tiredness and poor memory.

Calmative: calms the mind and nerves; for nervous disorders.

Cold, Coldness, Cold signs: lowered metabolism with symptoms of Coldness, clear to white bodily secretions, chills, body aches, poor circulation, pale complexion, lethargy, no thirst or sweating, frigidity, impotence, infertility, night time urination, frequent and copious urination, loose stools or diarrhea, undigested food in the stools, poor digestion, lack of appetite, achy pain in joints, slowness of speech, slow movements, low fever but severe chills, aversion to cold and craving for heat and hypo-conditions such as hypo-thyroidism, hypo-adrenalism and hypoglycemia.

Cools Blood: a function of herbs which clear Heat out of the Blood; symptoms include rashes, nosebleed, vomiting, spitting or coughing of blood, blood in the stool or urine, night fevers, delirium and hemorrhage.

Damp, Dampness: excessive fluids in the body with symptoms including feelings of heaviness, sluggishness, secretions that are turbid, sluggish, sinking, viscous, copious, slimy, cloudy or sticky, excessive leukorrhea, oozing, purulent skin eruptions, lassitude, edema, abdominal distention, chest fullness, nausea, vomiting, loss of appetite, lack of thirst and achy, heavy, stiff and sore joints.

Damp Heat: a condition of Dampness and Heat with symptoms of thick, greasy yellow secretions and phlegm, jaundice, hepatitis, dysentery, urinary difficulty or pain, furuncles and eczema.

Deficiency: a condition of weakness or lack of something, usually Qi, Blood, Fluids, Yin, Yang or Essence.

Deficient Heat: this is the same as Yin Deficiency.

Deficient Yang: see Yang Deficiency.

Deficient Yin: see Yin Deficiency.

Diuretic: eliminates excess fluids. Diuretics in Chinese medicine also enhance proper fluid metabolism by increasing absorption of fluids into the deep tissues of the body. Thus, contradictory symptoms of edema and dry skin can be eliminated together with diuretics.

Dryness: characterized by dehydration with symptoms of extreme thirst, dry skin, hair, mouth, lips, nose, throat, dry cough with little phlegm and constipation.

Essence: a highly refined fluid substance which provides the basis of reproduction, development, growth, sexual power, conception, pregnancy and decay in the body.

Excess: a condition of an accumulation of too much of something, either Yin, Yang, Heat, Cold or Fluids.

Excess Cold: a condition of too much Coldness in the body; see Cold.

Excess Heat: a condition of too much Heat in the body; see Heat.

Excess Yang: this is the same as excess Heat with symptoms of high fever, restlessness, red complexion, loud voice, aggressive actions, strong odors, yellow discharges, rapid pulse and hypertension.

Excess Yin: an imbalance of excessive fluids in the body with symptoms of edema, excessive fluid retention, lethargy, a plump or swollen appearance and overall signs of Dampness, and yet these people may have adequate energy.

Exterior: see external.

External: designates the location of an illness to be on the surface of the body; includes colds, flus, fevers, skin eruptions, sore throats and headaches.

False Yang: this is Deficient Heat, or Yin Deficiency, and results in emaciation and weakness with Heat symptoms; this type of Heat symptom occurs because the cooling moistening Fluids (Yin) are lacking and so is termed, "false Heat."

Heat, Hot, Heat signs: hyper-metabolism with symptoms of fever with little chills, restlessness, constipation, thirst, dark yellow or scanty urine, craving for cold, aversion to heat, burning digestion, infections, inflammations, dryness, red face, sweating, strong appetite, hemorrhaging and blood in vomit, urine, stool, nose or mucus, strong orders, sticky or thick yellow bodily excretions, irritability, scanty dark yellow urination, swollen, red and painful eyes or gums and red skin eruptions, and hyper-conditions such as hypertension.

Hot: overly active metabolism.

Interior: see Internal.

Internal: designates the location of an illness to be inside the body; includes conditions affection the Qi, Blood, Fluids and Internal Organs.

Jing: see Essence.

Meridians: the pathways along which Qi circulates to supply energy and nourishment to the Organs and the surface of the body.

Moves Blood: see regulates Blood.

Nervine: strengthens the nerves; for conditions of nervousness, anxiety, insomnia, emotional instability, pain, cramps, spasms, tremors, stress, muscle tension and epilepsy.

Organs: the Organs in TCM are different than in western medicine: Organs have energetic rather than physical functions; they are dynamic interrelated processes which occur throughout every level of the body. Yin Organs include the Heart, Lungs, Kidneys, Spleen and Liver; Yang Organs include the Small Intestines, Large Intestines, Urinary Bladder, Stomach and Gallbladder.

Qi: energy, life force; Qi circulates, protects, holds, transforms and warms.

Qi Deficiency: a lack of Qi or energy with signs of low vitality, lethargy, weakness, shortness of breath, slow metabolism, frequent colds and flu with slow recovery, low soft voice, spontaneous sweating, frequent urination, palpitations.

Regulates Blood: smoothes the flow of Blood in the body; symptoms of Blood imbalance include bleeding, hemorrhaging, excessive menstruation, localized stabbing pain, abdominal masses, ulcers, abscesses and painful menstruation.

Regulates Energy: smoothes the flow of Qi in the body; symptoms include dull aching pain, abdominal distention and pain, belching, gas, acid regurgitation, nausea, vomiting, stifling sensation in chest, pain in the sides, loss of appetite, depression, hernial pain, irregular menstruation, swollen, tender breasts and wheezing.

Sedative: sedate, calm the mind and spirit; for insomnia, anxiety, nervousness, irritability, fright and hysteria.

Seven Emotions: the seven emotions are a major cause of illness. They are: sadness, fright, fear, grief, anger, joy (overexcitability) and melancholy.

Shen: the overall spirit and mental faculties of a person, including enthusiasm for life, charisma and capacity to behave appropriately, be responsive, speak coherently, think and form ideas and live a life of joy and spiritual fulfillment.

Spirit: see Shen.

Stomach Heat: a condition of too much Heat in the Stomach with signs of bad breath, gum bleeding and swelling, mouth ulcers, frontal headaches, burning sensation in the stomach region and extreme thirst.

TCM: abbreviation for Traditional Chinese Medicine.

Tonification, Tonify: nourishes, strengthens, builds and improves the condition of either Qi, Blood, Yin or Yang in the body.

Wind: Wind causes movement with symptoms of spasms, twitches, dizziness, spasms, rigidity of the muscles, deviation of the eye and mouth, stiff or rigid neck and shoulders, tremors, convulsions, vertigo and sudden onset of colds, chills, fever, stuffy nose and headache.

Yang: the body's capacity to generate and maintain warmth and circulation.

Yang Deficiency: a condition of Coldness due to lack of the heating quality of Yang; symptoms include lethargy, Coldness, edema, poor digestion, lower back pain, the type of constipation caused by weak peristaltic motion and lack of libido.

Yin: the body's substance, including Blood and all other fluids in the body; these nurture and moisten the Organs and tissues.

Yin Deficiency: this includes Deficient Heat and results in emaciation and weakness with Heat symptoms such as night sweats, insomnia, a burning sensation in the palms, soles and chest, malar flush, afternoon fever, nervous exhaustion, dry throat, dry eyes, blurred vision, dizziness and nervous tension.

Zang Fu: the theory of the Organs; the hollow Organs (Fu) which transport and the solid Organs (Zang) which store.

General Index

Abdominal
  congestion/distension/fullness 318, 361
    Dampness and, 98, 106, 125, 133
    Deficient Qi and, 188
    Food Stagnation and, 137
    Purgatives and, 87
    Stagnation and, 141
  cramps/spasms 89, 342
  lumps/masses/tumors 26, 57, 171, 173, 226, 354
  pain
    Cold and, 178, 191, 212, 234
    Dampness and, 135
    Deficiency and, 190, 198, 239, 277, 306
    sharp, 347
    Stagnation and, 144
Abnormal
  discharge 49
  labor 401
  menstrual bleeding 60
  sex drive 51
  sweating 26, 229
  uterine bleeding 61
Abscesses 28
  chronic, 185, 265
  Dampness and, 96
  Heat and, 59, 72
  Internal ruptured, 55
  intestinal, 57, 69, 358
  Lung, 49, 100
  Phlegm and, 118
  Stagnation and, 93
  toxicity and, 70, 74, 81, 102, 195, 268
Acid regurgitation 147, 287, 296, 310, 316, 361
Acne 290, 359, 415
Aconite poisoning 83, 87, 175
Addiction
  tobacco, 74, 106, 118
Addison's disease 190, 278, 352

Agent orange disease 72
AIDS 189, 217, 218, 341
Albuminuria 352
Allergies 31, 114, 179
  respiratory 31, 34
  rhinitis and, 315, 391
Alopecia (baldness) 104, 110, 204, 210, 359, 417
Alterative 44, 95, 281, 289, 302
Alzheimer's disease 232
Amenorrhea 295, 347
  Blood Stagnation/Stasis and, 26, 57, 78, 103, 137, 158, 170
  Deficiency and, 213, 278
Amoebas 72, 75
Analgesic 301
Anemia 58, 186, 194, 206, 285, 288, 307, 312
  abdominal pain and, 304
  aplastic, 167, 323
Angina pectoris (heart pains) 112, 138, 148, 321, 331, 355, 368, 396
Anorexia 188, 312, 360, 374
Anthelmintic 344
Antibiotics 302, 334
  Antibacterial 44, 48, 56, 62, 68, 81, 130
  Antifungal 48, 56, 204
  Antimicrobial 69, 70, 134, 154
  Antiviral 44, 62, 68, 71, 81, 334
Antihyaluronidase 79
Antihypertensive 48, 50, 54, 280
  (See Hypertension)
Antiparasitic 275
Antipoison 83
Antispasmodic 30, 40, 106, 128, 155, 198, 254, 280, 291, 331, 350
Anxiety 160, 200, 226, 236, 241, 288, 370, 407
Appendicitis 69, 88, 286, 328
  acute, 358
Appetite
  insatiable, 222
  lack of, 318, 338

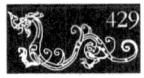

General Index

Coldness and, 178
Dampness and, 98
Deficiency and, 183, 236, 288, 367
Stagnation and, 137
promotion 26, 28, 180, 234, 361
Arrhythmia 282, 321
Arteriosclerosis 306, 331, 352, 395
Arthritic pain, acute 35
Arthritis
  Blood Stagnation and 154
  conditions of, 301
  Damp, Wind conditions and, 26 109, 161, 294
  Deficiency and, 101, 190, 311, 352
  Heat and, 69
  rheumatoid, 78, 101, 109, 161, 278, 368
  Wind and, 254
Ascariasis 231
Ascites 93, 94, 100, 106, 338, 350, 365
  due to cold 95
Asthenic conditions 368
Asthma 24, 294
  acute exacerbation of, 119
  bronchial, 388
  Deficiency and, 147
  Excess and, 46
  Heat and, 67
  Phlegm and 34, 134
  relieves, 257
Athlete's foot (see Tinea pedis)
Atherosclerosis 50, 395

Bad breath 63, 122, 134, 299
Back pain, lower 38, 109, 264, 285, 307, 316
  Deficiency and, 206, 226, 229, 238, 278, 304
Bed wetting 140
Belching 245, 287, 296, 330
  acid regurgitation and, 337

Stomach Cold and, 125, 147, 179
Stomach Heat and, 49, 130
Stagnation and, 138, 149
Bell's palsy 128, 321, 334
Berberine 64
Beriberi 304, 342
Bile 105, 161
Biliary calculus 338
Bites
  flea, 131
  insect, 76
  snake, 56, 76, 78, 82, 106, 128, 244, 268
  venomous, 81, 102, 105, 128, 258, 268
Black soya bean 42-3
Bladder infections (see Urinary Bladder)
Bleeding 83, 105, 194
  Coldness and, 176
  Deficiency and, 199
  disorders 82, 176, 224
  External, 77
  gums 77
  Heat in the Blood and, 42, 54, 84, 122
  in the lower burner 82
  mouth 77
  stop, 28, 150, 169, 235, 263, 286, 306, 362
Bloating 136, 138, 142, 144, 148, 337
Blood 37, 54, 56, 57, 112, 168, 176, 429
  and lymphatic purification 95
  and nutritive (ying) levels 56
  and ying stage fevers 54
  clots 152, 159, 232
  cooling the, 41, 88, 122, 124, 226, 429
  detoxify the, 35, 58, 62, 78, 83, 95
  Internal Heat and, 38, 47, 154, 224
    with symptoms of rashes and nosebleed 84

GENERAL INDEX

level 56-57
loss 185
pressure, high (see Hypertension)
reckless movement of, 56, 57, 61, 62, 72, 88, 166
spitting of, 63
stasis 57, 73, 88, 101, 152, 156, 160, 161, 162, 164, 165, 214
vomiting of, 38, 55, 57, 60, 62, 82, 88, 122, 151, 154, 166, 224
Blood Deficiency 41, 84, 155, 159, 167, 171, 180, 183, 190, 192, 205, 216, 223, 254, 305, 308, 327, 429
Blood, invigorates the 59, 61, 88, 137, 158, 213, 218
Blood, move/circulate the 25, 47, 57, 73, 82, 88, 91, 102, 113, 149, 155, 158, 201, 204, 217, 251, 265, 286, 293, 300, 305, 355
Blood, nourishes the 192, 215, 219, 223, 226, 236, 288, 292, 304, 306, 327, 359
Blood regulation 25, 102, 157, 181, 431
Blood Stagnation 26, 103, 109, 141, 192, 251, 293, 300, 310, 354, 360
 Internal Heat and, 74
 Lower Warmer and, 347
Blood tonics 192, 321, 367
Blood sugar level 56, 105, 135
 regulation of, 186
Body aches 43
Body heaviness 288, 317
Boils 29, 168, 186, 214, 218, 244, 322, 356
 Dampness and, 96
 Heat and, 46, 159, 302
 toxicity and, 195
Bones 109, 169
 broken 152
 strengthen, 226
 sinews and, 166, 173, 202, 209, 210, 217
Borborygmus 86, 106, 204, 318, 348
Breast 80, 108, 170, 173, 310

abscesses 108, 118, 119
diseases 70, 81, 82
lumps 70, 89
masses 145
Breathing difficulty 95
dyspnea (shortness of breath) 26, 41, 148, 183, 190, 216, 294, 312, 321, 343
Bronchiectasis 282, 332
Bronchitis 28, 33, 125, 128, 130, 131, 278, 283, 346, 388
 chronic 94, 123, 128, 130, 206, 213, 220, 297, 313, 332, 348, 352
Burning sensation in the palms, soles and chest 353
Burns 46, 49, 53, 58, 88, 90, 102, 154, 157, 169, 286, 414

Calmative 429
Calms
 and sedates the Spirit 244
 mind 109
 restless fetus 26, 28, 68
 shen 183
 Spirit 241-2
Cancer 36, 48, 54, 63, 70, 73, 78, 90, 95, 109, 123, 152, 258, 267, 271, 302, 385
 bladder, 81
 breast, 86
 Dampness and, 96
 esophageal, 320
 lung, 81, 332
 respiratory tract, 77
 throat, 81
 uterine, 86
Candida albicans, 262
Carbuncles 63, 88, 95, 159, 166, 186, 190, 244, 290, 322, 417
 Internal Heat and, 63
Cardiac
 disorders (see Heart also) 287
 edema 350
Carpal tunnel 346

General Index

Cataracts 52, 54, 336, 352, 418
Catarrhal jaundice 320
Cathartics 87
Cerebral vascular injury (see Stroke)
Chapped and bleeding hands 153
Chest
   congestion 40, 94, 116
   distension 84, 93, 125, 133
   fullness 41, 83, 134, 136, 149
   pain 66, 74, 148, 151, 152, 158, 160
   stifling feeling in, 36, 42, 119, 122, 126, 131, 142, 149
Chickenpox 58
Childbirth 59, 163
   difficult 214, 218
   pain 151
   postpartum inflammation and, 59
Chillblains 309
Chills 24, 26, 28, 29, 40, 42, 70, 84, 107
Cholagogues 62
Cholecystitis 66, 291, 316, 318, 322
Cholelithiasis (see Gallstones)
Cholesterol, serum 159
   lowers, 50, 83, 138, 153
Chong (Vital reproductive energy)
   Cold in the, 306
   regulate the, 295
Chorea 198
Circulates Qi 31
Circulation 109, 111
   Lung, 24
   promotes, 53, 109, 113, 192
   Spleen and Stomach, 28
   Yang, 25
Cirrhosis (see Liver)
Cock's crow diarrhea (see Diarrhea)
Cold 95, 110, 111, 129, 155, 174, 177, 180, 209, 213, 218, 429
   aversion/intolerance to, 36, 202, 209, 217, 294, 314, 319, 356
   Damp and, (see Damp Cold)
   Damp Phlegm 26
   disorders 309

dispersing/expel 25, 32, 42, 95, 146, 176, 208, 305, 307, 364
   External 26
   in summer 133
   in the Kidneys 146, 202
   in the lower back 177
   Internal 96, 97, 173, 176, 277, 319
   limbs 177
   Phlegm 34, 155
   phobia 279
   Stomach 27, 125, 178
   Wind Damp and, (see Wind Damp Cold)
Cold Blood Stagnation 26
Cold Qi Stagnation 148
Colds and flu's, prevent (see Common Cold)
Colitis 74, 81, 101
   acute, 303
Collapse
   of Yang 174
   revive from, 277
Colon
   spastic or irritable 378
Coma 61, 116, 173, 250, 260, 280, 284, 321, 339, 368
Common cold 279, 282, 287, 290, 301, 314, 387
   External conditions and, 23
   fever and headache with, 37, 38, 294
   frequent, 185
   Internal conditions and, 50
Concussion 355
Confusion 49
Congee
   coix, 101
   mung bean, 175
   rice, 186, 189
Conjunctivitis 38, 42, 44, 48, 61, 246, 322, 331, 360, 418
Consciousness
   impaired, 54
   loss of, 55, 251, 266, 286, 368
Constipation 35, 88, 108, 375

GENERAL INDEX

caused by Yin Deficiency 91
chronic 90, 269, 285, 292, 306, 364
Dryness and, 91, 111, 129, 131, 164, 200, 205, 219, 220
in the weak and elderly 91, 292
Internal Heat and, 50, 89, 318, 331, 339
laxatives and, 90, 358
lack of Fluids and, 222, 360
Qi or Blood Deficiency and, 215, 223
Stagnation and, 92, 134, 144, 288, 347
Contagious Heat diseases 81
Contraindications and Incompatibilities 21
Convulsions 54, 55, 65, 121, 126, 173, 241, 284, 321
associated with Heat 37, 244, 251
children and, 37, 254
due to warm febrile diseases 37
Wind and, 253
with mania 280
Corns 75, 231, 309
Cor Pulmonale 332
Coronary heart disease 112, 282
Cough 94, 104, 125, 231, 388
bloody, 53, 154, 207, 328
consumptive, 199
due to Deficiency 131, 184, 230
due to Lung Heat 38, 63, 77, 228
External conditions and, 24, 281
Internal Heat and, 46, 343
nonproductive, 191, 221, 316, 346
tuberculosis and, 207
with copious sputum 232, 297
with thick, yellow sputum 49
Crohn's disease 153
Cuts 286, 414
Cystitis 66, 99, 310, 322
Cysts 171, 293, 358, 403

Damp Cold 97, 217, 279
Damp Heat 96, 429
associated with dysentery 68
associated with Kidney Yin Deficiency, 97
conditions of, 58, 62, 98, 111
drain/dispersing, 47, 58, 70, 71, 96, 148, 154, 320, 322, 349, 362
in the Lower Burner 62, 65, 70, 97, 101, 104, 320
in the Urinary Bladder 100, 103, 310
Internal, 47
skin conditions and, 65, 76, 79, 109, 263, 367
sores and, 63
with symptoms of joint pain 85
Dampness 79, 80, 85, 125, 142, 185, 429
Deficiency and, 192
drain/eliminate/disperse, 29, 31, 62, 88, 124, 128, 149, 174, 235, 239, 252, 267, 297, 301, 304, 360, 368
Internal, 82
Spleen and, 133, 135, 137
Stagnation of, 99, 134, 300
Summer Heat and, 362
Wind and, 109
Deafness 66, 253, 336, 353, 419
Defensive Wei Qi 25
Deficient conditions, chronic 312, 325
Deficient Heat (see Yin Deficiency)
Dehydration 49, 183, 335
Delirium 47, 49, 52, 64, 116, 160, 284, 299, 358
Delivery of late or stillborn babies 251
Dementia 410
senile, 232
Demulcent 40, 100, 108, 223, 282, 335
Dental diseases 63, 189
Depression 44, 149, 249, 410
Dermatitis 59, 79, 290, 304, 415
Deviation of the eyes and mouth 334

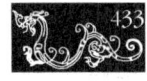

General Index

Diabetes
  insipidus 352
  mellitus 56, 60, 105, 135, 186, 201, 219, 278, 316, 336, 339, 353, 356, 369
Diaper rash 304
Diarrhea 229, 376
  acute 97
  chronic, 68, 231, 233, 241, 263, 352
  Cock's crow (daybreak), 205, 207, 230
  Coldness and, 178, 269
  Damp Heat and, 62, 235
  Dampness and, 96, 133, 174, 337, 368
  Deficiency and, 39, 82, 100, 236, 271
  dysentery and, 151, 154, 239
  food stagnation and, 139
  Internal Heat and, 303
Dietary restrictions 22
Digestion 26, 28, 34, 100, 139
  poor, 63
  promotes, 234, 337
Diphtheria 78, 82
Dissipates nodules 54
Diuretic 92, 94, 117, 275, 430
  External conditions and, 26
  Internal Heat and, 70
  Dampness and, 96
  Blood regulation and, 158
Dizziness 39, 41, 57, 65, 90, 112, 370
  Deficiency and, 37, 52, 66, 97, 195, 201, 229, 278, 316
  Heat and, 107
  Internal/External conditions 41
  Liver and, 65, 90, 167, 253, 288
  Wind Cold and, 158
Doctrine of Signatures 37
Dosage 17
Drains Excess heat 88
Drains Fire 49
Dreams
  disturbed sleep and, 241
  excessive, 294, 370

Dryness 38, 57, 87, 109
  Constipation and, 88, 296
  Deficiency and, 181, 227, 278
  moistening, 62, 120, 243, 311, 315, 360
  Stagnation and, 91
Dysenteric disorders 67, 76, 154
Dysentery 63, 69, 78, 81, 88, 106, 135, 151, 157, 284
  amoebic 76, 81, 235, 281, 303, 344
  bacterial, 281, 303
  bloody, 364
  chronic, 75
  Damp Heat and, 65, 72
  Deficiency and, 233
  food stagnation and, 144
Dysmenorrhea (painful menstruation) 34, 57, 78, 82, 88, 161, 293, 307, 347, 400
  Blood regulation and, 158
  Blood Stagnation and, 26, 34, 57, 78, 161
Dyspnea (shortness of breath) (see breathing difficulty)
Dysuria (burning urine) 108, 398

Ear
  hearing loss and, 195, 202, 210 (also see Deafness)
  infection of middle, 290, 322, 359
  ringing in the, 66
Earache 65, 418
Ecchymosis 58, 150
Eczema 40, 79, 205, 239, 264, 290, 294, 331, 352, 415
  Dampness and, 96
  Internal Heat and, 46
  weeping, 67, 304
Edema 123, 162, 172, 217, 261, 295, 399
  Blood Stagnation and, 163
  cathartics and, 92
  chronic, 105
  Dampness and, 97

General Index

Deficiency and, 174, 278, 304, 352, 365
External conditions and, 24
Internal Heat and, 49
leg 93, 106, 144
with lack of urination and Stagnant Qi 92
Emetic 106, 117
Emphysema 131, 207, 213, 217, 388
pulmonary, 282, 313
Encephalitis 46, 55, 284, 299, 318, 335, 369
Endogenous Liver Wind 280
Endometriosis 74, 293, 322
Entamoeba histolytica 72
Enteritis 82, 86, 106
chronic, 368
Enuresis 83, 204, 209, 293, 316, 339, 363
Ephedrine 25
Epidemic parotitis 335
Epilepsy 128, 160, 198, 241, 287, 336, 413
with profuse phlegm 160, 336
Epistaxis 55, 60, 63, 82, 154, 203, 356, 359
Erysipelas 69, 329, 415
Esophagus
constriction of, 320
spasm of the, 348
Essence 339, 430
augments/reinforce the, 202, 207, 216, 236
Deficiency of, 189, 196
nourish the, 299, 360
restrains, 48, 204, 217, 237
tonify the, 189, 192, 195, 211, 215, 229
Estrogen precursor 43, 86
Excess (Cold, Heat, Yang, Yin) 331, 430
Exhaustion 187, 189, 191, 335
fatigue and, 321
nervous, 320
sexual excess and 293

Expectorant 73, 94, 106, 117, 126, 130, 206, 220, 266, 329, 342, 347
External 430
Cold 23, 26, 28, 29, 44, 124
Heat 23, 44, 56, 71, 82, 124, 331
Internal and, 286, 341
Wind-Cold 26, 29, 33, 133, 197
Wind-Heat 36, 38, 44, 69, 129, 313, 333
Eye 23, 50, 135, 195, 211, 225
associated with heat 23, 47, 48, 54, 67, 164, 255
brightens the, 52, 53, 67, 72, 104, 198, 246
diseases 52
dry, 52, 336
inflammation 23, 63, 65, 66
External conditions and, 23
Internal Heat and, 50, 164
redness 23
Facial paralysis 29, 128
Fainting 83, 121
False
Heat 51
Yang 430
Fatigue 295, 312
chronic, 324
Deficiency and, 183, 239, 284
Fatty tumors 101
Fetus, restless 26, 28, 62, 155, 188, , 203, 226
Fever 23
acute, 318
chronic, 61, 194
Dampness and, 90
Deficiency and, 51, 56, 67, 194, 221, 238
excessive perspiration and, 46, 335
Heat in the skin, muscles and, 46
high, 46, 88, 126, 251, 280, 284, 302, 328, 356, 369, 440
severe, 357
Summer Heat and, 362
in children 59
in the night 84

General Index

intermittent 290
low-grade, 51, 56, 60, 67, 84
sore throat 46
Stomach Heat and, 318
Summer Heat and, 84
tidal 68, 219, 227, 289, 366
with associated eye problems 42
Fibroid cysts 88, 171, 293, 403
pelvic, 141
Fibromyalgia 309
Fire 56, 60, 65, 190
Deficient, 281, 295
drains, 46, 54, 87
in the upper burner 77
poison 78, 81
toxicity 56, 63, 68, 70, 73, 77, 81, 127, 195
Five Palm Heat 225
Flu 29, 69
Stomach, 139
Fluid 97, 100
congestion 93, 94, 188
drains, 94, 95
exhaustion of, 58
generates 49, 56, 61, 218, 220, 230, 321, 335
lack of, 91, 201, 215, 222, 243, 360
metabolism 101, 186
regulation of, 97, 101, 192
Stagnation 87, 93, 96, 116, 162, 293, 340
Food
allergies 46
aversion to, 296
poisoning 28, 262, 296
seafood, 26, 28, 35
shellfish, 262
Stagnation 91, 93, 134, 137, 143
constipation due to, 93, 261
due to Dryness 91
Forgetfulness 112, 183, 200, 226, 230, 323, 339
Four Treasures 180
Fractures 56, 169, 204

Frostbite 294, 307, 416
Fullness
of the abdomen 88
of the Stomach 296
Fungal
infections 42, 60, 66, 79, 81, 264, 304
ringworm 60, 90, 94, 235
Furuncles 65, 70, 72, 73, 95, 290, 417

Gallbladder 47, 65, 68, 105, 160
disease 62, 109, 378
Heat 309, 322
Gallstones (cholelithiasis) 102, 140, 160, 291, 318
Gangrene 309
Gastrectasis 350
Gastritis 279, 316, 337, 374
chronic, 297
Gastroenteritis 86, 324, 342
acute, 348
Gastrointestinal diseases 35
Hot or Cold Stagnation and, 348
Genistein (estrogen precursor) 43, 86
Genital itch 60, 66, 68, 77, 265, 322
Gingivitis 46, 77, 281, 369, 417
Glaucoma 336, 352
Globus hystericus 125, 348
Gobo 35
Goiter 48, 57, 117, 122, 195, 243, 327
Gonorrhea 63, 352
Greater Yang (see Tai Yang)
Gum
bleeding, 51, 77, 105, 154, 166, 210
disease 77, 331
painful, swollen, 51, 77, 265, 281

Halvah 224
Happiness herb 47
Headache 313, 406
acute, 406
chronic, 114
Dampness and, 133
Deficiency and, 166
frontal, temporal, 301, 369, 371

GENERAL INDEX

migraine, 30, 39, 128, 254, 301, 316, 406
  severe, 46, 317
  Wind Cold and, 24, 158, 254
  Wind Damp and, 110, 254
  Wind Heat and, 35
Healing
  bones 204
  injuries and fractures 56
  sores 91
Heart 56, 98, 138, 162
  cool the, 47, 54
  Deficiency and, 183, 241, 323
  disease 112, 137, 148, 162, 282, 321, 355, 365, 368 (also see Angina Pectoris)
  failure 278
  Fire 48, 63, 68, 103, 244, 292, 302
  Heat 51, 54, 109, 302
  nourish the, 226, 230, 236, 239, 246
  palpitations 26, 83, 98, 159, 168, 230, 241, 289, 304, 331, 349
  due to Deficiency 367, 370
  Yang Deficiency 174, 293
  Yin Deficiency 56, 220, 246
Heat 42, 89, 110, 430
  accompanied by swelling 89
  and accumulation of water 93
  caused by malnutrition in children 61
  clear, 35, 295, 320
    and calms spirit 47
    and Dampness 88, 93, 96, 133, 235
    and toxins 78, 80, 88, 244
    in the Blood 359
    Lung, 38
    Phlegm and, 118, 251
  delirium 47
  Deficient 327
  False (Yin Deficiency), 37, 111, 166, 199, 221, 289
    fever 49
    high fever 47

insomnia 47
Internal 44, 281, 286, 338
irritability and, 47, 49
muscle fever and, 61
Stagnation and 80, 172, 327, 358
thirst and, 49
Upper Burner and, 62, 68
Heat stroke 50, 69, 82, 84, 86, 100, 107, 335
Hematemesis 82
Hematuria (also see Urine, blood in), 154, 320, 356, 398
Hemiplegia 321, 334, 343
Hemophilia 218
Hemoptysis 316, 320, 332
Hemorrhage 150, 152, 170, 224
  uterine, 156
Hemorrhoids 65, 68, 72, 292, 306, 363
  external, 376
  internal, 377
Hepatic coma 356
Hepatitis 47, 62, 66, 70, 71, 78, 82, 107, 109, 111, 290, 322, 338, 379
  chronic, 286, 288, 333
Herbal
  contraindications & incompatibilities 21
  preparations, general, 15
Herbs conducting to Organ Meridians 14
Hernia 137, 143, 146, 148, 178, 208, 217, 286, 317
  due to Coldness 307
Herpes 80
  simplex 416
  zoster 66, 268, 322, 416
Hiccups 147, 150, 178, 245, 330, 375
High blood pressure 38, 98
High cholesterol 98
HIV 341
Hives 79
Hoarseness 320
Hookworm (see Worms)
How and when to take herbs 19

General Index

Hyperaldosteronism 352, 368
Hypertension 39, 83, 153, 163, 217, 280, 295, 306, 310, 322, 352, 393
   associated with menopause 209
   dizziness, headache and, 39
   fluid retention and, 349
   heart disease and, 137
   Liver Yang and, 37, 48, 132, 167, 203, 254
   relieve, 226
Hyperthyroidism 282, 327, 360, 382
   deficiency of iodine and, 361
Hypoadrenalism 368
Hypochondriac pain 354
Hypoglycemia (low blood sugar) 186, 323, 381
Hypotension 295, 395
Hypothyroidism 352, 368, 383
Hysteria 287, 291, 310, 407

Impetigo 83
Impotence 265, 269, 293, 316, 331, 403
   Deficiency and, 177, 202, 229
Incessant crying of babies 102
Increase flexibility 114
Increasing female libido 213
Infantile convulsions 252
Infection 70, 71, 74, 96
   fungal 42, 66, 81, 416
   hot 54, 68, 72
   inflammation and, 69, 104
   Lung 74
   of the Bladder or Kidneys 102
   urinary 81
   viral 71
Infertility 162, 265, 293, 316, 401
   Deficiency and, 202, 278
Influenza 38, 39, 43, 69, 71, 279, 389
Insect bites (see bites)
Insecticides 95
Insomnia 42, 98, 112, 226, 241, 283, 287, 290, 293, 299, 321, 363, 407
   after a prolonged fever 43
   Deficiency and, 183, 230, 236, 278, 370

Internal Heat and, 47, 159, 302
   sleepiness after meals and, 297
Internal 431
   Heat 331, 334, 338, 345
   warm the, 176, 279
Intestinal
   abscesses 69
   Heat 74, 87, 90, 306, 358
   inflammation 88
   obstruction 347
   parasites 72, 90, 260
   rumbling 106
   tuberculosis 368
   tumors 81
   wind 30
Intestines
   lubricate/moisten the, 35, 40, 44, 50, 59, 87, 164, 195
Irritability 40, 42, 43, 100, 103, 159, 287, 328
   Deficiency and, 199, 230, 236
   Internal Heat and, 44, 254
Irritable bowel syndrome 329, 360
Itching 29, 79, 103, 109
   anal, 265
   Damp-heat sores and, 66
   genital, 66, 68, 77, 265, 322
   relief from, 37, 66, 100, 109, 268
   skin and, 73, 79, 81, 114
   vaginal 72
      vaginitis 66

Jaundice 47, 62, 65, 70, 80, 84, 88, 96, 99, 104, 107, 109, 111, 160, 290, 320, 338
   fever and blood in the urine with, 47
Jing 192, 204
   consolidate the, 186
Joint 112
   inflammation of, 103, 116, 295
   pains 29, 34, 80, 81, 85, 167
      Bi 226
      Dampness and, 103, 206, 311
      Stagnant Blood and, 152
   warm the, 31

GENERAL INDEX

Kanpo 275
Keratitis 352
Kidney 146, 173, 176, 178, 209, 219
  augments the, 147, 237
  Deficiency 53, 104, 112, 173, 186, 189, 205, 210, 216, 236, 285
  Essence Deficiency 222, 235, 336, 363
  Fire 65
  infections (see Urinary tract)
  nourish the, 186, 195, 226, 236, 353
  stones 310, 352, 399
  tonics 115, 166, 189, 226, 229, 308, 368
  tuberculosis 366
  Yang Deficiency 34, 174, 177, 202, 264, 302, 316
  Yin Deficiency 37, 51, 65, 68, 97, 194, 199, 201, 223, 244, 278, 281, 332, 350

Lactation 70, 80, 103, 108, 170, 213
  contraindications during, (see individual herbs)
  increases, 70, 80, 108, 168, 173, 213
  insufficient, 70, 80, 103, 168, 170, 213, 216, 255, 262, 402
  stop, 138, 141
Laryngitis 79, 220, 332, 348, 392
Laxative 62, 87, 117, 285, 338, 364
Leeches 171
Legionnaire's disease 55
Leprosy 267
Lesser Yang diseases 40
Lesser Yin (Shao Yin) stage 277
Lethargy 319
Leukemia 309, 356
Leukopenia 112, 167
Leukorrhea (vaginal discharge) 49, 65, 83, 86, 98, 186, 211, 235, 281, 288, 363, 400
Lice (see Parasites)
Liver 64, 98, 160, 163
  cirrhosis 70, 78, 82, 94, 105, 380
  ascites and, 350
  Deficiency 38, 53, 104, 112, 199, 200, 216, 229, 370
  detoxifying function 290
  disorders 70, 98, 161, 306
  enlarged, 227
  Fire/Heat 54, 65, 67, 322
    rising 48, 62
  headaches and, 111
  heat and eyes 48
  Qi 138, 141, 149. 172, 206
    regulation of, 361
    Stagnation 36, 40, 145, 161, 198, 255, 288, 310
  Spleen disharmony and, 198, 288
  Stomach disharmony and, 283
  Wind 55, 65, 73, 81, 200, 253, 280, 291
  Wind Heat 37, 39
  Yang 50, 73, 81, 242
    calm, 50
    rising 37, 53, 62, 73, 81, 132, 166, 178, 203, 246
  Yin Deficiency 38, 50, 52, 60, 197, 200, 223, 226, 244, 246, 278, 281
Loose teeth 224
Lower Burner 70
Lumps 57, 69, 73, 118, 122, 124, 128, 243, 293
Lung 24, 116, 130, 153, 176
  bleeding in, 63, 157
  Cold in, 190
  Fire 51, 77
  Heat 38, 104, 118, 120, 130, 154, 156
    Deficiency and, 190
    Internal, 44
  infections 74
  lubricates the, 190, 220, 225
  Qi 78, 81, 124, 127, 186, 230
    Deficiency 183, 191, 205, 216, 232
  tonics 183
  warm the, 33, 176

General Index

Yin Deficiency 51, 118, 192, 228, 283, 332, 347
Lupus 350
  with arthritic symptoms 312, 357
  Yin Deficiency and, 366
Lymes disease 80
Lymph 56, 80, 95, 124
  circulation of, 293
Lymphadenitis (swollen lymph glands) 48, 69, 81, 123, 228, 290, 322, 328, 360, 397

Macular degeneration 232
Mal-development in children 202, 353
Malabsorption 83, 116
Malaria 75, 78, 81, 84, 86, 151, 268, 288
Male impotence 178
Malnutrition 52, 61, 62, 67, 140, 172
  childhood, 52, 67, 90
  Mammary glands 80, 95
  Mania 49, 52, 71, 268, 328, 410
Manic
  depression 242
  psychotic disorders 241
Masses caused by Blood Stagnation 162
Mastitis 69, 80, 118, 171, 290, 303, 401
Measles 28, 34, 36, 39, 41, 43, 58, 59, 81, 318, 343
  speed recovery of, 39
Meniere's disease 297, 317
Meningitis 46, 55, 284, 299, 318, 335, 369
Menopause 141, 209, 217, 295, 304, 352, 402
  hot flashes and, 198, 207, 295
Menorrhagia 63, 235, 306, 323, 400
Menstruation
  blocked/delayed, 101, 333
  Blood regulation and, 151, 158
  Blood Stagnation and, 151
  excessive, 57, 177, 190, 199, 226, 229, 289
  induce, 170, 173
  irregularity 36, 295, 310, 347, 354
    Deficiency and, 206, 288, 306
    Qi and, 145
    with depression and moodiness 41
  painful, 145, 147, 304, 354
  slow, 159, 161
Mental derangement 160, 161
Meridians 431
Methods of preparing and taking Chinese herbs 18-23
Migraine headaches (see Headaches)
Miscarriage 23, 28, 62, 136, 155, 211, 217, 401
  prevents, 306, 367
  threatened, 203
Mood swings 36
Morning sickness 26, 28, 125, 133, 136, 147, 316, 330, 402
Mother's milk 80
Mouth 81
  bitter taste in, 40, 41, 107, 309, 333
  bleeding in, 77
  dry 64, 201, 288, 299, 302, 333, 370
  inflammation in, 63, 89, 166
  sores 52, 77, 103, 244, 318
  sweet taste in, 134
  ulcers 52, 269 (also see Ulcers, aphthous)
Moxibustion 150, 155
Mucus and phlegm 27
Mumps 71, 75, 78
Muscular atrophy 206, 219, 412
Myocardial
  infarction 321
  ischemia 162
Myocarditis 282

Nasal
  congestion 26, 31, 33, 114, 282
  obstruction of passages 27, 32
  and pain 32

GENERAL INDEX

opening of passages and sinuses 27, 31, 33
polyps 268
Nasosinusitis 31
Nausea 27, 107, 130, 145, 156, 177, 374
   and vomiting 28, 116, 125, 142, 283
   Coldness and, 180, 234
   Dampness and, 133
   Deficiency and, 209
   Rebellious Qi and, 245
   relief of, 26
Neck lumps 57
Nephritic edema 78
Nephritis 94, 97, 162, 398
Nervine 293, 431
Nervous
   affections 198
   exhaustion 287, 293
   Stomach 365
Nervousness 175, 223
Neuralgia 287, 331, 412
   trigeminal, 279, 317, 321, 334
Neurasthenia 112, 282, 323, 352
Neurosis 200, 242, 287
Neutralize acidity 64, 83
Night blindness 52, 53
Night sweats 51, 61, 65, 186, 194, 218, 281, 311
   due to Deficiency 226, 230, 238, 278, 370
Nighttime urination (nocturia) 140, 352
Nocturnal emission 51, 65, 83, 199, 211, 229, 294, 327, 331
Nodules 267
   reduce, 54, 56, 81, 214, 218, 228, 259
   soften, 48, 123
Nosebleed 105, 245, 318
   Internal Heat and, 47, 122, 151, 166, 224, 302, 328
Nutrition 172
   improved 54

supplement 52, 123
Nutritive energy (see Ying)
Obesity 98, 331, 365
Ophthalmologic diseases 52, 290, 336
Orchitis (inflammation of the testicles) 404
Organ transplant rejection 232
Osteoarthritis 412
Otitis media (see Ear, infection)
Overindulgence in rich foods 296

Pain 25, 33, 68, 88, 95, 114, 143, 177
   abdominal 26, 32, 83, 180
      Blood Stagnation and, 160
      Dampness and, 135
      Qi and, 144
   arm and shoulder, 334
   neck and, 350
   back 109, 209, 217, 411 (also see Back pain)
   Bi, 31, 67, 107, 110, 146, 177, 206
      Blood regulation and, 154
      Dampness and, 109
      Syndrome 226
   chest 74
   chronic 27, 111
   Cold obstructing the channels and, 33
   Deficiency and, 206
   neck 412
   postoperative 74
   postpartum 74, 166, 170
   testicular, 178, 309
Palpitations (see Heart)
Pancreas, inflammation of (pancreatitis) 286, 328, 360
Parasites 61, 66, 109, 132, 148, 151, 157
   bacterial and amoebic dysentery 419
   expel, 94, 235, 260, 344
   food stagnation and, 93
   intestinal 72, 90, 104
   lice 266

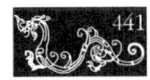

General Index

malarial, 85
scabies 79, 81, 94, 103, 328, 347, 358
vaginal 72, 75
worms 419 (also see Worms)
Pelvic inflammatory disease 304, 322, 328, 347, 358
Peristalsis, stimulate 87, 101
Peritonitis 69, 290
Perspiration, lack of 360 (also see Sweating)
Pharyngitis 320, 332
Phlegm 32, 78, 81, 95, 97, 104, 142, 153, 176, 219
  Cold, 34, 155, 176, 177
  Expel/resolve/transform, 55, 104, 116, 141, 154, 157, 208, 213, 218, 247, 252, 263, 269, 290, 297, 34, 361
  Heat 119, 122, 124, 160
    Lung, 38
  Hot 48, 79, 117, 123, 130, 132, 220, 264
  Stagnation of, 48, 57, 125
  thick, yellow, 38, 46, 51, 118, 120, 122
  transform, 116
Photophobia 52, 53, 54, 252
Placenta, retention of 293, 347
Planetary Herbology 7
Pleurisy (pleuritis) 46, 94, 287, 290, 342, 391
Plum-pit throat 134, 348
Pneumonia 71, 278, 287, 290, 343, 389
Pneumothorax 332
Poison ivy and oak 59, 103
Poison snakebite (see Bites)
Poisoning
  Aconite (Fu Zi) 83, 87, 175
  food (see Food)
Polyuria 398
Post-nasal drip 125
Pregnancy
  bleeding during, 226 (also see Uterine bleeding)

contraindications during, 23
  (also see specific herb)
Premature
  ejaculation 204, 206, 211, 215, 235, 316, 404
  graying of the hair 194, 201, 223
Premenstrual syndrome 141, 149
Processing of herbs 16
Prolapse
  of anus or uterus due to Deficiency of the Yang Qi 40
  of Internal Organs 185
  of rectum, uterus or veins 41
  uterine, 40, 41, 403
Prolapsed Qi 41
Prostate problems 310, 322, 405
Protozoas 72, 75
Pruritis 79, 415
  senile, 352
Psoriasis 79, 171, 204, 217, 304, 331, 415
Psychosis 292
Pterygium 42
Puerperal eclampsia 280
Pulmonary emphysema (see Emphysema)
Purgatives 87, 342
Purpura 304
  rashes and, 60
Pus 31, 74, 81, 100, 120, 128, 168, 173, 192
  drainage 57, 73
  expel, 269
  yellow, 79
Pyelitis 322

Qi 33, 50, 431
  circulation of, 25, 31, 33, 111, 113, 116, 146, 148, 155, 158, 161, 173, 203, 261, 363
  Deficiency 41, 142, 171, 180, 184, 190, 200, 241, 278, 300, 307, 431
  Heat in the, 369
  Rebellious, 124, 129, 134, 140, 177, 179, 245, 330

General Index

Stomach, 348
  regulates, 297, 329, 348, 364
  Stagnation 119, 142, 144, 146, 148, 160, 172, 251, 354
  tonics 92, 126, 183, 229, 239, 304, 311, 321, 335, 342, 367
  Wei, 23, 25, 185, 192, 293
Qi stage fevers 45, 53

Raises
  Qi 41
  Yang 41
Rapid pulse 71, 97
Rashes 28, 34, 35, 36, 41, 43, 44, 58, 79, 81, 84, 164, 249, 318
  urticaria, 304, 331, 352
Raynaud's disease 309
Reckless movement of Blood 54, 56, 60
Renal
  atrophy 349
  conditions 349
Respiratory
  conditions 314
  congestion 25, 31
  infections 68, 297, 316, 335
Restless mind 49
Restlessness 103, 159, 241, 246, 283, 299, 313, 335
  Deficiency and, 183
  Internal Heat and, 44
Retarded growth 353
Retinitis 336
Rheumatic
  complaints/conditions 26, 43, 78, 109, 113, 217, 271, 278, 301, 311, 365
  Coldness and, 29
  Dampness and 109, 115, 137, 159
  conditions 26, 43, 78, 109
  Heart 282, 355
  inflammations 69, 162
  pain 29, 35, 111, 168, 173, 258
  Wind Cold Damp 295

Rhinitis 27, 31, 168, 279, 301, 330, 359, 369
Rickets 202
Ringing in the ears 66
Ringworm (see Fungal infections)
Roundworm (see Worms)

Salivation, excessive 134
Scabies (see Parasites)
Schizophrenia 242, 336, 410
Sciatica 309, 411
Scrofula 70, 117, 122, 195 243, 327
Seafood poisoning (see Poisoning)
Sedate the mind 47
Sedative 63, 163, 167, 242, 251, 292, 320, 331, 370, 431 (also see Spirit, calm)
Seizure disorders 116, 160, 246, 291, 339
Seminal emission 204, 206, 209, 211, 216, 219, 235, 281
Sensitivity to light 50, 52
Septicemia 59, 299, 356
Serum cholesterol 50
Seven Emotions 431
Sexual excess 51, 65, 221, 293
Shen 432 (also see Spirit)
  calm the, 183, 189, 191, 242
Shortness of Breath (see Breathing difficulty)
Silicosis 332
Skin
  Dampness and, 101
  diseases 290, 304, 331 (also see specific type)
  dry, 221, 226
  External conditions and, 23
  Internal Heat and, 101
  irritations/sores 100, 252
  itching 37, 104, 114, 266
  rashes 71, 79, 328 (also see Rashes)
  Wind and, 158
  wrinkles 90
Sleeplessness 328
Snakebite (see Bites)

General Index

Sore throat 102, 252, 266, 320
   chronic, 55, 281
   External conditions and, 23
   Fire and, 190
   Internal conditions and, 44
   Stomach Heat and, 318
Sores
   chronic/non-healing, 57, 76, 153, 160, 165, 202
   Damp-Heat and, 62, 66, 93, 95, 109
   hot, 49, 59, 69, 79, 88, 91
   mouth, 47, 49, 63, 244
   open, 32
   Stagnation and, 95
   toxic 35, 59, 71, 73, 190, 267
Spasms 27, 61, 100, 126, 120, 269, 321
   associated with Heat 37
   back and neck, 40
   esophageal, 378
   Heat and, 37
   Liver Wind and, 198, 253
   Wind Dampness and, 111
Spermatorrhea (penal discharge) 49, 186, 204, 209, 211, 215, 235, 278, 281, 285, 316, 339, 363, 404
Spirit (Shen) 432
   calm, 47, 98, 99, 116, 200, 223, 228, 230, 239, 241, 246, 311
Spirochetes 80, 85
Spleen
   Dampness 82, 125, 134, 255, 279, 324, 337, 349
   Deficiency 39, 82, 86, 100, 133, 152, 237, 323
   enlarged, 227
   Qi 142, 149, 188
      Deficiency 289
      tonic 109, 135, 183
   strengthen the, 86, 98, 99, 100, 138, 145, 236, 317, 350
   warm the, 68, 136, 142, 176, 180, 234

Yang 204, 209, 212, 269, 350, 364
Sprains 27
Stagnation (also see specific type)
   all types 364
   relieve, 288
Steaming bone disorder 61, 68, 226, 281
Sterility 155
Stiffness
   of the joints 204
   of the neck 30, 280, 294
   and spine 29
Stimulant 106
Stings 81
   bee, 105
Stomach
   Coldness 176, 179, 234, 316
   Dampness 279
   Fire 46, 51, 63, 351
   Heat 39, 45, 122, 124, 130, 132, 156, 220, 222, 299, 339, 351
   inflammation 41
   harmonize the, 139, 296
   pains 70, 316
   Qi Deficiency 101, 349
   Tonics 98, 113, 186, 318
   Yin Deficiency 220, 222
Stones 75, 81
Stools
   blood in, 231, 268, 363
      Internal Heat and, 28, 88, 154, 199, 224
   dark black, 356
   dry, hard, 87, 220, 292, 327, 347
   loose, 142, 324, 326, 368
   soften, 91, 92
Stroke 29, 126, 250, 284, 321, 368
   Heat and sun, 335
   recovery from, 306, 334
Summer Heat 82
   Dampness and, 33, 35, 104, 133
   expel, 49, 99, 335, 362
Sweating 24, 82
   abnormal, 26, 226
   Deficiency and, 238

General Index

excessive/profuse, 25, 46, 184, 229, 243, 321, 335
   lack of, 24, 351
   promote, 32, 34, 44, 345
   spontaneous, 186, 188, 229, 294, 313, 324, 365
   stop, 185
Sweet cravings 351
Swelling
   due to Heat and toxicity 68
   eye, 88
   gland, 44, 80, 118, 124, 128, 228, 258
   hot, 43
      and damp, 62
   joint, 106, 135
   reduces, 28, 31, 33, 72, 95, 118, 125, 163, 170, 214, 218
   testicle, 66, 170, 173, 338, 350
   throat, 35
   whole body, 43
Syphilis 80, 81

Tapeworm (see Worms)
Tear ducts and inflammation 42
Tearing, excessive 50, 52, 255
Tetanus 128, 258
Thirst 107, 120, 156, 291, 313, 335
   Deficiency and, 183, 278, 360
   extreme, 46, 56, 221, 299
   Internal Heat and, 46
   lack of, 277, 299, 319
Throat 23
   dry, 219, 288
      due to Yin Deficiency 221
   inflammation of, 89
   sore, (see Sore throat)
Thrombocytopenia 323, 384
Thyroid glands 48, 123
Thyroiditis 328
Tineas pedis (athlete's foot) 42, 231, 260, 267, 294, 304, 416
Tinnitus 97, 232, 295, 336, 419
   Deficiency and, 194, 199, 201, 210, 216, 223, 226, 245, 281, 304, 353

Tiredness 218
Tonsillitis 75, 78, 359
Toothache 417
   due to Cold 32, 115
   due to toxins 41
   due to Stomach Fire 46, 299, 318
   due to reckless flow of Blood 166
Tonification 432
Torn ligaments 210
Toxic 74
   skin conditions 68
   swellings 32, 35, 74, 78, 80
Toxicity 70, 251, 306
   Blood, 72
   Excess and, 88
   Fire/Heat and, 78, 127, 195, 284
   Internal 74
   relief of, 54, 75, 79, 81, 190, 258, 267, 271, 334
   skin 36, 265
Trauma 37, 58, 78, 83
Tremors 30, 54, 246, 253
Trichomonas 60, 66, 72, 265
Trigeminal neuralgia (see Neuralgia)
Triglycerides 83, 159
Trikatu 173, 179
Triphala 233
Triple Warmer 53
Tuberculosis (TB) 123, 125, 131, 153, 189, 217, 290, 321, 332, 346, 359, 390
   cough and, 207
   Deficiency and, 278
   hemoptysis and, 220
   intestinal, 368
   Kidney, 366
Tumors 43, 57, 95, 99, 101, 123, 126, 171, 214, 267
   cancer 48, 258
   intestinal, 81

Ulcerative colitis 377
Ulcers 95, 159, 170, 239, 267
   aphthous, 360 (also see Mouth sores)

General Index

chronic, 185
duodenal, 323, 333, 361
peptic, 297, 306, 309
Stomach, 153, 331
venereal, 322
Upper Burner Heat 62
Uremia 284, 356
Urethritis 310, 322
Urinary
 bladder 24, 47, 66, 100
 calculus 320, 331
 stones 78, 100, 102, 108, 205, 310
  Damp Heat causing, 166
  dispel/dissolve, 105, 140, 217
 retention 350
 tract 75, 81
  infection 42, 101, 108, 122, 362, 397
   acute, 302
   chronic, 281, 295
   due to Internal Heat 47
   pregnancy and, 67

Urination 74, 75, 104, 105, 106, 107
 burning/hot, 49, 122, 156, 398
 difficult, 43, 47, 84, 93, 98, 302
 diminished, 82, 84, 93, 101, 105, 187, 291
 excessive/copious, 207, 398
 frequent, 83, 98, 146, 150, 229, 232, 292, 339, 363
 due to Deficient Yang 202
 incontinence/inability to hold, 146, 163
  due to Deficiency 184, 229
 inhibited, 98
 painful, 59, 76, 88, 98, 100, 103, 108, 122, 156, 166, 289, 320
 promotes, 96, 261
 scanty, 84, 97, 103, 108
Urine
 bloody, 101, 162, 166, 302, 358
  Internal Heat and, 47, 224
  stops, 154
 clear, 202, 207

cloudy, 109
copious, 207
dark, 64, 84, 97, 100, 101, 103, 302
red, 302
yellow, 49
Urticaria (see Rash)
Uterine bleeding
 abnormal, 28, 61, 83, 235, 289
 Cold and, 202, 176
 Deficiency and, 185, 199, 203, 229, 278, 323
 due to Internal Heat 154, 156, 226
 pregnancy and, 204, 226
 Stagnation and, 162
Uterine inflammation 358
Uterine prolapse 40, 41, 403

Vaginal
 discharge 235, 264
  due to Dampness 135, 166
  due to Deficiency 178, 202, 230, 232
  due to Internal Heat 49
 douche 60
 itching 58, 65, 72, 152, 265
 parasites 72, 75, 260
 yeast infection (see Candida albicans)
Vaginal trichomonas 72, 104, 151
Vaginitis 72, 76
Veins
 prolapse of, 41
 varicose, 397
Veneral infections 320
Vertigo 195, 200, 216, 224, 245, 253, 321
Vision
 blurred, 37, 52, 167, 195, 223, 245, 256
 impairment of, 53, 135, 199, 211, 217, 224
 improving, 53, 135, 201, 211, 221, 228, 238, 336, 418
 spots in, 38, 52, 224
Vitamin B12 193

General Index

Vitiligo 204, 217
Vocal polyps 332
Voice loss 77, 233
Vomiting 27, 40, 49, 63, 86, 231, 374
  after drinking water 350
  blood 47, 49, 54, 55, 57, 60, 62, 82, 88
  clear fluids 297
  Damp Heat and, 86
  Dampness and, 134
  Internal Cold and, 27, 125, 147, 178, 234
  Internal Heat and, 27, 47, 63, 122, 130, 151, 221, 224
  Lesser Yang diseases and, 40
  Liver Spleen disharmony and, 177
  Rebellious Qi and, 142, 245
  Spleen Qi Deficiency and, 212, 318
  Stagnation and, 145

Warming
  and circulating Qi in the Middle Burner 26
  the center 26, 28
  the channels 26, 32
  the joints 31
  the meridians 174
  the Spleen and Kidneys 176
  the Stomach and Spleen 34
  the Yang
Warts 75, 81, 94, 95, 96, 101, 231
Wasting diseases 189, 342
  and thirsting disorders 56
  due to Deficiency 183, 230
Water
  accumulation in the chest 94
  metabolism 100
  regulation of, 97, 100
  retention 93
    associated with Excess 95
Weight reduction/control 123, 188
Wet dreams 65, 363
Wheezing 107, 233
  Dampness and, 134
  Deficiency and, 183, 230

Internal Cold and, 24
Internal Heat and, 156
Phlegm and, 95, 116, 140
Whooping cough 129
Wind 24, 30, 66, 79, 103, 110, 128, 254, 432
  aversion to, 26, 294
  disperse, 30, 39, 41, 116, 119, 126, 161, 222, 259, 268, 300, 304, 363, 369
  External, calms, 365
  Internal 30, 222
  intestinal, 30
Wind-Cold 25
  common cold and, 42, 111
  Deficient conditions and, 294
  disperse, 127, 158, 282, 315
  summer 33
Wind-Damp 109, 291
  Bi pain and, 67, 100
  cramping and, 39
  disperse, 109, 166, 173, 226, 295, 345
  heavy feeling in the limbs and, 39
  numbness and 39
  obstruction and, 39, 67, 255
  skin ailments and, 79
Wind-Damp-Cold 110, 264
  conditions/diseases 26, 30, 210, 339, 351
  invasion of, 135, 345
  painful obstructions 29, 30, 31, 32, 252
  Stagnation 311
Wind-Damp-Heat 67, 107
Wind-Heat 35
  chills and, 38
  common cold and, 42
  disperses, 36, 37, 38, 39, 41, 69, 109, 255, 343
  External, 28, 119, 129, 222
  eyes and, 36, 37, 39, 50
  fever 35, 38, 42, 69, 70
  headache and, 36, 38, 41
  influenza and, 38, 69

General Index

Internal, 50
irritability and, 42
Liver channel and, 37
loss of voice 37
skin ailments and,
  measles, 35
  rashes, 35
sore throat and, 35, 36, 37, 38, 41, 69
Wind-stroke 254
Winston, David 42
Worms 152, 235, 260, 286
  expel, 344
  in the liver 286
  hookworm, 261
  pinworms, 131
  roundworm 90, 231, 235, 262
  tapeworm 151, 235, 261
Wounds 46, 77, 154, 157, 165, 169, 239, 286

Yang 432
  anchor the, 311
  ascending, 48
  brightness channels 31
  collapse of 173, 180
  obstructed, 25
  Tai, 24, 29, 314, 328
    conditions 351
  vitalizing, 32
  warming the, 31, 33, 178
Yang Deficiency 278, 309, 432
  Coldness and, 173
  Dampness and, 174, 296
  Spleen/Stomach, 40
Yang Ming 45, 53, 369
Yang tonics 202, 277, 285, 295, 315, 325
Yin 37, 432
  nourishing the, 44, 51, 53, 56, 91, 218, 226, 280, 282, 292, 295, 299, 321, 327, 349, 360
Yin Deficiency 180, 295, 327, 353, 360, 432

Yin Essence, nourishing 365
Yin tonics 181, 218
  Blood and, 199
Ying 25, 85, 185, 293
  clears Heat from, 299

Zang Fu 432

Index of Herbs by Latin Name

Abutili seu Malvae 108
Acanthopanax Gracilistylus 112
Achyranthis Aspera et Longumfolia 77
Achyranthis Bidentata 166
Acori Graminei 252
Actinolitum 212
Agastache Rugosa 132
Agrimonia Pilosa 151
Ailanthi Altissimae 235
Akebia Trifoliata 102
Albizziae Julibrissan 248
Alisma Orientalis 97
Allium Fistulosi 32
Allium Sativus 262
Allium Tuberosi 211
Alpinae Oxyphyllae 208
Alpinia Officinarum 179
Alumen 263
Amomum Villosum (Kravanh) 136
Anemarrhena Asphodeloides 50
Angelica Dahurica 31
Angelica Pubescentis 110
Angelica Sinensis 192
Aquilaria Agallocha 147
Arctium Lappa 35
Areca Catechu 144, 261
Arillus Euphoria Longanae 200
Arisaema Consanguineum (Arisaematis) 126
Aristolochia Debilis (Aristolochia) 131
Aristolochia Fangchi 107
Artemisia Annua 84
Artemisia Anomala 168
Artemisia Argyi 155
Artemisia Capillaris 107
Asarum Sieboldi 33
Asparagi Cochinchinensis 219
Asteris Tatarici 129
Astragalus Complanati 211
Astragalus Membranaceus 185
Atractylodes Lancea 135
Atractylodes Macrocephala 187

Bambusai in Taeniis 122
Belamcanda Chinensis 78
Benzoinum 251
Biota Orientalis 154, 248
Bletilla Striata 153
Bombyx Batryticatus 258
Borax 264
Borneol 251
Boswellia Carterii 165
Brucea Javonica 75
Buddleia Officinalis 52
Bupleurum Chinense 40
Buthus Martensi 257

Calculus Bovis 55
Calcitum 49
Calomelas 268
Camphora 266
Cannabis Sativa 91
Carapax Amydae Sinensis 227
Carthamus Tinctorius 164
Cassia Obtusifolia 50
Celosia Argentea 53
Chaenomelis Lagenaria 114
Chicken Gizzard's Skin 140
Chrysanthemum Indicum 73
Chrysanthemum Morifolium 37
Cibotii Barometz 209
Cimicifuga Foetida 41
Cinnabaris 244
Cinnamomum Cassia 25, 176
Cistanches Deserticolae 215
Citri Reticulatae 142
Citri Reticulatae Viride 143
Citrullus Vulgaris 84
Clematis Chinensis 113
Cnidii Monnieri 264
Codonopsis Pilosula 184
Coix Lachryma-jobi 100
Commiphora Myrrha 165
Concha Haliotidis 255
Concha Ostreae 243
Coptidis Chinensis 63
Cordyceps Sinensis 207
Coriandrum Sativum 34

Index of Herbs by Latin Name

Corni Officinalis 229
Cornu Cervi Parvum 202
Cornus Saigae Tataricae 256
Corydalis Yanhusuo 159
Crataegus Pinnatifida 137
Crinis Carbonisatus Hominis 155
Croton Tiglii 95
Cryptotympana Atrata 36
Cucurbitae Moschatae 262
Curculiginis Orchioidis 209
Curcuma Longa 160, 161
Cuscutae Chinensis 211
Cynanchi Baiwei 59
Cynomorium Songaricum 215
Cyperus Rotundus 144

Daphne Genkwa 94
Daucus Carota 261
Dendrobium Nobile (Dendrobii) 221
Desmodium Styracifolium 101
Dianthus Superbus 101
Dictamni Dasycarpi 79
Dioscorea Hypoglauca 108
Dioscorea Opposita 186
Diospyri Kaki 147
Dipsaci Asperi 203
Dolichoris Lablab 86
Drynariae Fortunei 210

Ecliptae Prostratae 224
Eleutherococcus Senticosus 112
Elsholtziae Splendens 32
Ephedra Sinica 24
Ephedrae Sinensis 238
Equiseti Hiemalis 42
Epimedii Grandifolrum 206
Eriobotrya Japonica 130
Eucommiae Ulmoidis 203
Eugenia Caryophyllata 178
Eupatorium Fortunei 133
Euphorbiae Kansui 93
Euryales Ferocis 236
Evodia Rutaecarpa 177

Foeniculum Vulgaris 178

Forsythia Suspensa 69
Fraxini Rhynchophylla 67
Fritillaria Cirrhosa 117
Fritillaria Thunbergii 118
Fructificatio Tremellai Fuciformis 225

Gardenia Jasminoidis 47
Gastrodiae Elatae 254
Gecko 207
Gelatinum Corii Asini 199
Gentiana Macrophylla 111
Gentiana Scabra 65
Ginkgo Biloba 232
Glehniae Littoralis 220
Glycines Germinatum 85
Glycyrrhizae Uralensis 190
Gypsum Fibrosum 45

Haematitum 245
Hailong 213
Hippocampus 214
Hirudo seu Whitmania 171
Hordeum Vulgaris Germinatus 138
Houttuynia Cordata 74
Hydnocarpi Anthelminticae 267

Immaturus Citri Aurantii 143
Imperata Cylindrica 156
Inula Japonica 125
Isatis Tinctoria 70, 71

Juglandis Regiae 205
Juncus Effusi 102

Kochia Scoparia 103

Lasiosphaera seu Calvatiae
 (Fructificatio) 76
Lateralis Aconiti 173
Ledebouriella Divaricata 30
Leonurus Heterophyllus 162
Lignum Pini Nodi 115
Lignum Sappan 170
Ligusticum Chuanxiong 158
Ligusticum Sinense 31

Index of Herbs by Latin Name

Ligustri Lucidum 224
Lilium Brownii (Lilii) 222
Lindera Strychnifolia 146
Liquidambar Orientalis 252
Liquidambar Taiwaniana 167
Lithospermi seu Arnebiae seu
    Macrotomia 58
Lobelia Chinensis 105
Lonicera Japonica 68
Lophatherum Gracilis 51
Loranthus Parasiticum 225
Lumbricus 257
Lycii Barbarum 198
Lycii Chinense (Radicis) 60
Lycopus Lucidum 163
Lygodium Japonica 75

Magnetitum 244
Magnolia Liliflorae 27
Magnolia Officinalis 134
Manitis Penta-Dactyla 168
Massa Fermentata 139
Melia Toosendan 148, 260
Mentha Haplocalycx 36
Millettia Reticulata 167
Minium 269
Mirabilitum 89
Momordicae Cochinchinensis 265
Momordicae Grosvenori 227
Morinda Officinalis 205
Morus Alba 38, 112, 201
Myristacae Fragrantis 233
Myrrha 165

Nelumbinis Nucifera
    48, 82, 156, 236
Nidus Vespae 267
Notopteryguim Incisum 29

Olibanum 165
Ootheca Mantidis 240
Ophiopogonis Japonici 219
Oryza Glutinosa 238
Oryza Sativa Germinatus 139
Os Draconis 242

Os Sepiae Seu Sepiellae 239

Paeonia Lactiflora 197
Paeonia Rubra 163
Paeonia Suffruticosa 57
Panacis Quinquefolii 218
Panax Ginseng 183
Panax Notoginseng 152
Pasta Acaciae seu Uncariae 265
Patrinia Villosa et Scabiosaefolia 73
Pericarpium Papaveris 234
Pericarpium Punicae Granati 234
Perillae Frutescens 28, 130
Peucedanum Praeruptorum
    (Peucedani) 119
Pharbitidis Nil 92
Phaseolus Radiatus 83
Phellondendron Amurense 64
Phragmites Communis 49
Phytolacca Acinosa 94
Picrorhiza Scrophulariaflora 67
Pinellia Ternata 124
Piper Longum 179
Placenta Hominis 216
Plantaginis Asiatica 104
Plastrum Testudinis 226
Platycodum Grandiflorum 127
Polygalae Tenuifoliae 247
Polygonatum Odorati 222
Polygonatum Sibiricum 189
Polygonum Avicularis 104
Polygonum Multiflorum 195, 249
Polyporus Umbellatus 99
Poria Cocos 98
Portulaca Oleracea 76
Prunella Vulgaris 48
Prunus Armeniaca 128
Prunus Japonica 92
Prunus Mume 231
Prunus Persica 164
Pseudobulbus Shancigu 267
Pseudostellaria Heterophylla 188
Psoraleae Corylifoliae 204
Pteria Margaritifera 246
Puerariae Lobatae 39

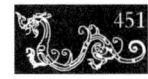

Index of Herbs by Latin Name

Pulsatilla Chinensis 72
Pumice 122
Pyritum 169

Quisqualis Indicae 260

Raphanus Sativus 140
Realgar 268
Rehmannia Glutinosa 56, 194
Rheum Palmatum (Rhei) 87
Rhinoceri Unicornis 54
Rosa Laevigatae 237
Rosa Rugosa 149
Rubi Chinigii 237
Rubia Cordifolia (Rubiae) 157

Saccharum Granorum 191
Salvia Miltiorrhiza 159
Sanguis Draconis 169
Sanguisorba Officinalis 153
Santali Albi 148
Sargassii Pallidum 123
Saussurea Lappa 145
Schisandrae Chinensis 230
Schizonepetae Tenuifolia 28
Scolopendra Subspinipes 258
Scrophularia Ningpoensis 56
Scutellaria Baicalensis 62
Scutellaria Barbata 78
Secretia Moschus 250
Sesami Indicum 223
Smilacis Glabrae 79
Sojae Praeparatum 42
Sophora Flavescentis 66
Sophora Tonkinensis et
    Subprostrata 77
Spirodela Polyrrhiza 43
Stalactitum 213
Stephania Tetrandra 106
Stellaria Dichotomae 61
Stemona Sessifolia (Stemonae) 131
Strichopus Japonicus 214
Strychni 270
Succus Bambusae 121
Sulfur 269

Talcum 99
Taraxacum Mongolicum 70
Terminaliae Chebulae 233
Testis et Penis Otariae 212
Thallus Algae (Laminaria) 123
Torreyae Grandis 261
Tribuli Terrestris 255
Trichosanthes Kirilowii 119, 120
Tritici Levis 239
Trogopterori seu Pteromi 172
Tussilago Farfarae 129
Typha Angustifolia (Pollen Typhae)
    151
Typhonium Giganteum 127

Uncariae Rhynchophylla 253

Vaccaria Segetalis 170
Vespertilionis Murini
    (Excrementum) 52
Viola Yedoensis 72
Viscum Coloratum 225
Viticis Rotundusfolia 39

Xanthium Sibiricum 114

Zea Mays 105
Zingiberis Officinalis 26, 176
Zizyphus Jujuba 189
Zizyphus Spinosae 246

Index of Herbs by Chinese Name

Ai Ye 155
An Xi Xiang 251

Ba Dou 95
Ba Ji Tian 205
Bai Bu 131
Bai Fu Zi 127
Bai Guo 232
Bai He 22
Bai Ji 153
Bai Ji Li 255
Bai Jiang Cao 73
Bai Mao Gen 156
Bai Mu Er 225
Bai Shao 197
Bai Tou Weng 72
Bai Wei 59
Bai Xian Pi 79
Bai Zhi 31
Bai Zhu 187
Bai Zi Ren 248
Ban Bian Lian 105
Ban Lan Gen 71
Ban Xia 124
Ban Zhi Lian 78
Bei Sha Shen 220
Bei Xie 108
Bi Ba 179
Bian Dou 86
Bian Xu 104
Bie Jia 227
Bing Lang 261
Bing Pian 251
Bo He 36
Bu Gu Zhi 204

Cang Er Zi 114
Cang Zhu 135
Ce Bai Ye 154
Chai Hu 40
Chan Tui 36
Che Qian Zi 104
Chen Pi 142
Chen Xiang 147
Chi Shao 163

Chuan Bei Mu 117
Chuan Lian Zi 148
Chuan Shan Jia 168
Chuan Xiong 158
Chun Pi 235
Ci Shi 244
Cong Bai 32

Da Feng Zi 267
Da Fu Pi 144
Da Huang 87
Da Qing Ye 70
Da Suan 262
Da Zao 189
Dai Zhe Shi 245
Dan Dou Chi 42
Dan Shen 159
Dan Zhu Ye 51
Dang Gui 192
Dang Shen 184
Deng Xin Cao 102
Di Fu Zi 103
Di Gu Pi 60
Di Long 257
Di Yu 153
Ding Xiang 178
Dong Chong Xia Cao 207
Dong Kui Zi 108
Dou Juan 85
Du Huo 110
Du Zhong 203

E Guan Shi 213
E Jiao 199
Er Cha 265

Fan Xie Ye 89
Fang Feng 30
Fei Zi 261
Fu Hai Shi 122
Fu Ling 98
Fu Pen Zi 237
Fu Ping 43
Fu Xiao Mai 239
Fu Zi 173

Index of Herbs by Chinese Name

Gan Cao 190
Gan Jiang 176
Gan Sui 93
Gao Ben 31
Gao Liang Jiang 179
Ge Gen 39
Ge Jie 207
Gou Ji 209
Gou Qi Zi 198
Gou Teng 253
Gu Sui Bu 210
Gu Ya 139
Gua Lou 119
Gua Lou Ren 120
Guang Fang Ji 107
Gui Ban 226
Gui Zhi 25

Hai Dai 123
Hai Gou Shen 212
Hai Ma 214
Hai Piao Xiao 239
Hai Shen 214
Hai Zao 123
Han Fang Ji 106
Han Lian Cao 224
Han Shui Shi 49
He Huan Pi 248
He Shi 261
He Shou Wu 195
He Ye 82
He Zi 233
Hei Zhi Ma 223
Hong Hua 164
Hou Po 134
Hu Huang Lian 67
Hu Lu Ba 208
Hu Sui 34
Hu Tao Ren 205
Hua Shi 99
Huang Bai 64
Huang Jing 189
Huang Lian 63
Huang Qi 185
Huang Qin 62

Huo Ma Ren 91
Huo Xiang 132
Ji Nie Jin 140
Ji Xue Teng 167
Jiang Can 258
Jiang Huang 161
Jie Geng 127
Jin Qian Cao 101
Jin Sha Teng 75
Jin Yin Hua 68
Jin Ying Zi 237
Jing Jie 28
Jiu Zi 211
Ju Hua 37
Jue Ming Zi 50

Ku Lian Gen Pi 260
Ku Shen 66
Kuan Dong Hua 129
Kun Bu 123

Lai Fu Zi 140
Lian Qiao 69
Lian Xin 48
Lian Zi 236
Ling Yang Jiao 256
Liu Huang 269
Liu Ji Nu 168
Long Dan Cao 65
Long Gu 242
Long Yan Rou 200
Lu Dou 83
Lu Feng Fang 267
Lu Gen 49
Lu Hui 90
Lu Lu Tong 167
Lu Rong 202
Luo Han Guo 227

Ma Bo 76
Ma Chi Xian 76
Ma Dou Ling 131
Ma Huang 24
Ma Huang Gen 238
Ma Qian Zi 270

Index of Herbs by Chinese Name

Mai Men Dong 219
Mai Ya 138
Man Jing Zi 39
Mang Xiao 89
Mei Gui Hua 149
Mi Meng Hua 52
Ming Fan 263
Mo Yao 165
Mu Bie Zi 265
Mu Dan Pi 57
Mu Gua 114
Mu Li 243
Mu Tong 102
Mu Xiang 145
Mu Zei 42

Nan Gua Zi 262
Niu Bang Zi 35
Niu Huang 55
Niu Xi 166
Nu Zhen Zi 224
Nuo Dao Gen Xu 238

Ou Jie 156

Pei Lan 133
Pen Tsao 9
Peng Sha 264
Pi Pa Ye 130
Pu Gong Ying 70
Pu Huang 151

Qian Cao Gen 157
Qian Dan 269
Qian Hu 119
Qian Niu Zi 92
Qian Shi 236
Qiang Huo 29
Qin Jiao 111
Qin Pi 67
Qing Fen 268
Qing Hao 84
Qing Pi 143
Qing Xiang Zi 53
Qu Mai 101

Quan Xie 257

Ren Shen 183
Rou Cong Rong 215
Rou Dou Kou 233
Rou Gui 176
Ru Xiang 165

San Qi 152
Sang Ji Sheng 225
Sang Piao Xiao 240
Sang Shen 201
Sang Ye 38
Sang Zhi 112
Sha Ren 136
Sha Yuan Ji Li 211
Shan Ci Gu 267
Shan Dou Gen 77
Shan Zha 137
Shan Shu Yu 229
Shang Lu 94
She Chuang Zi 264
She Gan 78
She Xiang 250
Shen Qu 139
Sheng Di Huang 56
Sheng Jiang 26
Sheng Ma 41
Shi Chang Pu 252
Shi Di 147
Shi Gao 45
Shi Ju 221
Shi Jue Ming 255
Shi Jun Zi 260
Shi Liu Pi 234
Shu Di Huang 194
Shui Zhi 171
Song Jie 115
Su He Xiang 252
Su Mu 170
Suan Zao Ren 246
Suo Yang 215

Tai Zi Shen 188
Tan Xiang 148

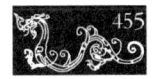

Index of Herbs by Chinese Name

Tao Ren 164
Tian Hua Fen 120
Tian Ma 254
Tian Men Dong 219
Tian Nan Xing 126
Tu Fu Ling 79
Tu Niu Xi 77
Tu Si Zi 211

Wang Bu Liu Xing 170
Wei Ling Xian 113
Wu Gong 258
Wu Jia Pi 112
Wu Ling Zhi 172
Wu Mei 231
Wu Wei Zi 230
Wu Yao 146
Wu Zhu Yu 177

Xi Gua 84
Xi Jiao 54
Xi Xin 33
Xi Yang Shen 218
Xia Ku Cao 48
Xian He Cao 151
Xian Mao 209
Xiang Fu 144
Xiang Ru 32
Xiao Hui Xiang 178
Xin Yi Hua 27
Xing Ren 128
Xiong Huang 268
Xu Duan 203
Xuan Fu Hua 125
Xuan Shen 56
Xue Jie 169
Xue Yu Tan 155

Ya Dan Zi 75
Yan Hu Suo 159
Yang Zi Shi 212
Ye Jiao Teng 249
Ye Ju Hua 73
Ye Ming Sha 52
Yi Mu Cao 162

Yi Tang 191
Yi Yi Ren 100
Yi Zhi Ren 208
Yin Chai Hu 61
Yin Chen Hao 107
Yin Yang Huo 206
Ying Su Ke 234
Yu Jin 160
Yu Li Ren 92
Yu Mi Xu 105
Yu Xing Cao 74
Yu Zhu 222
Yuan Hua 94

Ze Lan 163
Ze Xie 97
Zhang Nao 266
Zhe Bei Mu 118
Zhen Zhu Mu 246
Zhi Mu 50
Zhi Shi 143
Zhi Zi 47
Zhu Li 121
Zhu Ling 99
Zhu Ru 122
Zhu Sha 244
Zi Cao 58
Zi He Che 216
Zi Hua Di Ding 72
Zi Ran Tong 169
Zi Su Ye 28
Zi Su Zi 130
Zi Wan 129

Index of Chinese Herbal Formulas

Achyranthes and Rehmannia Combination
    (Restore the Left Pill - Zui gui wan) 278
Aconite and Asarum Combination (Ma huang fu zi xi xin tang) 278
Aconite, Ginger and Licorice Combination (Si ni tang) 277
Aconite, Ginseng and Ginger Combination (Fu zi li zhong wan) 279, 326
Anemarrhena, Phellodendron and Gehmannia Formula
    (Zhi bai di huang wan) 195, 280
Anemone Combination (Bai tou weng tang) 281
Antelope Horn and Uncaria Combination
    (Ling yang gou teng tang) 280
Apricot Seed and Perilla Formula (Xiang su san) 281

Baked Licorice Combination (Zhi gan cao tang) 282
Bamboo and Poria Combination (Wen dan tang) 283, 298
Bezoar Resurrection Pills (An gong niu huang wan) 283
Big Pearl for Internal Wind (Da ding feng zhu) 283
Blood Replenishing Decoction (Ji chuan jian) 285
Blue Fairy Pills For Lower Back Pain (Qing e wan) 285
Bruise Relieving Powder (Qi li san) 286, 414
Bupleurum and Cinnamon Combination (Chai hu hui zhi tang) 287
Bupleurum and Dang Gui Formula
    (Xiao yao san or Rambling Powder) 287
Bupleurum and Dragon Bone Combination
    (Chai hu jia long gu mu li tang) 288
Bupleurum and Peony Combination (Jia wei xiao yao san) 289, 273
Bupleurum and Schizonepeta Formula (Shi wei bai du tang) 289
Bupleurum and Zhi Shi Formula
    (Si ni san or Frigid Extremities Powder) 286
Bupleurum, Cinnamon Twig and Ginger Combination
    (Chai hu gui zhi gan jiang tang) 290
Bupleurum Formula (Yi gan san) 290

Cannabis Seed Pills (Ma zi ren wan) 291
Capillaris Combination (Yin chen hao tang) 291
Cinnabar Sedative Pills (Zhu sha an shen wan) 292
Cinnamon and Dragon Bone Combination
    (Gui zhi long gu mu li tang) 292
Cinnamon and Poria Combination (Gui zhi fu ling wang) 58, 293
Cinnamon Combination (Gui zhi tang) 293
Cinnamon Twig Paeonia and Anemarrhena Decoction
    (Gui zhi shao yao zhi mu tang) 26, 294
Circuligo and Epimedium Combination (Er xian tang) 295
Citrus and Crataegus Formula
    (Bao he wan or Preserve Harmony Pill) 296

Index of Chinese Herbal Formulas

Citrus and Pinellia Combination
   (Er chen tang or Two Cured Decoction) 296
Clear the Nutritive Decoction (Qing ying tang) 298
Clear the Stomach Powder (Qing wei san) 299
Clematis and Stephania Combination (Shu jing huo xue tang) 299
Clove and Persimmon Calyx Combination (Shi di tang) 300
Cnidium and Green Tea Combination (Chuan xiong cha tiao san) .. 300
Coix Combination (Yi yi ren tang) 301
Conduct the Heart Fire Downward (Dao chi san) 301
Coptis and Cinnamon Formula (Jiao tai wan) 302
Coptis and Rhubarb Combination (San huang xie xin tang) 306
Coptis and Scutellaria Combination (Huang lian jie du tang) 302
Dang Gui and Arctium Combination (Xiao feng san) 303
Dang Gui and Evodia Combination (Wen jing tang) 305
Dang Gui and Gelatin Combination (Jiao ai tang) 306
Dang Gui and Jujube Combination (Dang gui si ni tang) 307
Dang Gui and Peony Formula (Dang gui shao yao san) 304
Dang Gui Decoction for Frigid Extremities (Dang gui si ni tang) 309
Dang Gui, Dipsacus and Tian Qi Ginseng Combination (Shu jin san). 307
Dang Gui Four Combination (Si wu tang) 194, 195, 273, 308
Dang Gui, Gentiana and Aloe (Dang gui long hui wan) 308
Dianthus Formula (Ba zheng san) 310
Disperse Vital Enerby in the Liver Powder (Chai hu su gan san) 310
Dragon Bone and Oyster Shell Combination (Long gu mu li tang) .. 311
Du Huo and Loranthes Combination (Du huo ji sheng tang) 311

Eight Precious Herbs (Ba zhen tang) 312, 325
Ephedra, Aconite and Asarum Combination
   (Ma huang fu zi xi xin tang) 315
Ephedra and Ginkgo Combination (Ding chuan tang) 313
Ephedra, Apricot, Gypsum and Licorice Decoction
   (Ma xing shi gan tang) 313
Ephedra Decoction (Ma Huang Tang) 314
Eriobotrya and Ophiopogon Combination (Qing zao jiu fei tang) ... 315
Eucommia and Rehmannia Combination
   (You gui wan or Restore the Right) 316
Evodia Combination (Wu zhu yu tang) 178, 316

Five Peel Decoction (Wu pi yin) 317
Forsythia and Rhubarb Combination (Liang ge san) 317
Four Major Herbs Decoction (Si jun zi tang) 99, 184, 318
Frigid Extremities Decoction (Si ni tang) 319

Index of Chinese Herbal Formulas

Gardenia and Poria Combination (Wei wu lin san) 319
Gardenia and Prepared Soybean Decoction (Zhi zi dou chi tang) 320
Gasping Formula (Xiang sheng po tai luen) 320
Gastrodia and Uncaria Combination (Tian ma gou teng yin) 321
Generate the Pulse Powder (Sheng mai san) 321
Gentiana Combination (Long dan xie gan tang) 322
Ginseng and Astragalus Combination (Bu zhong yi qi tang) 41, 324
Ginseng and Dang Gui Ten Combination
 (Shi quan da bu tang) 325
Ginseng and Ginger Combination
 (Li zhong wan or Regulate the Middle Pill) 326
Ginseng and Longan Combination (Gui pi tang) 201, 322
Ginseng and Zizyphus Combination (Tian wang bu xin tang) 326
Ginseng, Poria and Atractylodes Posder (Shen ling bai zhu san) 323
Goiter Pills (Xiao lei wan) 327
Gypsum Combination (Shi gao tang) 328

Increase Body Fluids Decoction (Zhen yi tang) 328
Inula Flower and Hematite Decoction (Xuan fu dai zhe tang) 329

Jade Screen Powder (Yu ping feng san) 185, 329

Kaki Combination (Ding xiang shi di tang) 330

Ledebouriella dna Platycodon Formula (Fang feng tong sheng) 330
Licorice, Sprouted Wheat and Jujube Date Decoction
 (Gan mai da zao tang) 331
Lily Bulb Decoction to Consolidate the Lungs
 (Bai he gu jin tang) 331
Lindera Decoction
 (Jia wei wu yao tang or Augmented Lindera Decoction) 333
Lindera Formula for Regulating Qi (Wu yao shun qi wan) 333
Liver Strengthening Decoction (Yi guan jian) 332
Lonicera and Forsythia Combination (Yin qiao san) 334
Lotus Stem and Ginseng Combination (Qing shu yi qi tang) 335
Lycium, Chrysanthemum and Rehmannia Combination
 (Qi ju di huang wan) 336

Magnetite and Cinnabar Sedative (Ci zhu wan) 336
Magnolia and Ginger Formula (Ping wei san) 336
Magnolia and Hoelen Combination (Wei ling tang) 337
Major Bupleurum Combination (Da chai hu tang) 338
Major Rhubarb Combination (Da cheng qi tang) 338
Mantis Egg-case Powder (Sang piao xiao san) 339

INDEX OF CHINESE HERBAL FORMULAS

Minor Bluegreen Dragon Decoction (Xiao qing long tang) 176, 315, 340
Minor Bupleurum (Xiao chai hu tang) 341
Minor Cinnamon and Paeonia Combination (Xiao jian zhong tang) . 342
Minor Pinellia and Poria Combination
  (Xiao ban xia jia fu ling tang) 342
Minor Rhubarb Combination (Xiao cheng qi tang) 342
Modified Du Huo and Loranthes Combination
  (Du huo ji sheng tang) 312
Morus and Chrysanthemum Combination (Sang ju yin) 343
Morus and Lycium Formula (Xie bai san) 343
Mume Formula (Wu mei wan) 343

Nine Herbs with Notopterygii Decoction (Jiu wei qiang huo tang) ... 344
Notopteryguim and Tumeric Combination (Chuan bi tang) 345

Ophiopogon and Trichosanthes Combination (Mai men dong yin zi) . 346
Ophiopogon Combination (Mai men dong tang) 346

Persica and Rhubarb Combination (Tao he cheng qi tang) 347
Pinellia and Magnolia Combination (Ban xia hou po tang) 347
Pinellia Combination (Ban xia xie xin tang) 348
Polyporus Combination (Zhu ling tang) 349
Poria, Cinnamon, Atractylodes and Licorice Combination
  (Ling gui zhu gan tang) 349
Poria Five Herbs Formula (Wu ling san) 99, 350
Pueraria Combination (Ge gen tang) 350
Pueraria, Scute and Coptis Combination
  (Ge gen huang qin huang lian tang) 303

Rehmannia and Gypsum Combination (Yu nu jian) 351
Rehmannia Eight Combination
  (Jin gui shen qi wan or Ba wei di huang wan) 177, 295, 352
Rehmannia Six Combination (Liu wei di huang wan) 58, 65, 195, 202, 353
Remove Blood Stagnation Below the Diaphragm Decoction
  (Ge xia zhu yu tang) 354
Remove Blood Stagnation in the Chest Decoction
  (Xue fu zhu yu tang) 355
Replenishing the Yang (You gui wan) 356
Rhinoceros and Antelope Horn Formula (Zi xue dan) 357
Rhinoceros and Rehmannia Combination (Xi jiao di huang tang) ... 356
Rhubarb and Mirabilitum Combination (Tiao wei cheng qi tang) 358
Rhubarb and Moutan Combination (Da huang mu dan pi tang) 358

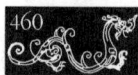

Index of Chinese Herbal Formulas

Schizonepeta and Forsythia Combination (Jing jie lian qiao tang) 358
Schizonepeta and Ledebouriella Combination
  (Jing fang bai du san) 359
Scrophularia and Ophiopogon Combination (Zeng ye tang) 360
Seaweed Decoction (Hai zao yu hu tang) 360
Six Major Herbs (Liu jun zi tang) 53, 298, 361
Six to One Powder (Liu yi san) 361
Small Thistle Decoction (Xiao ji yin zi) 362
Sophora Flower Powder (Huai hua san) 362
Spermatorrhea Pills (Jin suo gu jing wan) 363
Spleen Warming Decoction (Wen pi tang) 364
Stagnation Relieving Pills (Yue qu wan) 180, 364
Stephania and Astragalus Combination (Fang ji huang qi tang) 365
Sweet Wormwood and Tortoise Shell Formula
  (Qing hao bie jia tang) 366

Threatened Abortion Powder (Tai shan pan shi san) 366
Two Effective Ingredients (Er miao san) 367

Vitality Combination (Zhen wu tang) 367

Warm and Activate the Circulation of the Heart Pill
  (Guan xin su he wan) 368
White Tiger Decoction (Bai hu tang) 368

Xanthium Powder (Cang er san) 369

Zizyphus Combination (Suan zao ren tang) 370

INDEX FOR CHAPTER 3
TREATMENT OF SPECIFIC DISEASE

Abnormal labor 401
Acne 415
Allergic rhinitis 391
Alopecia (baldness) 417
Amenorrhea 399
Angina pectoris (heart pains) 395
Anorexia 374
Anxiety 407
Arteriosclerosis 394
Atherosclerosis 394
Arthritis 412
Athlete's foot 416

Back pain 411
Bronchial asthma 388
Bronchitis 388
Burns 414

Cancer 385
Carbuncle 417
Cataracts 418
Change of life (Climacteric) 402
Cirrhosis 380
Colitis, ulcerative 377
Colon
   spastic or irritable 378
Common cold 387
Conjunctivitis 418
Constipation 375
Cough 387
Cuts 414
Cysts 403

Deafness 419
Dementia
   pre-senile 410
   senile 410
Depression 410
Dermatitis 415
Diabetes mellitus 381
Diarrhea 376
Dysentery 419
Dysmenorrhea (painful menstruation) 399

Dysuria (burning urine) 398

Earache 418
Eczema 415
Edema 398
Emphysema 388
Epilepsy 413
Erysipelas 415

Fibroids 403
Flatulence 373
Frostbite 416
Furuncle 417

Gallbladder disease 378
Gastritis 374
Gingivitis 417

Headaches
   acute 406
   chronic 407
Heart disease 392
Hematuria (blood in the urine) 397
Hemorrhoids
   external 376
   internal 377
Hepatitis 379
Herpes
   simplex 416
   zoster 416
Hiccups 375
Hypertension 392
Hyperthyroidism 382
Hypoglycemia (low blood sugar) 381
Hypotension 394
Hypothyroidism 383
Hysteria 407

Impotence 403
Indigestion 372
Infections
   fungus 416
Infertility 400
Influenza 389
Injuries 414

Index for Chapter 3
Treatment of Specific Disease

Insomnia 407
Insufficient lactation 402

Kidney stones 398

Laryngitis 392
Leukorrhea (vaginal discharge) 398
Lupus erythematosus 383
Lymphadenitis (swollen lymph glands) 396

Malignancies 385
Mania 410
Mastitis 401
Memory weakness 410
Menopause 402
Menorrhagia 400
Migraine 406
Miscarriage 401
Morning sickness 402
Muscular atrophy 412

Nausea 374
Neck pain 412
Neuralgia 412
Nephritis 397

Orchitis (inflammation of the testicles) 404
Osteoarthritis 412

Pain
  back, 411
  neck, 412
Parasites
  bacterial and amoebic 419
  worms 419
Peptic ulcer 374
Pleurisy 390
Pleuritis 390
Pneumonia 389
Premature ejaculation 404
Prostate problems 405
Pruritis 415
Psoriasis 415

Polyuria 397

Rheumatic arthritis 412

Schizophrenia 410
Sciatica 411
Shingles 416
Skin 415
Sore throat 392
Spasm
  esophageal 378
Spermatorrhea (penile discharge) 404
Stomachache 373
Stress 407

Temporal frontal headaches 371
Thrombocytopenic purpura 384
Tinea pedis (athlete's foot) 416
Tinnitis 419
Toothache 417
Tuberculosis 389

Ulcerative colitis 377
Upper respiratory allergies 390
Urinary tract
  bleeding 397
  infection 396
Urination
  burning, 398
  excessive, 398
Uterine prolapse 403

Varicose veins 395
Vision
  improving, 418
Vomiting 374

Worms 419
Wounds 414

Herbs and other natural health products and information are often available natural food stores or metaphysical bookstores. If you cannot find what yo need locally, you can contact one of the following sources of supply.

Sources of Supply:

The following companies have an extensive selection of useful products and a long track-record of fulfillment. They have natural body care, aromatherapy, flower essences, crystals and tumbled stones, homeopathy, herbal products, vitamins and supplements, videos, books, audio tapes, candles, incense and bulk herbs, teas, massage tools and products and numerous alternative health items across a wide range of categories.

WHOLESALE:

Wholesale suppliers sell to stores and practitioners, not to individual consumers buying for their own personal use. Individual consumers should contact the RETAIL supplier listed below. Wholesale accounts should contact with business name, resale number or practitioner license in order to obtain a wholesale catalog and set up an account.

Lotus Light Enterprises, Inc.
PO Box 1008 N
Silver Lake, WI 53170 USA
262 889 8501 (phone)
262 889 8591 (fax)
800 548 3824 (toll free order line)
Website: www.lotuslight.com
email: lotuslight@lotuspress.com

RETAIL:

Retail suppliers provide products by mail order direct to consumers for their personal use. Stores or practitioners should contact the wholesale supplier listed above.

International
PO Box 489 N
Twin Lakes, WI 53181 USA
800 643 4221 (toll free order line)
262 889 8581 office phone
EMAIL: internatural@internatural.com
WEB SITE: www.internatural.com

Web site includes an extensive annotated catalog of more than 14,000 items th can be ordered "on line" for your convenience 24 hours a day, 7 days a week.

BIOMAGNETIC and Herbal Therapy
by Dr. Michael Tierra

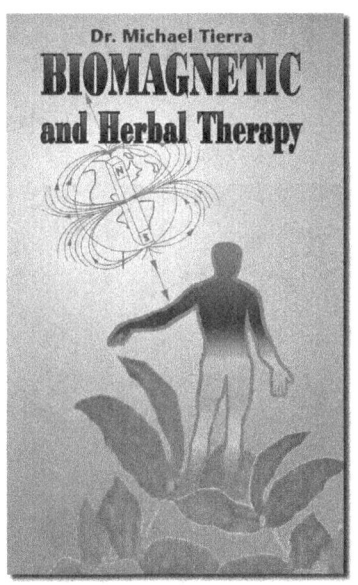

$10.95 | 96pp
5.375" x 8.5" | tradepaper
ISBN: 978-0-9149-5533-7

Magnetic energy is the structural force of the universe. In this book the respected herbalist, Dr. Michael Tierra, enlightens us on the healing influence of commercially available magnet for many conditions and describes the sometime miraculous relief from such problems as joint pain, skin diseases, acidity, blood pressure, tumors, kidney, liver and thyroid problems, and more. Magnetizing herbs, teas, water and their usage in conjunction with direct placement of magnets for synergistic effectiveness is presented in a systematic, succinct and practical manner for the benefit of the professional and lay person alike. Replete with diagrams and appendices, this is a "how to do" practical handbook for augmenting health and obtaining relief from pain.

The paradigm of health in the future is based on energy flow. This paradigm reaches back to the ancient healing arts of the traditional Chinese, the Ayurvedic and the Native American cultures. It is connected to the work of Hippocrates, the "father" of Western medicine, in ancient Greek culture, and found its way through the herbal and homeopathic science that has flourished in Europe over the last few hundred years.

Dr. Tierra is the author of the all-time best selling herbal *The Way of Herb* as well as the synthesizing work *Planetary Herbology*. He is a practicing herbalist and educator in the field with a background of studies spanning the Chinese and Ayurvedic, the Native American and the European herbal traditions.

Available at bookstores and natural food stores nationwide OR order your copy directly be sending $24.95 plus $2.50 shipping/handling ($.75 s/h for each additional copy ordered at the same time) to:

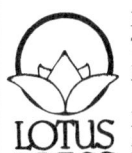

LOTUS PRESS | PO Box 325, Twin Lakes, WI 35181, USA
Toll Free Order Line: 800.824.6396 | Office PH: 262.889.8561 | Office FAX: 262.889.8591
Email: lotuspress@lotuspress.com | Web Site: www.LotusPress.com

Lotus Press is the publisher of a wide range of books in the field of alternative health, including Ayurveda, Chinese medicine, herbology, aromatherapy, Reiki and energetic healing modalities. Request our *free* book catalog.

Planetary Herbology
by Dr. Michael Tierra, C.A., N.D.

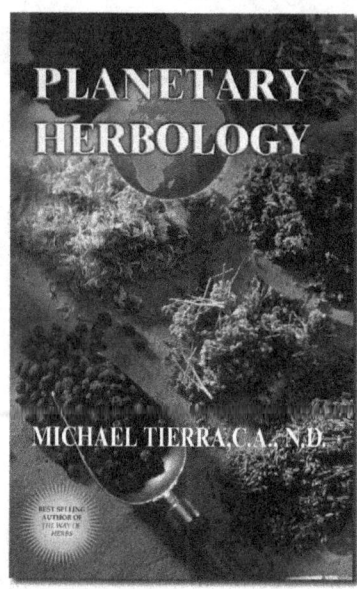

$19.95 | 485 pp
5.5" x 8.5" | paper; charts
ISBN: 978-0-9415-2427-8

Lotus Press is pleased to bring to you a practical handbook and reference guide to the healing herbs, a landmark publication in this field. For unprecedented usefulness in practical applications, the author provides a comprehensive listing of the more than 400 medical herbs available in the west. They are classified according to their chemical constituents, properties and actions, indicated uses and suggested dosages. Students of eastern medical theory will find the western herbs cross-referenced to the Chinese and Ayurvedic (Indic) systems of herbal therapies. This is a useful handbook fror practitioners as well as readers with a general interest in herbology.

Michael Tierra, C.A., N.D., whose very popular earlier book *THE WAY OF HERBS,* led the way to this new major work. He is one of this country's most respected herbalists, a practitioner and teacher who has taught and lectured widely. His eclectic background studies in American Indian herbalism, the herbal system of Dr. John Christopher, and traditional oriental systems of India and China, contributes a special richness to his writing.

Available at bookstores and natural food stores nationwide OR order your copy directly be sending $24.95 plus $2.50 shipping/handling ($.75 s/h for each additional copy ordered at the same time) to:

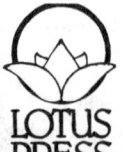

LOTUS PRESS | PO Box 325, Twin Lakes, WI 35181, USA
Toll Free Order Line: 800.824.6396 | Office PH: 262.889.8561 | Office FAX: 262.889.8591
Email: lotuspress@lotuspress.com | Web Site: www.LotusPress.com

Lotus Press is the publisher of a wide range of books in the field of alternative health, including Ayurveda, Chinese medicine, herbology, aromatherapy, Reiki and energetic healing modalities. Request our *free* book catalog.

The Definitive Text on Chinese Herbal Medicine in 2 Volumes!

CHINESE TRADITIONAL HERBAL MEDICINE, VOL. 1 & 2
by Michael Tierra, O.M.D. and Lesley Tierra, L.Ac.

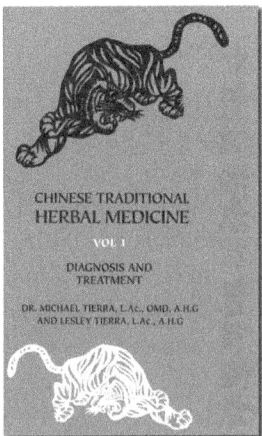

VOLUME I: Diagnosis and Treatment
ISBN: 978-0-9149-5531-3 | $22.95 | 418pp

This first volume focuses on theory, principles, diagnostic methods and treatment modalities that are an essential part of the practice of Traditional Chinese Medicine (TCM). It provices background and theoretical framework for the reader to both understand the viewpoint and apply the principles of TCM.

VOLUME II: Materia Medica and Herbal Resource
ISBN: 978-0-9149-5532-0 | $29.95 | 480pp

This Materia Medica and Herbal Resource has been organized and developed to make Chinese herbology accessible to the Western reader or practitioner. The book also include extensive treatement of disease conditions. There are a number of useful index listings including Latin name, Chinese name, Chinese herbal formulae, disease condition and general index.

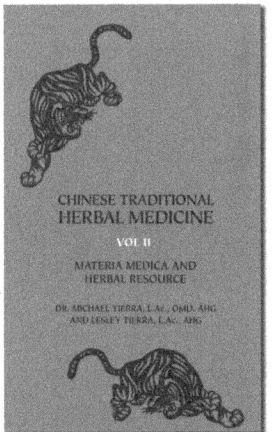

Also Available in a TWO VOLUME SET!
ISBN: 978-0-9149-5539-9 | $51.95 | 898pp *(total)*

ailable at bookstores and natural food stores nationwide OR order your copy directly be sending $24.95
 is $2.50 shipping/handling ($.75 s/h for each additional copy ordered at the same time) to:

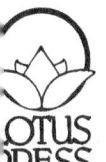

LOTUS PRESS | PO Box 325, Twin Lakes, WI 35181, USA
Toll Free Order Line: 800.824.6396 | Office PH: 262.889.8561 | Office FAX: 262.889.8591
Email: lotuspress@lotuspress.com | Web Site: www.LotusPress.com

Lotus Press is the publisher of a wide range of books in the field of alternative health, including Ayurveda, Chinese medicine, herbology, aromatherapy, Reiki and energetic healing modalities. Request our *free* book catalog.

the way of AYURVEDIC HERBS

A Contemporary Introduction and Useful Manual for the World's Oldest Healing System

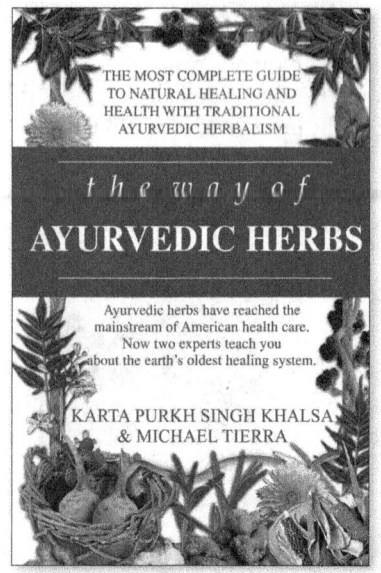

Ashwaganda for stamina and vitality... arjuna for heart health... dandelion for breast wellness... gokshura to reach a sexual peak. Traditional Ayurveda, using the principles of the tree doshas, constitutional body typing and highly individualized therapies, is the oldest continuously practiced healing system on Earth. Over those many centuries, generations of Ayurvedic scholars and physicians have reviewed, inspected, dissected and refined the system to perfect a highly effective form of health, balance and healing. Now, two of the world leading Ayurvedic herbalists, both leaders of the holistic health renaissance, and who, together, bring a total of over 75 years of practice to the work, heave crafted a manual for making Ayurveda understandable and eminently, practically useful. *The Way of Ayurvedic Herbs* is more than an herb manual. It is a life path to well-being.

THE WAY OF AYURVEDIC HERBS
Karta Purkh Singh Khalsa & Michael Tierra
ISBN: 978-0-9409-8598-8 | $24.95 | 400 PAGES

Available at bookstores and natural food stores nationwide OR order your copy directly be sending $24.95 plus $2.50 shipping/handling ($.75 s/h for each additional copy ordered at the same time) to:

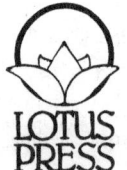

LOTUS PRESS | PO Box 325, Twin Lakes, WI 35181, USA
Toll Free Order Line: 800.824.6396 | Office PH: 262.889.8561 | Office FAX: 262.889.859
Email: lotuspress@lotuspress.com | Web Site: www.LotusPress.com

Lotus Press is the publisher of a wide range of books in the field of alternative health, including Ayurveda, Chinese medicine, herbology, aromatherapy, Reiki and energetic healing modalities. Request our *free* book catalog.

Treating Cancer
with HERBS

Dr. Michael Tierra, L.Ac., N.D., AHG

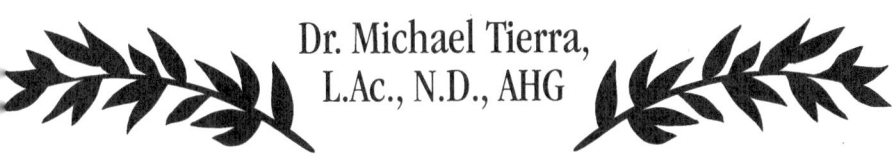

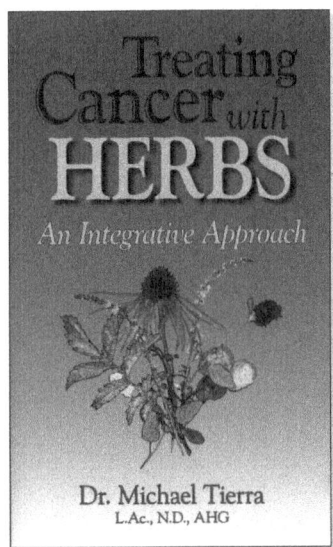

Treating Cancer with Herbs
ISBN: 978-0-9149-5593-1
$27.95 • 528pp • Paperback

"Michael Tierra's commitment to healing and the needs of human beings–particularly those who have received the devastating news that they have cancer– for sensitive, honest and open-minded health care is evident throughout this book. His impassioned plea for the medical system to begin to address the health of individuals, not of diseases (or profit motives) rings crystal clear, and his focus on prevention as the appropriate primary goal of the health care system should be heard by all health professionals working directly with patients as well as those setting cancer research agendas in the new millennium."

– **Avia Romm,** President of the American Herbalists Guild

"Valuable insights from an herbalist who actually practiced the art for 30 years. While most books report over and over on what others have done, Michael was working with patients and learning what actually works."

– **Christopher Hobbs,** author of *Medicinal Mushrooms, Peterson Field Guide to Western Medicinal Plants* and *Herbs and Foundations of Health*

Available at bookstores and natural food stores nationwide OR order your copy directly be sending $24.95 plus $2.50 shipping/handling ($.75 s/h for each additional copy ordered at the same time) to:

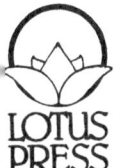

LOTUS PRESS | PO Box 325, Twin Lakes, WI 35181, USA
Toll Free Order Line: 800.824.6396 | Office PH: 262.889.8561 | Office FAX: 262.889.8591
Email: lotuspress@lotuspress.com | Web Site: www.LotusPress.com

Lotus Press is the publisher of a wide range of books in the field of alternative health, including Ayurveda, Chinese medicine, herbology, aromatherapy, Reiki and energetic healing modalities. Request our *free* book catalog.